My Office Is Killing Me!

JEFFREY C. MAY

My Office Is Killing Me!

The Sick Building Survival Guide

The Johns Hopkins University Press • Baltimore

Note to the reader: This book is not intended to provide medical or legal advice. The services of a competent professional should be obtained whenever medical, legal, or other specific advice is needed. The author makes no warranty, either express or implied, regarding the recommendations offered or the practices described; nor does the author assume liability for any consequences arising from the use of the content of this book.

Printed in the United States of America on acid-free paper
2 4 6 8 9 7 5 3 1

The Johns Hopkins University Press
2715 North Charles Street
Baltimore, Maryland 21218-4363
www.press.jhu.edu

Library of Congress Cataloging-in-Publication Data
May, Jeffrey C.
My office is killing me! : the sick building survival guide / Jeffrey C. May.
p. cm.
Includes bibliographical references and index.
ISBN 0-8018-8341-5 (hardcover : alk. paper) — ISBN 0-8018-8342-3 (pbk. : alk. paper)
1. Sick building syndrome—Popular works. 2. Indoor air pollution—Health aspects—Popular works. I. Title.
RA577.5.M39 2006
613′.5—dc22 2005028334

A catalog record for this book is available from the British Library.

CONTENTS

PREFACE

Growing numbers of people are suffering symptoms caused by poor indoor air quality. Many of them feel isolated, ignored, or frustrated. They are surrounded by co-workers and friends who may not believe them, because they themselves are not affected by the conditions. My advice is to believe what your body is telling you and take steps to improve your health.

I have taken thousands of air and dust samples, looking for clues as to why building occupants may be coughing, wheezing, or experiencing allergies, headaches, or eye irritation. Whether one person or a dozen people are suffering, I have often seen connections between such health symptoms and what is in the air or settled dust. And nearly always, if the sources of indoor air quality (IAQ) problems can be identified and removed, people's health symptoms abate. Some professionals refer to the field as *indoor environmental quality,* or IEQ, because this newer term encompasses more than just problems with the air. I am sticking, however, to the term *indoor air quality.*

I am neither a physician nor a microbiologist. The advice I offer in this book is based on my training as a chemist and on my experiences as a building consultant and a certified indoor air quality professional. If you are suffering symptoms that you suspect may be caused by conditions indoors, see a physician who specializes in environmental or occupational medicine.

Still, reading this book may help you understand the connections between your symptoms and the spaces in which you work. (This book addresses problems in nonmanufacturing environments.) I encourage you to start at the beginning of the book and move through the chapters in order, because the discussion in each section builds on what has come before. Parts I and II describe IAQ problems that have arisen in particular buildings and how people's lives have been affected, and in some cases devastated, by exposures to indoor contaminants. Part III defines some air- and dust-sampling techniques and highlights some IAQ guidelines and standards (which change over time), developed by organizations such as the American Society of Heating, Refrigerating, and Air-Conditioning Engineers (ASHRAE) and agencies such as the National Institute of Occupational Safety and Health (NIOSH). I also discuss the content of some IAQ test reports.

Such reports list contaminants carried through a building by airflows. Principles of science dictate how air moves, and so I explain those principles as well. I have a passionate interest in science. When I see the vibrant colors of fall foliage, I am reminded of the chemical processes occurring in the dying leaf that lead to the unfolding yellow and red pigments. When I appreciate the infinite variety of cloud shapes in the sky, I muse on how the interaction of energy and matter creates weather patterns. The clarity and elegance of science speak to me the way the brush strokes of a painting or the lines of a poem speak to others.

Even if you were confused in the past by chemistry or physics, I hope you will now take the time to savor the science in the book, because understanding scientific principles will help you be a more effective advocate for the quality of the air in your indoor environment.

ACKNOWLEDGMENTS

I would like to recognize some of those who helped me complete this work. Thanks to David Bearg, who gave me the first feedback and many helpful hints, to James Scott and Thad Godish, who responded to urgent calls for help, and to David Gordon for his comments. I was honored to meet Joellen Lawson and Kathy Sperrazza, two fighters who provided their stories, which greatly enrich the book. The book is also enriched by the unsung efforts of people like Barbara Herskovitz and Cynthia Coulter Mulvihill—pioneers in mining media stories about indoor air quality and sharing them on the Internet. Thanks also to Lew Harriman and Wagdy Anis for their photographic contributions, to Joan Parker for her insight and firsthand knowledge, to Charlotte Leslie for sharing her experiences, and to Dr. John Santilli for his commitment to victims of poor IAQ.

Finally, words cannot express my gratitude to Connie May, my life partner, for all the grueling hours we spent together working on this manuscript (and others!). I will have to lose Scrabble and gin rummy games for decades to repay her for her monumental efforts.

My Office Is Killing Me!

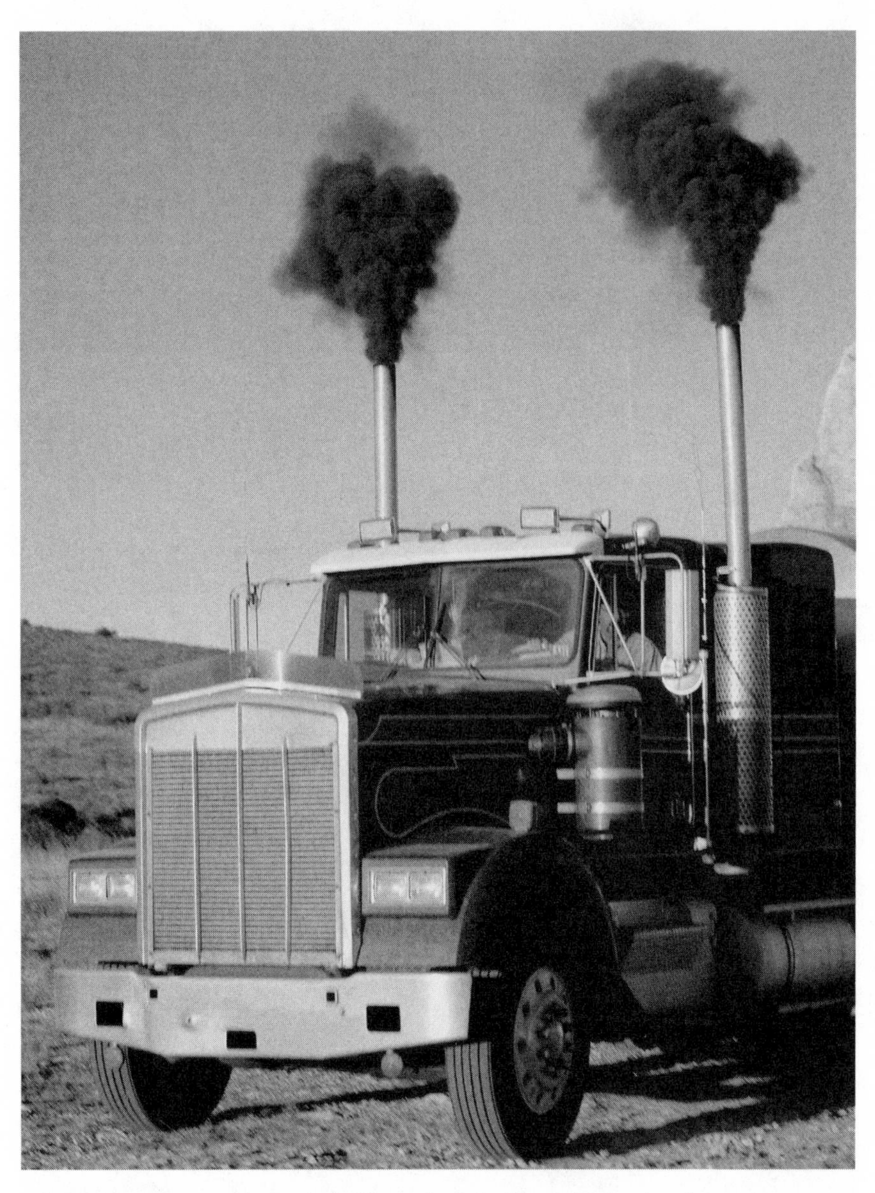

Whether moving on a road or parked at the back of a building, this diesel truck is emitting too much soot. This is one vehicle you do not want idling at the loading dock under your building's fresh-air intake. *Getty Images, Photodisc*

PART I

The Basics

Why might a diesel truck idling at the loading dock in back of a building give someone on the fifth floor a headache? Part I discusses how construction techniques, human behavior, and the laws that govern the flow of energy and matter can help spread contaminants indoors in ways we might not consider.

CHAPTER

1

Poor Indoor Air Quality

A Health Concern

We spend most of our lives indoors. We work behind expansive glass facades. We commute in cars, trains, and planes; shop in enclosed malls; and exercise in health clubs. Our toddlers play in subterranean day care centers. Our children learn in sealed schools, and then, rather than playing outdoors, they become couch potatoes at home. Thus much of what we all breathe is indoor air, which can be very different from outdoor air. As you will see in this book, indoor air may be polluted with irritants, allergens, and even toxins. And if you live, work, or study in such a contaminated space, your health may suffer.

Exposures to contaminants may be chronic (occurring over a long period of time) or acute (when one or more people in the same place are suddenly overcome by either minor or serious symptoms). In either case, when people experience symptoms unexpectedly, they may panic and behave in ways that others may label irrational. In this way, sufferers and nonsufferers can become adversaries. In addition, sufferers may cite radon gas, electromagnetic waves, or emissions from a power plant five miles away as a cause of their symptoms, rather than a heating and cooling system contaminated with concealed mold, carpets full of hidden bacteria, or fresh-air intakes that are sucking in invisible sewer or combustion gases.

When serious indoor air quality (IAQ) problems arise, misunderstandings regarding the sources of contamination, as well as conflicting reports and opinions, denials of wrongdoing, and assertions of blame, hinder the balanced approach and decisive action required to arrive at commonsense solutions.

THE UNIVERSITY OF MASSACHUSETTS BOSTON

In 1994 an indoor air quality crisis occurred on the 175-acre harbor campus of the University of Massachusetts Boston. Over a period of several weeks, more than fifty people at the university experienced symptoms indoors. Some of the symptoms were serious enough to require emergency medical treatment. In hindsight, the causes of the exposures may seem banal and the behavior of some campus constituencies extreme, but the accusations that were made and the conflicts that occurred were painfully disruptive to the community.

The story began shortly before noon on January 26, when eight students and employees reported feeling nauseated and complained of burning lips and tight throats, after which they were taken to a local hospital. Events unfolded as follows:

> *Thursday, January 27.* The campus was closed to the twenty-one thousand students and faculty while representatives from the local department of public health investigated.
>
> *Friday, January 28.* The campus was reopened after city officials assured university chancellor Sherry Penney that the buildings were safe. Within hours, twenty-seven people sought medical assistance. One of them was Cheryl Cummings, bookstore manager. Disoriented, with her throat constricting, she was administered oxygen at an emergency center set up outside the administrative building.
>
> The administration closed the campus through the weekend as a precaution to protect people's health and to allow for extensive testing. Emergency crews and environmental consultants were mystified, but city officials thought that perhaps potentially toxic gases, including methane, were rising out of the landfill on which the campus had been built. Some feared that, if present in high enough concentrations, the methane could blow up a campus building. (Methane gas is a by-product of waste degradation by soil microbes and is explosive when mixed in the right proportions with air.) Newspapers published stories about the toxic sludge buried under the campus. University officials insisted that the dump had been capped and that the venting system prevented contaminants from entering the buildings.

The week of January 31. On the following Monday, the campus was reopened for faculty members, management, staff, and nonunion employees. Nancy Sullivan, the steward with the union, recommended that member-employees stay away. Representatives from the Boston health and fire departments were at the site to respond to any further incidents.

That afternoon, a hastily organized cluster of concerned faculty, staff, and students gathered at an administration building for an anticipated meeting with university officials, only to find out that the appointment had been canceled. The group defied the orders of campus police to disband, and, locking arms, they marched toward the administration building. State police were called to assist. An angry confrontation ensued and continued until provost Fuad Safwat came outside coatless, apologized for missing the meeting, and said that officials were trying to figure out whether the campus was safe enough for classes to resume.

Tuesday's classes were canceled, but faculty and nonunion staff were nonetheless expected to report to work. Union representatives accused the administration of using employees as human guinea pigs and called on the university to close the entire campus until testing was completed. Seven more students and employees sought medical treatment for sore throats, dizziness, and compromised motor skills. Rumors of sabotage began to circulate.

On Wednesday the university chancellor met with Boston health department and hospital officials to discuss whether classes should resume the following day. On Thursday two more employees sought medical treatment, bringing the total reported number of medical complaints to sixty-two in a week and a half. The campus remained closed to students.

The week of February 7. Students returned to campus on Monday, a few wearing surgical masks. Six more employees were treated for what was suspected to be IAQ problems. Environmental consultants rushed in to take air samples. No major contaminants were reported; nonetheless, university officials laid out an action plan to expand health functions, hire a full-time industrial hygienist, and establish an oversight committee. The campus remained open.

On Tuesday ten more people needed medical treatment, and two were hospitalized. Three of those stricken were students working at the campus radio station, WUMB, located adjacent to the lower level of a parking garage. The station's ventilation system had been shut off for air quality testing, so combustion gases from the adjacent garage had infiltrated (leaked into) the station.

On Wednesday two employees and two students sought medical treatment, but no one was hospitalized. On Friday four more people fell ill.

The week of February 14. On Monday university officials expressed the view that the crisis was tapering off. Administrators were hopeful that the worst was over, and indeed, in the weeks that followed, most students and staff returned to the business of education.

What Really Happened?

As mentioned earlier, when the crisis began, the primary culprit was believed to be methane gas, but investigators early on concluded that no methane emanating from the landfill was ever present indoors. Other suspected causes included problems with the heating system and the sanitary waste system. David Gordon and other indoor air quality investigators took dozens of air samples to unravel the mystery. They found trace amounts of a solvent called *methylene chloride* (the main ingredient in paint strippers), with the highest concentration being detected in a large basement room.

It was subsequently discovered that on the first day of the crisis, January 26, an employee had spent a break from her work in the basement storage room, stripping the finish off a couch. The label instructed her to use the stripping product only in a well-ventilated area. In the room was a large grille that emitted a throaty hum. Thinking this was an exhaust, the employee placed the couch close to the grille and set to work. Unfortunately, the grille was a return for the heating system, and toxic fumes that included methylene chloride and toluene (both solvents; see chapter 5) were sucked in and distributed throughout the building.

During the emergency evacuation that followed, the employee dutifully left the building without having a clue that she had caused the problem. The campus was closed the following day. When it reopened on Friday, the employee again took advantage of a work break to continue stripping the couch, precipitating the second evacuation of the building. And her building wasn't the only one affected in the days that followed. One IAQ problem may have been initiated by the use of epoxy-based spray paint. Another may have been caused when an employee mixed chlorine bleach and ammonia, creating toxic fumes.

These chemicals and odors might not have been such problems if the buildings had had adequate amounts of fresh air to dilute these contaminants (see chapter 7). Unfortunately, the fresh-air intakes for the ventilation systems had been closed for years, to save the money that would have been spent to condition (heat or cool) outdoor air, so contaminated air was recirculated rather than exhausted and replaced by fresh air. No doubt this money-saving step had been responsible for many of the complaints about indoor air quality voiced over the years. (Early in the crisis, an economics professor accused the administration of poor management, saying that faculty concerns about IAQ problems had been ignored for at least eight years.)[1]

The university promised to take steps to improve the indoor air quality. For example, vice chancellor Jean MacCormack banned the indoor use of cleaning products and paints by all employees except designated contractors. Eliminating the sources of odors and irritants was essential, but improvements also had to be made to the ventilation systems, including increasing the supply of fresh air indoors at an estimated additional heat cost for that academic year alone of nearly $600,000.[2]

Despite evidence that many of the health symptoms people suffered could be traced to identifiable causes, some observers of the crisis still wondered whether hysteria was at the root of the commotion. Physicians recognize that some illnesses are indeed psychogenic (emotional rather than physical in origin), and outbreaks of mass psychogenesis do occur when people, often within sight of each other, experience in a domino fashion common symptoms such as vomiting or fainting.* In my opinion, however, symptoms caused by indoor air polluted with invisible chemicals or allergens are too often discounted as psychogenic. Sometimes these symptoms are discounted because IAQ investigators fail to identify the sources of contamination. Asthma (difficulty breathing caused by inflammation and constriction of the airways in the lungs)

* *Psychosomatic* generally refers to symptoms experienced by a single individual and *psychogenic* to symptoms experienced by several individuals or by a group, although some medical professionals use the words interchangeably.

was once thought to be psychosomatic, because heightened emotional states can make symptoms worse. Now we know that asthma is indeed a genuine, often allergy-related, disease. Yet even today another illness called *angioedema* (an acute, sometimes life-threatening swelling of tissues) is considered a hysterical affliction, even though it has the hallmarks of a severe allergic reaction.

A VARIETY OF SYMPTOMS

Our perception of air quality can be quite subjective. To many, the air outside on a crisp fall day may seem pure and clean, but to someone with ragweed allergy, that air might be problematic. Similarly, if indoor air contains irritants and allergens, not everyone will be affected, but if enough people experience symptoms, the building may be considered to have "poor indoor air quality."

Whether one person is affected or many, sufferers may experience a variety of symptoms, some minor, others alarming.

Irritation

The surfaces on the body where irritation most commonly occurs are the skin, the eyes, the lips, and the mucous membranes that line the respiratory system, including the throat and nose. People suffering irritation may experience rashes, watery eyes, and a cough.

Allergic Symptoms

Allergic reactions require a history of exposures, occurring over weeks to years, and the development of antibodies within the immune system. Indoor exposures to allergens from organisms such as mold and mites depend on the concentrations of contaminants present as well as on the amount of time the person spends in the space. But generally, symptoms worsen with continued, chronic exposure.

People first may cough or sneeze, or their eyes and noses may run. Sometimes they have breathing difficulties or related chronic sinus or respiratory infections, in part because of excessive fluid production. Depending on their level of susceptibility and family medical history, some individuals may develop asthma. Others may complain of headaches, joint pain, and chronic fatigue.

Allergic reactions are caused by the immune system's "memory," which stores an individual's unique history of exposure to allergens. Anyone can be affected by a toxin, however, depending upon the toxin involved and the levels of present and future exposure (although some people, such as those with compromised immune systems, may be particularly susceptible).

Toxicity

Chemical vapors from some cleaning compounds and solvents can be toxic. A number of toxic gases (carbon monoxide, nitrogen dioxide, hydrogen cyanide; see chapter 5) can be severely debilitating, or even lethal, because of how they react with and interfere with body metabolism. Lead dust is toxic and can be generated when paint containing lead pigments is sanded or otherwise disturbed during renovation work. Ingestion, rather than inhalation is the primary route for lead poisoning; nonetheless, inhalation of lead paint dust can be hazardous, particularly to pregnant women and to children under the age of six.

Under certain growing conditions, some molds (fungi) can produce toxins called *mycotoxins*, and many people are concerned about exposures to such "toxic molds." Without sophisticated chemical analysis, however, the question of whether a mold is toxic has no easy answer. Some mold species, but not all, produce mycotoxins, and then only under certain conditions that are not fully understood and thus cannot be predicted. The mold *Aspergillus ochraceus* grows in damp dust and can produce the mycotoxin ochratoxin-A. Among other potentially toxic genera (groups) of molds, two types, *Stachybotrys* and *Fusarium*, can produce spores containing mycotoxins. One of these mycotoxins, called T-2 (one of several trichothecenes, a type of mold toxin produced by *Stachybotrys chartarum*, the so-called toxic black mold), has been developed for use in chemical warfare, because it causes blistering, hemorrhaging, and, in high enough exposures, death.

Exposure to high levels of inhaled mycotoxins can be very harmful. Even inhaling low levels of mycotoxins may have an impact on the immune system and on very localized areas of the lung where they land. At this point, though, there is no consensus in the medical community on the impact of indoor exposures to low levels of mycotoxins through inhalation of spores; nonetheless, all molds should be treated with caution.

And mycotoxins are not the only toxins molds contain. Mold spores are surrounded by a cell wall. Depending on the mold species, this protective wall

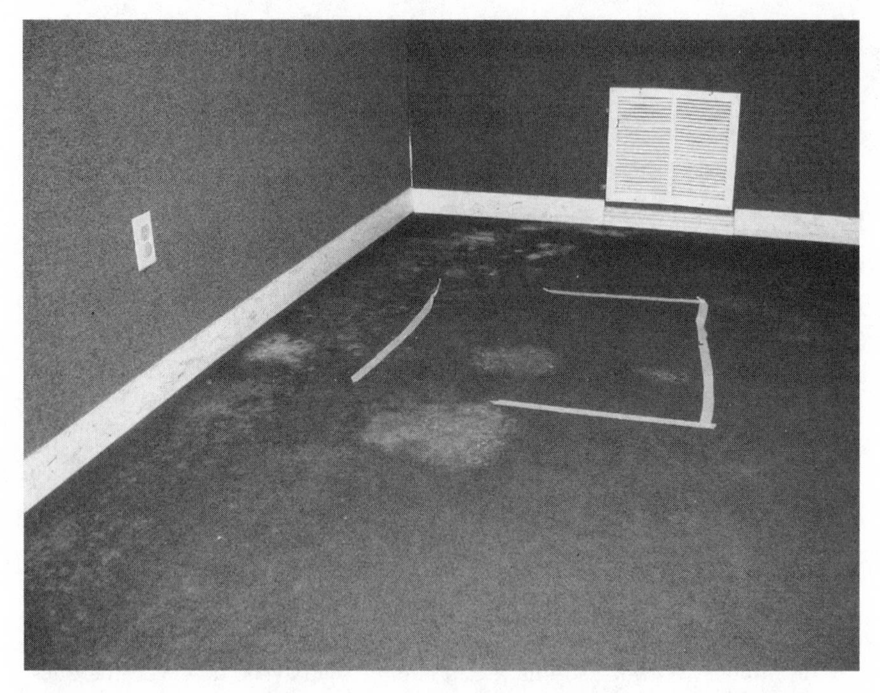

FIGURE 1.1. *Aspergillus* mold in a basement playroom carpet. The splotches near the tape on the floor are large colonies of mold, most likely growing in spilled food. A day care was about to occupy this space. *May Indoor Air Investigations LLC*

may contain a variety of allergenic or toxic substances, but nearly all species of mold contain *glucans:* structural components of the fungal cell wall. Inhalation of glucans is believed to cause tissue inflammation that may contribute to respiratory symptoms.

Still, I think focusing too much on whether a mold is "toxic" or whether there might be mold "toxins" (mycotoxins) in your blood draws attention away from a more important concern: a potential allergic response to mold exposures. In fact, a recent study reported that just over half of sixty-five patients who felt they had suffered from toxic-mold exposures were in fact allergic to mold.[3]

A severe reaction to very high levels of inhaled organic dust (bioaerosol) is called *organic dust toxic syndrome* (ODTS). This relatively rare flu-like illness causes symptoms that include extreme shortness of breath, chest tightness, and fever. Sufferers are usually hospitalized but recover completely from an acute episode. Farmers and other agricultural or sanitation workers are particularly susceptible to ODTS, because they may be exposed to thick clouds of bioaerosol arising from heavily contaminated dry materials such as moldy hay, manure, or other waste products. Glucans (one of the components in the cell walls of fungi) may play a role in ODTS.

Cancer

Cancer can be defined as the uncontrolled reproduction of cells and growth of tissues. Some carcinogens (substances that cause cancer) are naturally present in the environment, while others are man-made.

Naturally occurring carcinogens include radon gas, asbestos, and aflatoxin-A. Radon is a carcinogenic, gaseous, inert element produced by the natural radioactive breakup of uranium in soil and rock (see chapter 5). Asbestos is a noncombustible mineral once used in pipe insulation, joint compound, ceiling panels, floor tiles, plaster, fireproofing, and other construction products. You cannot tell if a product contains asbestos unless it is so labeled. People are often upset to discover any asbestos-containing material in their environment, but generally, as long as the material is left undisturbed, asbestos fibers will not become aerosolized (airborne). Aflatoxin-A is a mycotoxin produced by the fungus *Aspergillus flavus* and is commonly found on moldy peanuts and grains (it can also grow on damp paper). Because aflatoxin-A can cause liver cancer if consumed regularly over a long period of time, its presence in human and animal foods is regulated, and contaminated food may not be sold.

Man-made carcinogens include pesticides, some of which (such as chlordane) were used for many years indoors. Polychlorinated biphenyls (PCBs), also man-made, were once used as the oil in electrical transformers because of their high heat stability and insulating properties. Though PCBs have been banned from use, many pieces of electrical equipment still contain these oils, and accidents such as leaks and fires continue to be sources of exposure to these carcinogens.

Aflatoxin-A is not the only mycotoxin produced by *Aspergillus* molds. The mold *Aspergillus versicolor* is commonly found growing in musty, damp buildings. This mold produces sterigmatocystin, a mycotoxin that may cause liver damage and is carcinogenic. In one study of residential carpet dust,[1] almost 20 percent of the dust samples contained low concentrations (about 3 parts per billion, or ppb) of sterigmatocystin, and nearly all the carpet dust sampled yielded toxigenic (toxin-producing) fungi colonies. Another mycotoxin, ochratoxin-A, produced by the mold *A. ochraceus* and by some species of the mold *Penicillium,* causes kidney damage and is also carcinogenic. This mycotoxin was found at concentrations of from 8 to 20 ppb in dust samples taken from contaminated residential carpeting in three water-damaged buildings in Texas.[2] For comparison, the regulatory limits for various mycotoxins in food are in the approximate range of 5 to 300 ppb.

1. S. Engelhart et al., "Occurrence of Toxigenic *Aspergillus versicolor* Isolates and Sterigmatocystin in Carpet Dust from Damp Indoor Environments," *Applied and Environmental Microbiology* 68, no. 8 (August 2002): 3886–90.
2. E-mail from John Richard, scientist at Romer Labs.

IS IT SICK-BUILDING SYNDROME OR A BUILDING-RELATED ILLNESS?

When occupants experience a cluster of certain symptoms indoors, and the symptoms do not point to a specific disease, the illness is sometimes referred to as *sick-building syndrome (SBS)*. Symptoms due to SBS usually abate within hours or days (say, over a weekend) after sufferers leave the building and reappear when they reoccupy the building.

Chemical sensitivity, also referred to as *multiple chemical sensitivity (MCS),* is a hypersensitivity to organic compounds (compounds that contain carbon) such as solvents, fuels, combustion products, pesticides, and fragrances (see chapters 3 and 7). People suffering from chemical sensitivities describe symptoms such as headache, fatigue, muscle pain, and a variety of neurological symptoms (including "brain fog," or an inability to think clearly).

Many people believe that multiple chemical sensitivity is caused by any of the following:

—Exposures to pesticides
—Long-term exposures to combustion products
—Either short-term exposures to high concentrations or long-term ex-

TABLE 1.1. Percentages of women suffering symptoms in fifty-six BASE buildings and in eighty NIOSH HHE buildings

Symptom	In BASE buildings	In NIOSH HHE buildings
Dry, itching, or irritated eyes	22	35
Unusual tiredness, fatigue, or drowsiness	18	31
Headache	20	30
Stuffy or runny nose or sinus congestion	15	24
Sneezing	14	21
Sore or dry throat	7	19
Cough	6	11
Dry or itchy skin	6	11
Difficulty remembering or concentrating	6	11
Dizziness or lightheadedness	4	11
Chest tightness	2	7
Shortness of breath	3	6
Wheezing	2	4

Source: Adapted from J. Spengler et al., eds., *Indoor Air Quality Handbook* (New York: McGraw-Hill, 2001), table 3.11, p. 3.20, and table 3.14, p. 3.24.

Note: The women experienced symptoms at least once a week over a four-week period. Their symptoms improved when they were away from work. (Men generally experience symptoms at approximately half the rate that women do.) The symptom data from the BASE Study are based on questionnaires collected from just over twenty-five hundred men and women working in offices. (In the BASE Study, the EPA continues to conduct monitoring of healthy buildings all over the country.) The NIOSH Health Hazard Evaluation (HHE) data are based on surveys from just under twenty-five hundred men and women queried in the course of NIOSH investigations of problem workplaces.

posures to low concentrations of volatile organic compounds (called *volatile* because they evaporate at room temperature; see chapters 4 and 5)

Some physicians think that chemical sensitivity is psychosomatic.[4] Others believe that it is a legitimate illness.[5] Because MCS is an illness without a widely accepted medical diagnosis, it is still considered by most physicians to be a sick-building syndrome.

Specific diseases that can be diagnosed and identified as caused by building conditions are referred to as *building-related illnesses (BRIs)*. Examples of BRIs include occupational asthma, hypersensitivity pneumonitis (a lung disease also referred to as extrinsic allergic alveolitis), and humidifier fever, all related to exposures to indoor bioaerosol: airborne particulate matter arising from living things such as bacteria, mold, plants (pollen), and animals (pet dander). Legionnaires' disease is also a BRI, because it is caused by a specific organism present in cooling towers (part of many large buildings' air-conditioning systems), hot-water piping, and hot tubs (see chapter 7).

Because of the range and inconsistency of symptoms associated with both

In a letter to Senator Frank Lautenberg, Timothy Coyle, the assistant secretary of the U.S. Department of Housing and Urban Development, wrote that "MCS is a disability entitling those with chemical sensitivities to reasonable accommodation under Section 504 of the Rehabilitation Act of 1973."[1] The U.S. Army Medical Evaluation Board also certified several Persian Gulf war veterans with diagnoses of MCS.[2] And MCS is recognized as a syndrome (code T78.4) in the modified German version of the World Health Organization's International Statistical Classification of Diseases and Related Health Problems.[3]

1. MCS Referral and Resources, www.mcsrr.org/fedmcsgroup/fedmcsrec.html.
2. Ibid.
3. German Institute of Medical Documentation and Information, ICD-10-SGB-V, version 3.1, November 2000.

The CDC (Centers for Disease Control and Prevention) estimates that there might be eighteen thousand cases of Legionnaires' disease a year in the United States. Some epidemiologists, however, think that there could be as many as one hundred thousand cases a year because the disease may be incorrectly diagnosed as pneumonia, and some studies suggest that 5–10 percent of Americans have serologic (blood serum) evidence of past exposure to *Legionella* bacteria.

building-related illnesses and sick-building syndrome, doubts about the validity of building-related health concerns often arise in the minds of nonsufferers and sufferers alike, as well as in the minds of physicians who treat them. Some frustrated doctors suggest that sufferers consult psychiatrists, but in my experience, when people complain of SBS symptoms, there are usually IAQ problems present.

WHAT IS THE TRUE COST?

Ignoring health complaints of building occupants can prove to be expensive. The money that the University of Massachusetts Boston saved annually by reducing the amount of fresh air introduced into the buildings was possibly exceeded by the cost of lost work time, hospitalizations, and legal and consulting fees resulting from the university's IAQ problems. It is difficult to attach a dollar figure to the harm done to the school's reputation and to the relationships among its constituents, but this damage too represents a loss.

David Bearg, an indoor air quality professional, estimates that the annual cost of an employee is about one hundred times greater than the energy cost to keep a building heated, cooled, and ventilated for that one person.[6] If an employer saves an energy cost of $1 a day by reducing the ventilation in a building, and an employee who is paid $100 a day misses a day of work because of illness, the employer's net loss is $99 (the salary is paid to the employee even if he or she is out sick).

In the mid-1990s, William J. Fisk of the Indoor Environmental Department at Lawrence Berkeley National Laboratory in California estimated that the financial benefits of improving indoor air quality included a "potential annual savings and productivity gains in 1996 dollars of $6 to $14 billion from reduced respiratory disease; $2 to $4 billion from reduced allergies and asthma; $15 to $40 billion from reduced symptoms of sick building syndrome; and $20 to $200 billion from direct improvements in worker performance that are unrelated to health. In two calculations, the potential financial benefits of improving indoor environments exceed costs by factors of 9 and 14."[7] The dollar amounts of these savings would be even greater today.

Ironically, we started to build "tight buildings" in the 1970s because people became interested in protecting the Earth's resources. Yet in preserving fuel, we sometimes place a higher value on the conservation of energy sources than on the preservation of human health.

SOME PRACTICAL STEPS

- If you think you are experiencing symptoms inside a building and you feel better when you are away from the space, believe what your body is telling you and see your doctor.
- Keep a daily log of your symptoms—where and when they occur—along with any other relevant information, such as the activities going on in the space around you.
- Avoid using solvents indoors unless there is plenty of ventilation. Follow manufacturer's directions and use an appropriate respirator if required.

CHAPTER

2

Shelter in the Storm

Think of any building and then try to imagine what would be there in its absence: space. The *building envelope* encloses the space, lets in light, keeps the heated or cooled (conditioned) air within, and keeps the rain, snow, and wind out. If the building envelope fails to prevent the entry of water, a host of indoor air quality problems can develop, which I discuss later in this chapter and in the chapters that follow. For now, let's examine some of the ways in which buildings can be vulnerable to conditions in the exterior environment.

DEFICIENT DRAINAGE

In one older urban office building I investigated, the owner complained that water entered one wall of the basement after heavy rains. He and I went to look at the condition of the asphalt pavement and concrete sidewalk in the wide alley on that side of the building. There was a downspout coming down the side of the six-story building from the roof and entering the sidewalk to drain roof water into the sewer system. The concrete was cracked, and the asphalt was caving in near the pipe. The owner noted that the asphalt had been patched numerous times by the city. Oddly enough, he never made any association between his basement water problem and the cave-ins. Most likely there was a broken section of pipe below grade (below ground level), and water was leaking into the soil beneath the pavement. During heavy rains, water would erode the soil and wash it into the city sewer, undermining the support for the asphalt surface above. At the same time, some of the water would flow into the basement through foundation cracks.

I investigated another building, a university museum that was fairly new, in which exterior water leaked into the basement library during winter rains when there was snow on the ground, or during rain storms in any season when the wind blew from the northeast. (In New England, some of the strongest storms with the heaviest wind and rainfall are called *nor'easters.*) The ground around the building was entirely paved with concrete walkways, stairs, and parking spaces. Whenever concrete is used outdoors at grade (at ground level, as for sidewalks or patios), it is installed with control joints: small gaps to direct shrinkage cracks. And just as soil around a building should be sloped away from it, not level, concrete surfaces around a building should be sloped toward drains to carry away rainwater.

The concrete surfaces around this museum were pitched correctly toward drains, but I wanted to see if water would flow into the control joints. I squirted water from a bottle into several of the joints. The water eventually overflowed, with the exception of one joint, located at the edge of the patio and the beginning of a sloped walkway. This crack seemed a little wider than the others. No matter how much water I squirted into that joint, the crack never filled. I then ran a hose to increase the water flow and asked the museum guard to let me know if water entered the basement library. I assumed it would take hours for the water to migrate to the lower level, but within minutes the guard came out to the patio to tell me that water was trickling down the foundation walls and onto the library floor.

Because the crack was at a high point, not much water poured in during normal rain. That part of the building faced east, however, and when the wind blew from the northeast, wind-driven rain would pour down the exterior wall in torrents, drain into the crack, and leak from there into the basement. In the winter, snow and ice on the ground would prevent water flow from draining away from the crack, and again, rainwater would be directed into the crack.

I recommended a temporary solution—caulking all the control joints—which solved the immediate problem. In the end, though, the university spent many thousands of dollars tearing up the entrance patio and re-waterproofing the foundation concrete, because the facilities director felt that a caulked joint was not sufficient protection.

FROM THE BOTTOM UP

When a building is being constructed, a location is chosen and a foundation prepared. Some foundations (most of which in newer buildings are made of concrete) go deep into the earth and enclose many levels of below-grade parking or even retail spaces. Other foundations are only one or two levels deep. Some buildings, including many modern school buildings, are constructed over shallow crawl spaces (spaces in which you can't stand up straight) and supported by piers in the middle. Crawl spaces can have dirt or concrete floors. Some buildings are constructed directly on the ground (at grade) on a layer of concrete that rests on crushed stone and soil, with deeper "footings" at the perimeter (this kind of construction is called *slab on grade*).

Picture a hole being dug for a building foundation. At first, the spaces between the soil particles are filled with air. Then, as the digging goes deeper and deeper, the bottom of the hole may eventually fill with water (the way a hole fills with water when you are digging in the sand at the beach). At this point the excavating crew has reached the *water table,* where water instead of air fills the spaces between the soil particles. Geological considerations such as the soil type, the incline of the terrain, and the proximity to ledge, mountains, and bodies of water, as well as weather patterns and the recent history of rainfall, help determine the depth at which the water table lies in any specific location.

The layer of soil above the water table where the spaces between the soil particles are filled with air is called the *vadose zone.* It is preferable to have a building foundation sit entirely in the vadose zone, because the foundation is not meant to be like the hull of a ship, partially submerged in the water table. Those buildings with basements, parking garages, or living or work spaces below the water table must hold back the water that would otherwise enter the space in its effort to reach its own level. (The exteriors of many foundation walls are usually treated with or covered by water-impervious coatings to prevent the movement of soil moisture through the concrete, but more significant design modifications are necessary for foundations that are continuously below the water table.)

Creeping Seeping

Water in the water table may be part of an *aquifer.* An aquifer is like a very slow-flowing subterranean stream, and it can carry contaminants that have either accidentally leaked into the soil from buried tanks or been intentionally (and illegally) disposed of on or in the soil above the aquifer.

The Hillside School in Needham, Massachusetts, had an air quality problem because of pollutants carried by the aquifer beneath the building. A foul odor inside the building was causing headaches among students and faculty. Extensive air testing revealed elevated levels of trichloroethylene (TCE), a degreaser that may cause liver cancer. When investigators sampled the air in the crawl space under the building, they found even higher levels of TCE, suggesting that the solvent vapor was entering the building from the soil. Behind the school was a hill, and at the top was an industrial park that included an electronics manufacturer. Sampling wells were placed at various locations in the soil behind the school and near the industrial park where investigators found the highest concentrations of the solvent. Solvent from the industrial park percolated down (penetrated) the soil and reached the aquifer, and as the aquifer flowed toward the school, it carried the solvent with it. Vapor then diffused through (moved through instead of with) the air in the vadose zone into the crawl space, and from there it infiltrated the classrooms above.

All the students and faculty were relocated among a number of schools in the city's school system while a cleanup was undertaken. The town spent approximately $100,000 on remediation efforts, and the manufacturer blamed for the contamination spent another $100,000. Still, some teachers said they would not return to the building even after the source of the contamination was mitigated, and a number of families chose to transfer their children permanently to other school buildings. As is often the case with air quality problems, relationships were disrupted and mistrust ensued.

Concrete Quandary

Concrete itself can cause problems. Fluid concrete about to be poured is a slushy mixture of water and minerals that includes Portland cement and an aggregate consisting of sand and stone, along with air bubbles and small amounts of various additives. Some of the water combines chemically with

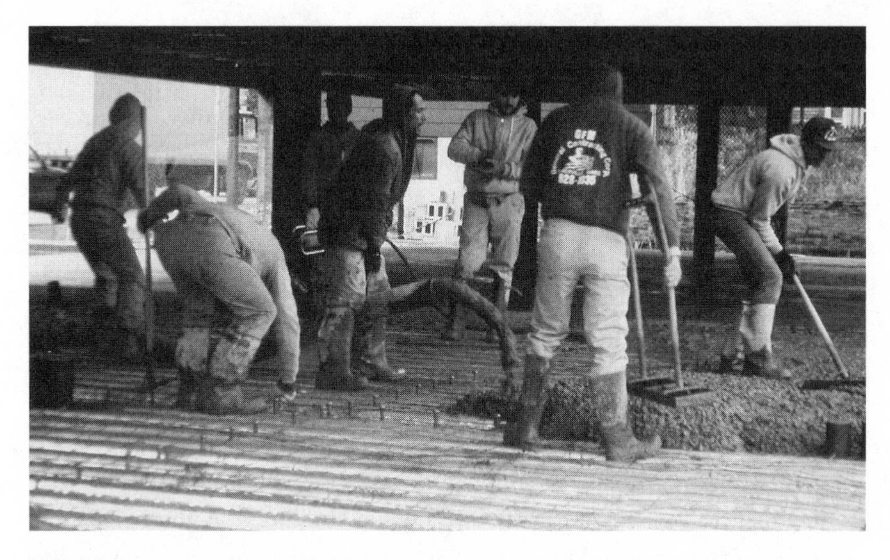

FIGURE 2.1. Pouring a concrete slab. The worker in the center is holding a large hose that is pumping out concrete. Other workers are spreading the concrete. Excess moisture from the mix will evaporate as the concrete hardens, but this will not affect the inside of the building, because there are no walls yet. However, a vapor barrier must be located beneath the concrete to prevent soil moisture from moving through the slab after the concrete has cured and the building has been enclosed. *Jeffrey C. May*

the cement and hardens with it to form solid concrete. The excess water either drains out or evaporates from the concrete surface when it is exposed to air. If a building is enclosed before the excess water in the concrete has evaporated, conditions of elevated humidity can develop within and lead to microbial growth on biodegradable materials (see chapter 4). I investigated an office building with exposed concrete walls. The odor from the additives in the concrete was causing two employees to experience sick-building symptoms. Aluminum foil–backed drywall was installed in front of the concrete, and their symptoms abated.

Wet concrete is a very thick ooze, and contractors sometimes add more water to increase its flow. Too much water in the wet mix results in a weaker concrete. Concrete shrinks as it cures (dries). If it is weak to begin with, the concrete will not have sufficient tensile strength when it dries and may develop cracks after it hardens.

Moisture Invasion

Some of the moisture that leaks through foundation cracks or diffuses through the concrete (even hard concrete is partially porous) comes from the water table, but much of it is the result of poor control of rainwater.

When it rains, water soaks slowly through the soil where the particles are densely packed (clay-like soil) and rapidly where there are many interconnected pores (sandy soil). The soil around the foundation of any building has been excavated and replaced, so it tends to be more porous than the surrounding native soil, making it easier for rainwater to penetrate. Rainwater can also enter the soil through the fissures (cracks) that develop through erosion where there are concentrated water flows, such as under roof water runoffs or in pavement low points.

In frigid climates, when the ground has long been frozen, rainwater cannot drain easily, because the soil is like an impervious sheet of ice. Unfortunately, the water *can* drain into the foot or so of soil around the building, where heat loss from the foundation has prevented the ground from freezing. Even when the rainfall is not that heavy, there may be inadequate roof overhang or improperly discharging roof water systems (gutters and downspouts). And sometimes the grading (slope of the surface soil) is either level or pitched toward rather than away from the building, thus directing rainwater toward the foundation wall.

Any combination of soil porosity, the tendency of shrinkage cracks to form in soil, inadequate rainwater dispersal, and incorrect grading can lead to water problems in below-grade levels. Even in a building constructed on a slab, soil moisture will soak into the concrete unless a water or vapor barrier is present under the slab.

BONES AND SKIN

The building—sometimes one story, made of wood; sometimes ten stories, made of steel or concrete—rises up above the foundation or slab. The outside of the building consists of exterior walls and a roof; the inside, of interior walls, floors, and ceilings. The exterior, perimeter walls support some of the weight, but the weight of the interior of most large building has to be supported by vertical posts, piers, or columns. Like the foundation, the bottoms

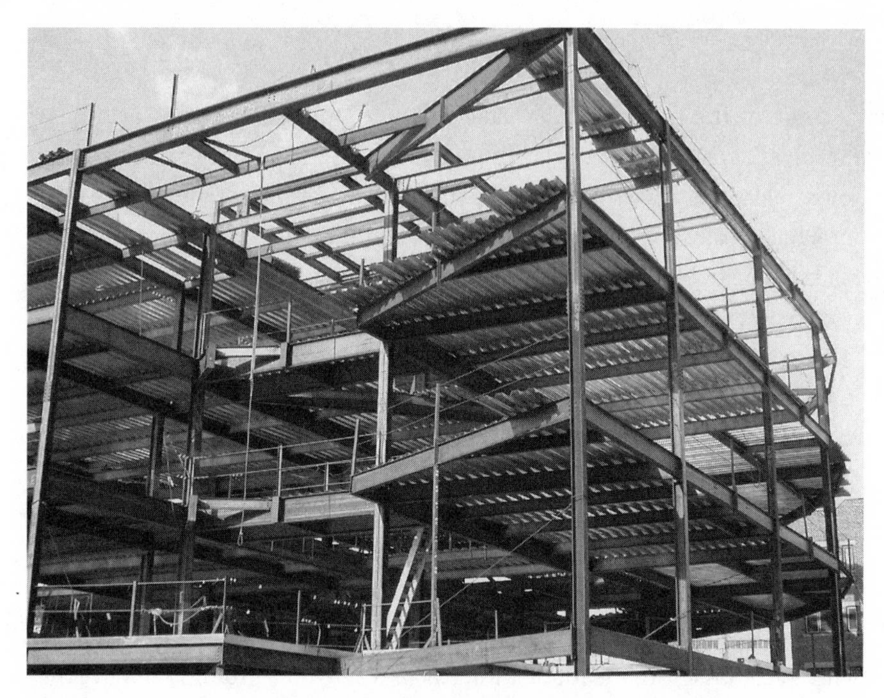

FIGURE 2.2. The steel "skeleton" of a building. These steel beams (girders) and columns will support the weight of the floors and walls of the building. The floors are partially covered with steel pans that will serve as the form for the concrete floors. At this point, the "indoor" air quality of this building is the best it will ever be! *Jeffrey C. May*

of these vertical supports are embedded in and supported by the earth. Before a building's "skeleton" is completed and covered with its exterior "skin," you can still see through the structural "grid" to the space within.

Water and moisture problems that can occur in a building depend to some extent on how the space is enclosed. If the building is single story, with a full basement, and is spread out over a wide area (like the "footprint" of many newer school buildings), much of the building consists of the roof, and about half of the interior is below grade. Roofs (especially flat ones) are prone to leaks, and basements are subject to ground water penetration and condensation problems. In such a building, a roof leak can damage the ceiling of any or every room on the ground level, depending on where the leak occurs. Foundation leaks and condensation can also damage building materials in finished, below-grade space and foster microbial growth, leading to air quality problems both below grade and in the rooms above, if bioaerosol is carried upward on airflows.

In a twenty-story building, the ground level may be directly affected by the basement and the top floor by the roof, but in between are eighteen floors that to some extent are isolated from the bottom and top of the building (except for such connections as elevator shafts and stairwells). Yet the exterior of a tall building has more exposure overall to strong winds and wind-driven rain than the exterior of a lower building does.

Whether horizontal (the roof) or vertical (the walls), any exterior surface hit by rain is vulnerable to water intrusion.

Leaking Walls

Roof water flowing directly down exterior walls can over time damage the cladding—the exterior skin of the building—by corrosion or decay. In addition, no exterior articulation, such as horizontal trim, drip edge, or window and door sills, should be dead flat or pitched toward the vertical wall, because wind-blown rain can then enter the joints where the horizontal and vertical surfaces meet and drip down behind the cladding. Leaks can also damage ceilings, walls, and trim. Very often, after a painted surface gets wet, the paint will crack and peel because of the swelling and shrinking of the surface beneath the paint. If water soaks into wooden floorboards, the boards will swell, cup, and possibly loosen. Water can also dampen carpeting, which can then acquire a musty smell.

During the renovation of a faculty dining room at a New England univer-

EIFS (exterior insulation and finish system) is a cladding that became popular in the 1960s. As originally applied in Europe, the system consisted of approximately 2-inch-thick panels of insulating foam adhered to the exterior masonry of existing buildings (as opposed to new construction). A coating of synthetic stucco was applied to a fiberglass mesh attached to the foam, and then the stucco was coated with a finish. In the United States, the system was initially used in new construction and applied over drywall (a substrate containing two layers of biodegradable paper). Because the foam insulation is impervious to moisture, any water that penetrated through gaps or cracks in an incorrectly installed EIFS could not evaporate. The trapped moisture led to mold growth in the drywall beneath the EIFS and ultimately to failure of the cladding.

sity, shortly before the varnish was to be applied to the smooth-sanded oak window trim inside, a nor'easter descended. Heavy wind-blown rain sheeted down the exterior brick of the sixty-year-old building, and horrified workers watched as water dripped onto the unfinished interior window trim.

I was asked to find out how and why the rain had entered the building. On a sunny day, I placed my ladder against the exterior brick above a window, and as students and faculty passing by looked on curiously, I squirted water from a small plastic bottle onto a vertical mortar joint several courses of brick above the suspect window. The water soaked into the mortar and moved by *capillary action* (a physical force that draws water into small gaps between fine solids, such as fibers and crystals) along the surface of the mortar until it came to the horizontal mortar joint, at which point it followed the mortar to the right and left. Additional water followed the same path, spreading steadily down the vertical joints and across the horizontal joints. The water traced a pattern on the brick wall that looked like the outline of a jagged pyramid.

Two brick courses above the window, there was a long horizontal crack between the mortar joint and the brick. The water flow entered this crack by capillary action. I applied more water to the face of the brick, and it started to drip onto the oak trim indoors. That crack could potentially have ruined some beautiful woodwork!

A horizontal capillary crack is not necessarily a problem unless there are significant water flows down the side of the building in that location. Water does not enter larger cracks by capillary action, but in conditions of wind-driven rain, air pressure differences between the outside and inside of the building (which I discuss further in chapter 4) will push water into those cracks.

Leaky Roofs

Any roof can develop leaks. Most people picture a roof as *gabled* (A-shaped). Some larger buildings have either gable or similarly shaped roofs that shed rainwater to the outside edges, but most larger buildings, including newly constructed schools, have flat roofs. No roof should be dead flat; in fact, *flat roof* is a misnomer, because any well-designed roof, even if called flat, will be pitched to direct rainwater to one or more drains.

Water should never pond on a flat roof, because most traditional roof materials, if continuously wet, will weaken or deteriorate, particularly at the

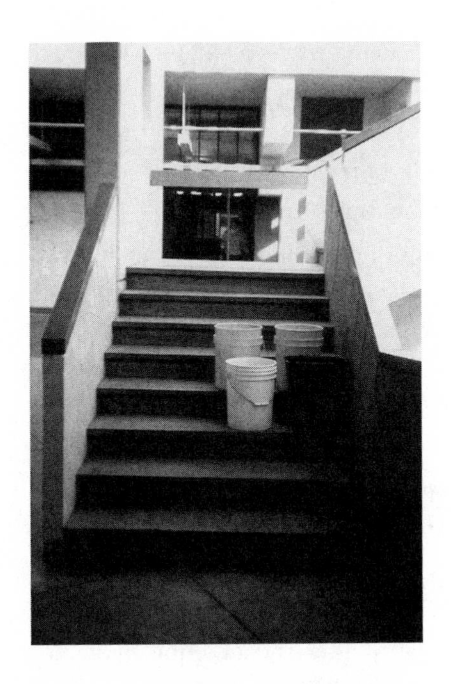

FIGURE 2.3. Buckets in college. In the nearby lecture halls in this modern university building, knowledge filled the students' heads. On the stairway outside the lecture halls, water filled the buckets on rainy days. The leaks originated at skylights where all the outside "weep" (drain) holes had been inadvertently caulked, forcing the rainwater to flow inside. *May Indoor Air Investigations LLC*

seams. (The thawing and freezing of puddles also stresses the surfaces of roofing materials.) Flat roofs may have small holes for a variety of reasons—say, a nail puncture or a gap where some wires or pipes are penetrating. As long as water moves quickly across a small hole like this, there may be little or no leakage. But if water ponds over the hole, a substantial leak can develop. This is why drains on flat roofs must not become clogged, which in turn means that tree branches should not extend over a flat roof, because they shed leaves and twigs that can clog a drain.

From Tar and Gravel to Membrane

Years ago most flat roofs had *tar-and-gravel roofing*. A concrete or wood surface was covered with asphalt-impregnated roof paper, and hot tar (asphalt) was mopped out on top. Then a second and sometimes a third layer of roof paper was covered with tar, and finally, gravel was spread out over the uppermost tar surface. This type of flat roof lasts a long time, sometimes up to thirty years.

You can tell that a tar-and-gravel roof is nearing the end of its useful life when large bubbles (blisters) appear to be growing out of the surface. These bubbles usually form because water has leaked into small spaces between layers of the roofing material. The trapped water is warmed and then turned to vapor by heat from the sun. Water vapor takes up about a thousand times as much space as the liquid from which it came, so as the water in the roofing material turns to vapor, a bubble builds up, stretching the tar and paper like the skin of a balloon. At night the vapor cools and condenses back to liquid, but the bubble doesn't shrink because the cooled tar and paper retain their expanded shape, and air replaces the vapor. In cold weather, stepping on such a bubble will break it open because the cold asphalt is brittle.

When tar-and-gravel roofing starts to leak, the surface is sometimes scraped and recoated with more tar and gravel. The process of applying tar is messy, though, and pollutes the air with choking smoke from the heated asphalt. Today a newer type of material called *membrane roofing* is often installed over an old tar-and-gravel roof. Sometimes the old roofing material is removed before the membrane is applied. More often, some of the gravel is scraped off, oriented strand board (OSB), a rigid synthetic board made from wood chips and glue, is screwed down on top of the old tar roofing, and a roofing membrane is glued down on top.

Some membrane roofing is not adhered to the surface beneath and must be covered with *ballast* (smooth river stones, not sharp crushed stones that can create holes), to prevent the membrane from ballooning in strong winds. Occasionally, despite the presence of ballast, wind will cause the membrane to balloon in one corner. A bulge can then rise up from the surface and push the stones away. If the bulge becomes large enough, the stones will roll to one end or side of the roof, and the entire membrane will "inflate," eventually ripping and allowing massive amounts of rainwater into the building envelope. It is therefore essential to have adequate stone ballast on the roof and to inspect the roof surface periodically.

Membrane Moisture

Since roofing membranes only come in certain widths, most such roofs have overlapping seams that are glued together. Water can leak in at the seams if the adhesive deteriorates. One type of membrane roofing is made of thermoplastic such as vinyl and has seams that are melted together rather than glued. Roofs covered with thermo-plastic membrane are less likely to leak at the seams, but thermo-plastic membrane can become brittle in cold weather and

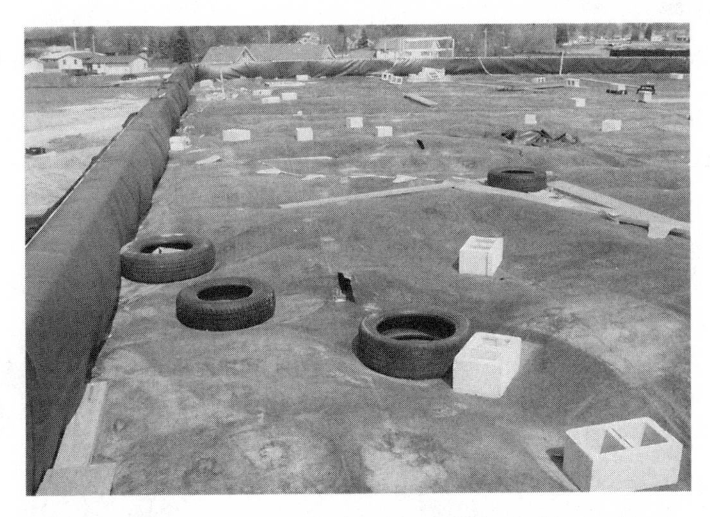

FIGURE 2.4. A billowing roof membrane. Stone ballast had not yet been spread on this membrane roofing. The temporary ballast (tires and cement blocks) was not able to hold the roofing down when the wind started to blow, and the membrane billowed. *Benchmark, Inc.*

thus be easily cracked. A walkway is often installed across thermo-plastic roofing, to protect the membrane when contractors need access to mechanical systems located on the roof (see chapter 7).

Membrane roofing can leak where stack pipes protrude up through the roofing material. Nails, screws, branches, and even icicles can also puncture the membrane, potentially leading to water entry. I was once up on a flat membrane roof, on top of a one-level auditorium that extended beyond a gable roof several stories above. The roofing was full of small slits. Icicles formed at the edge of the gable roof above and from there would fall like a shower of spears, puncturing the membrane roofing below. One type of membrane roofing, EPDM (ethylene-propylene-diene monomer), is made from a kind of synthetic rubber, similar to that used for tire inner tubes. EPDM is soft and only about sixty-thousandths of an inch thick, and can thus be easily punctured.

When water leaks through gaps or holes in membrane roofing, the OSB beneath eventually softens and decays, but as long as the new holes are not in the same places as the old ones, the older roofing material under the OSB continues for a while to keep the water out of the building envelope. Despite its fragility, however, membrane roofing can be patched, EPDM as easily as a rubber tire.

DISTANT AND LOCAL SOURCES OF POLLUTANTS

Though it can cause mold problems (see chapter 4), water in and of itself is not a contaminant. Depending on a building's placement and its mechanical systems, however, contaminants *can* enter the envelope from both below ground (as with the Hillside School) and above ground from distant sources of pollutants, such as highways, waste facilities, mulch farms, construction sites, farm harvesting or fertilizing, and power plants.

In a surprising example of long-range transmission of allergens in Barcelona, Spain, occurring between 1981 and 1987, emergency room physicians were puzzled by the periodic peaks in hospital admissions due to asthma. Researchers ultimately associated the cluster of hospitalizations with the offloading of soybeans in the city's harbor. The epidemic ended after bag filters were installed at the offending silos.[1] In another example of long-range transmission of particulates, fires in Quebec, Canada, consumed thousands of acres of forest in July 2002, and smoke rose up into the atmosphere and was carried with airflows to other parts of the continent. The sky was whitened over much of the East Coast, and the color of sunlight turned from yellow to orange. I was in Vermont at the time, and the air was hazy, even at ground level; sometimes I could catch a whiff of the smoke, even indoors. During this period researchers from the Johns Hopkins Bloomberg School of Public Health recorded as much as a thirtyfold increase in outdoor fine particulate matter (see chapter 6).[2]

> The atmosphere is constantly carrying particles—some living, some that come from living things, some visible, some invisible—from one part of the Earth to another. These riders, gliders, floaters, and hitchhikers include pollen, mold spores, and spiders. Blue mold infects tobacco plants in Cuba, where the spores become airborne with wind and are then carried in the atmosphere over the Caribbean and the Atlantic Ocean, as well as the Gulf of Mexico, to the mainland of the United States. Tracking the invisible plumes of spores has been very important in helping to protect American tobacco crops from infection. Before the advent of the spore-monitoring network, tobacco farmers spent a lot of money treating their crops regularly with fungicides as a protective measure. Now most farmers only treat when they are warned that the spores are on their way from Cuba to the United States.

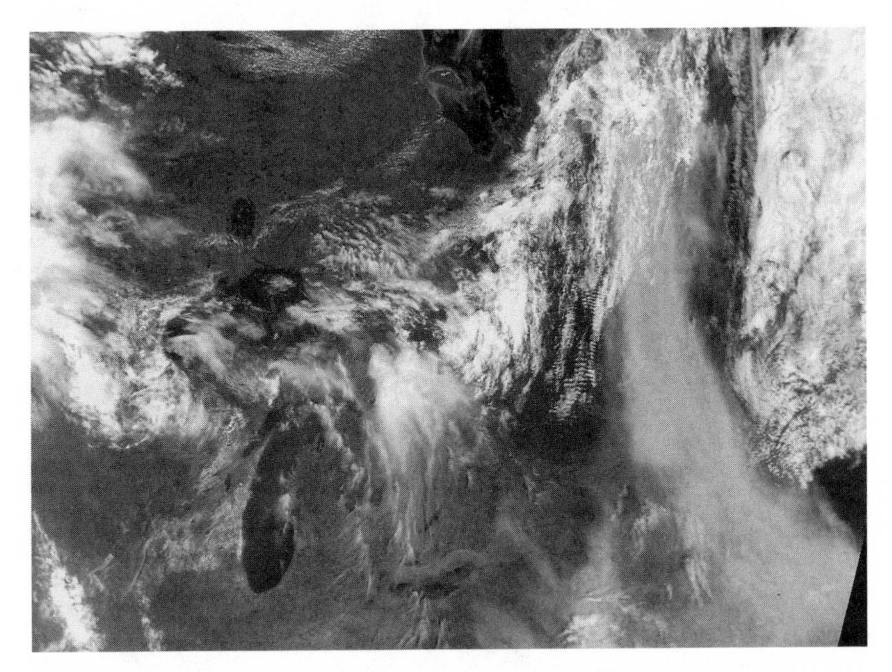

FIGURE 2.5. Smoke from Quebec forest fires. This satellite image depicts southeastern Canada and the northeastern United States. Lake Michigan is visible at the lower left, looking like an elongated black teardrop. The white structures in the atmosphere are clouds, and the gray area is smoke from the forest fires in Quebec. The plume of smoke is narrow at the source and widens as it spreads south and east. *NASA*

Significant indoor contamination is more often due to local sources than to distant ones. Nearby demolition or construction projects can send plumes of contaminants—concrete and masonry dust, paint droplets and solvent vapor from spray-painting—into the air that flows into other buildings. The exhaust from a neighborhood laundromat can contain fabric softeners, fragrances, and enzymes that affect individuals who are sensitized to such chemicals. During morning and evening rush hours, carbon monoxide concentrations due to automobile traffic can increase in cities or near major highways. Tire particles, soot, smoke, and smog can also infiltrate a building located in a high-traffic area. And cars entering and exiting a below-grade parking garage, as well as trucks idling at the back of a building, can emit combustion products.

Recently I joined a number of other building investigators at a professional conference held in a hotel. Suddenly the irritating odor of diesel fumes entered the meeting room. Some participants became frightened, thinking there was a fire in the building. But the smell had another source. Most large buildings have emergency power-generating equipment that can provide electricity in a power failure. Such equipment—often diesel fueled and located at the exterior, adjacent to the building—is tested periodically, to ensure that it is in operable condition. While it was being tested, the equipment in this hotel produced noxious combustion products, and the fumes flowed into our meeting room. Within minutes, hotel employees moved us to another space.

Air quality problems within a building caused by outside sources of pollutants can be difficult to solve, because the problems are intermittent and depend on wind direction and speed as well as on weather and traffic conditions. In addition, the sources of the problems are not under anyone's immediate control. Nonetheless, when investigating what might be contaminating the air we breathe inside a building, it is important to consider conditions in the exterior environment.

SOME PRACTICAL STEPS

- During or after a heavy rain, scrutinize the ceilings located immediately under the roof as well as the interior side of perimeter walls, under windows, and in the basement to see if rainwater is getting into the building. Don't forget to look behind heavy furniture or file cabinets that are up against exterior walls. Keep a log of any occurrences of water intrusion.
- Be aware of any activities around or near your building (spray-painting, renovation or construction projects, heavy traffic, incineration, power generation, manufacturing or industrial activity, pesticide use) that may be producing contaminants that can infiltrate the building.
- Research the history of the building. Might there be contaminants in the soil from prior industrial, manufacturing, or agricultural use?

CHAPTER

3

Diseased Decor

To make use of the space within the building envelope, the interior must be partitioned into rooms by floors, walls, and ceilings. Then depending on how the rooms will be used, floor coverings, lighting, furniture, and office equipment are added. While most buildings are "healthy," anything that is applied or brought into a building has the potential of being the source of an indoor air quality problem.

WALLS

An *exterior wall* faces the backside of the building envelope on one side and the inside of a room on the other. An *interior wall* partitions a space into two rooms. Walls may consist of paneling, concrete blocks, or, in older buildings, several layers of plaster applied over metal mesh or wood lath. Most walls, however, consist of drywall, which is then either primed and painted directly (or skim-coated with plaster first) or covered with wallpaper. Drywall is made of gypsum (a white mineral material) and paper, with the gypsum sandwiched between two layers of paper. The paper is made of cellulose and other organic materials that can be degraded by some fungi; thus a drywall ceiling or wall is a potential source of nutrients for mold growth if the requisite moisture (from liquid water or high humidity; see chapter 4) is present. You might also see mildew growing on the surface of plaster or cement walls, but in this case the mildew is most often subsisting on the nutrients in the dust settled on the wall surface.

In some buildings mildew growth may have already begun in the paper of the drywall before or after its installation, if the drywall was piled up outside in the rain or if the building interior was exposed to the weather or to leaks before it was completed. One type of mold, *Stachybotrys chartarum* (referred to as *toxic black mold*), is so common on drywall that some air quality professionals think that the paper becomes contaminated with mold spores during the manufacturing process. To minimize the chances of mold growth in drywall, one manufacturer has begun to sell drywall with the gypsum sandwiched between fiberglass mats instead of paper. Another manufacturer sells drywall made with paper that contains mildewcide.

Materials applied to wall surfaces (paint, wallpaper) can *off-gas* (emit into the air) solvents or chemicals that were mixed in with the coating to preserve the product. I am aware of several instances in which homes and offices began to smell months after being painted. It was theorized that a fungicide in the paint reacted with ozone in the air to produce a foul sulfurous odor, strongest on warm days and in bright sunlight. In other buildings, mildewcide intended for exterior use had been added to the paint used in interior spaces. Long after the solvent evaporated from the paint, small amounts of the fungicide continued to produce odors irritating to the buildings' occupants. I think that mildewcides that continue to vaporize should not be used in indoor paint.

In apartment and commercial buildings, vinyl cove molding is often applied to the base of a wall to protect the wall from being damaged at floor level. The off-gassing of solvents from the cove-molding adhesive has been a problem for those who are sensitized.

WINDOWS

Nonmetallic window treatments or insect screens may off-gas a burned-plastic odor, particularly when heated by the sun. I was once in a museum in which the stairwell skylights were covered with shades made from this material. The entire upper floor had an odor characteristic of heated and burned plastic. The simplest way to determine if a heated vinyl fiberglass product is off-gassing is to remove the item, ventilate the room, and see if the odor goes away. If insect screens are a problem, aluminum screening can be substituted for vinyl fiberglass. Plastic window shades (blinds, scrim, screen) can also off-gas.

CEILINGS

In some buildings, the concrete slab serves as the floor for one level and the ceiling for the level below. In most wood-frame buildings (buildings in which the skeleton is made of wood; see chapter 2), horizontal wooden joists hold up the floor above, and the drywall ceiling for the room below is attached to wood strips perpendicular to the bottoms of the joists. A third type of ceiling, called a *drop* or *suspended ceiling,* is common in many schools and offices. Drop ceilings consist of movable tiles suspended below a *ceiling plenum* (the space between the drop ceiling and the floor structure above, through which air can flow back to the building's heating or cooling system; see chapter 7). The tiles are supported in place by a metal grid attached to framing members or suspended from wires connected to the structural floor above.

Ceiling Tiles

Suspended ceiling tiles are composites consisting of either fiberglass (a material made of glass fibers held together by adhesive) or fiberglass mixtures containing cellulose. A *composite* is a blend (a mixture) of materials that has properties different from and usually better than the properties of the individual components. For example, roads are paved with a composite of asphalt and stones. If asphalt alone were used, it would heat up and soften in the sun. The stones make the paving stiffer, particularly when hot.

Ceiling tiles that contain cellulose can be contaminated with bacteria that grow in the process water used to manufacture the tiles. I heard about one office in which occupants were complaining about an odor of vomit in a bathroom. No one could figure out where the odor was coming from. Investigators discovered that one of the workers was bulimic and regularly used the same bathroom for her regurgitations. The bathroom was thoroughly cleaned, but the odor persisted. The ceiling was removed and the smell went away. The ceiling tiles were contaminated with bacteria that produced butyric acid, a chemical that has the odor of vomit.

For obvious reasons, ceiling tiles used in office buildings cannot be combustible.

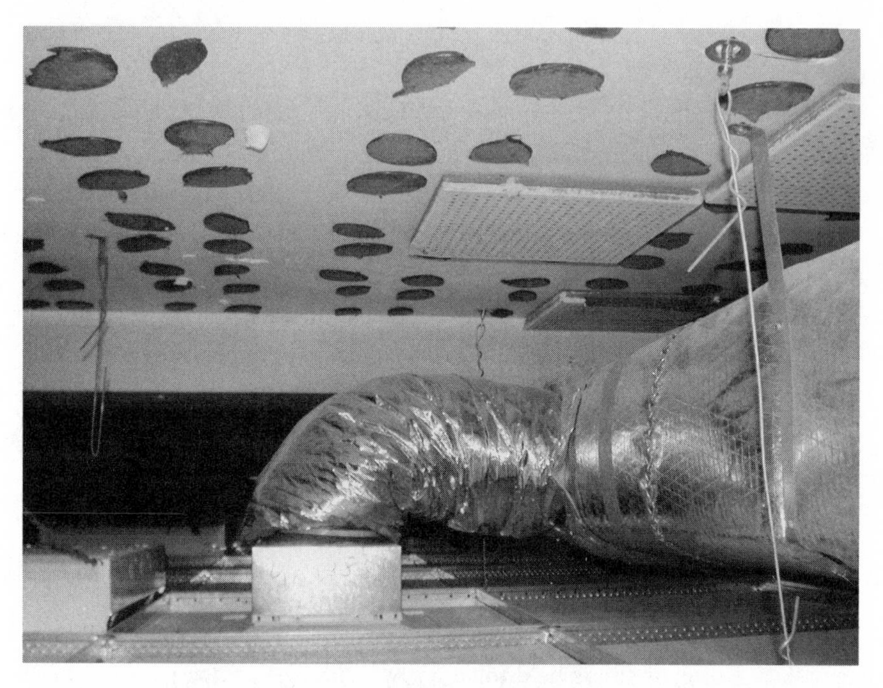

FIGURE 3.1. Inside a ceiling plenum in an older building. At the bottom of the photograph is a suspended ceiling. The wires at the right and left support the ceiling grid that holds the ceiling tiles. At the top of the photograph is the older, original plaster ceiling with oval flattened dollops of adhesive that once held acoustical tiles, two of which are still visible. At the center of the photograph is a supply duct. Immediately to the left is the top of a fluorescent light fixture (a metal box). This ceiling plenum tells a story: The original ceiling could have become damaged, so acoustical tiles were glued on. Those tiles probably became loose, and a suspended ceiling was installed. The space between the original ceiling and the suspended ceiling then served as a return for the mechanical system. *May Indoor Air Investigations LLC*

Ceiling Lights

Ceiling lights face the room and don't appear to do much other than provide light; however, they can sometimes create odor problems if the base for an incandescent (not fluorescent) fixture is made from defective nylon plastic. When heated, the plastic gives off a smell like dead fish caused by one of the chemicals (hexamethylene diamine) used to make the plastic.

FLOORS

Floors in a smaller building may be plywood (sometimes covered with a thin layer of concrete) with wood flooring or carpeting on top. A structural floor in a bigger building is usually concrete, covered with either carpet, resilient or vinyl tile, or sheet goods (the same composite in vinyl tiles but applied in a roll).

Sheet Goods and Floor Tiles

Most older sheet goods or floor tiles (those manufactured before 1950) were composites of asphalt and an inorganic material, such as stone dust or asbestos, that gave the composite such physical properties as toughness and rigidity.

Asbestos is no longer used in construction, because it has been found that the inhalation of asbestos fibers can cause mesothelioma (cancer of the lung pleura). However, asbestos-containing composites were used in construction for many years, and for various purposes. Asbestos was added to joint compounds to impart strength to the dried plaster. The steel columns and girders of many tall buildings were encapsulated in asbestos to insulate the steel structure from the heat of a fire. Without this protection, the steel would more readily soften when exposed to intense heat and then fail (by sagging). Asbestos was used in this way in the lower floors of the World Trade Center towers (see chapter 6). When the two buildings collapsed, asbestos fibers became airborne and settled in the dust and debris that collected within a half-block of ground zero.[1]

Flooring containing asbestos (asbestos composite tile, or ACT) was installed in many older hospitals and schools and was subsequently covered with carpeting. Intact ACT flooring is not a source of significant asbestos exposure, though caution must be exercised when ACT is burnished (polished). Damaged asbestos-containing composites are considered hazardous when disturbed and must be contained or removed from buildings and disposed of professionally, under the strictest containment conditions.

The U.S. Environmental Protection Agency's Asbestos Hazard Emergency Response Act (AHERA) regulates the procedures for asbestos inspection, sampling, and remediation, as well as the requirements for training and accreditation of asbestos inspectors, contractors, management plan developers, and workers. AHERA was originally developed as a set of regulations for schools, but the Asbestos School Hazard Abatement Reauthorization Act (ASHARA) applied some of AHERA's regulations to the handling of asbestos in public and commercial buildings.

Vinyl Flooring

Some modern vinyl flooring is a composite of vinyl plastic (vinyl with plasticizer added), a fibrous material such as cellulose to give it strength, and fillers such as limestone dust. (Pure vinyl is a crystal-clear, brittle solid, but the addition of plasticizer makes the vinyl soft. Think of the mixture as a gel, like a gelatin dessert: a semirigid dispersion of a solid within a liquid.) This kind of flooring is called *VCT,* or *vinyl composite tile.* In one basement office, a strong chemical odor appeared several years after the installation of a new VCT floor. The odor was traced to the degradation of the plasticizer into a chemical that had permeated the concrete floor. (Concrete can be very alkaline and thus hastens the breakdown of plasticizer.)

Another type of vinyl flooring is a multilayered *laminate* (a layered material), with a thin top layer of clear vinyl, a thick middle layer of color-containing vinyl composite with cellulose fibers, and a bottom layer of paper. I looked at one sample of discolored vinyl tile that had been returned to the installer, who wanted to know if the discoloration was caused by mold growth. Mold doesn't grow readily on plastic, but when I looked at the sample under the microscope, I could see that instead of being a solid film, the top layer of clear vinyl was perforated with holes, like a slice of Swiss cheese, perhaps to give the surface a mottled look or because of some defect in the manufacturing process. Water penetrated the holes when the floor was mopped, supplying moisture for mold growth in the discolored cellulose in the composite below.

Carpeting

Some people swear by carpeting. It is not slippery; it is comfortable to walk on, absorbs sound, and can be pleasing to look at. It is also easier to install and replace than a wood floor and is usually less costly. Carpeting is an ideal floor covering, but unless it is manufactured, installed, and maintained properly, carpeting can be a significant source of a variety of IAQ contaminants.

Typical carpeting consists of a pile of more or less vertical fibers, either synthetic (in commercial buildings, generally nylon, acrylic, polyester, or polypropylene) or natural (generally wool or cotton). When the carpet is manufactured, the pile is either mechanically fastened or glued to the horizontal backing.

With both synthetic and natural carpeting, irritating solvents and other chemical residues from the manufacturing process can be released into the air, including a semivolatile chemical, 4-phenylcyclohexene or 4-PC. The source of 4-PC is the "latex" (synthetic styrene-butadiene rubber) adhesive in the carpet backing. (*Latex*, in this context, does not refer to the sap from rubber trees that poses a threat to those with latex allergy.)

When 4-PC and other chemicals in carpeting off-gas, they can be inhaled and lead to a variety of neurological symptoms (and even to chemical sensitivity), though not everyone is affected. Usually a new carpet will off-gas for only a few days or weeks, but some carpeting will off-gas for months. The off-gassing is so irritating in some buildings that the carpeting has to be replaced. Carpet manufacturers have worked hard to minimize the off-gassing of chemicals (see chapter 9) such as styrene and formaldehyde (the latter is no longer used in carpet manufacture).

I am sensitive to some of the chemicals that off-gas from new carpets. When I had to choose a new carpet for a stairwell in my home, I carefully sniffed the loose end of the roll from which my piece was going to be cut. In the showroom, the carpet piece seemed odorless, yet when the carpet was installed the stairwell reeked of "new-carpet odor." We opened the door leading from the staircase to the exterior and operated two fans for weeks to air out the space, but the smell persisted. It was months before I could walk up the stairs without holding my breath. (Had I been employed in a space with this carpet and not been able to relocate, I would have had to quit my job.)

At one time most carpets were treated with an antistain compound called perfluorooctane sulfonate (PFOS). DuPont was the only manufacturer of this chemical. Around the year 2000, researchers began to find minute concentrations of PFOS in the blood of everyone tested. Even though no one was aware of any ill effects caused by this chemical, DuPont stopped manufacturing PFOS.

One of the mysteries about the ubiquitous presence of PFOS in human blood was its mode of entry: skin, ingestion, or inhalation? In many of the air samples I have taken in buildings with carpets, I have found high concentrations of microscopic clumps, looking like lumpy sausages, that I suspect had rubbed off the carpet fibers and that may have contained PFOS. These clumps were under 20 microns in size and were thus inhalable (see chapter 6), so perhaps inhalation *is* one of the ways in which PFOS is introduced into the human body.

The *volatility* (tendency to evaporate) of a solvent is related to its *boiling point,* or the temperature at which the solvent boils. The lower the temperature at which a solvent boils, the more apt the solvent is to evaporate at room temperature. Solvents in paint strippers and paints smell strongly at first and then dissipate over a few days as they evaporate, whereas the chemicals in other thicker building materials may take weeks or months to off-gas, if the chemicals embedded within have higher boiling points.

The rate at which the solvents off-gas is also affected by the temperature of the room, because the tendency to evaporate increases with temperature. In addition, the rate of off-gassing depends on the surface area of the material (how much of the surface is exposed to air). A carpet that is rolled up will off-gas much more slowly than a carpet that is spread out, and solvents in paint will evaporate more quickly once applied to the wall than when sitting in an open can.

Wool rugs can also be irritating to some people. Wool fibers are hairs consisting of a thin outer layer called the *cuticle* that surrounds a thicker cylindrical bundle of fibrous structures called the *cortex.* Just as human hairs can develop split ends, wool hairs can develop split ends when people walk across a wool carpet's surface, and bits of the cuticle and cortex break off and become aerosolized. Under the microscope, a cortex fragment has the shape of a broken pea pod, and a wool cuticle has the shape of a tiny shard of smashed china. Both a wool cortex fragment and a wool cuticle are about the size of a small mold spore and thus are respirable (see chapter 6). People may cough when they inhale wool aerosol, and some, particularly those who wear contact lenses, may find that the aerosol causes eye irritation. I also believe that wool carpeting will occasionally acquire microbial contaminants in the manufacturing process because of bacterial, yeast, or fungal growth in the processing water. In humid weather, wool carpeting sometimes has an animal-like odor that some people find unpleasant.

Some carpet manufacturers advertise their products as "hypoallergenic," which I take to mean that the carpeting doesn't support the growth of mold and bacteria. This label could be applied to just about any synthetic carpet, because nylon and polypropylene do not readily support microbial growth. On the other hand, any dust in the carpet is biodegradable and can be a source of nutrients for mold, bacteria, and yeast. And pollen, pet dander, or dust mite

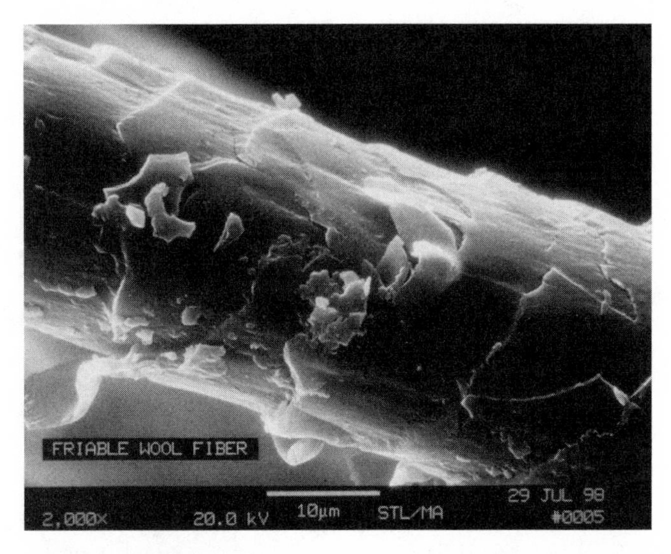

FIGURE 3.2. Wool cuticle (SEM 2,000×). This SEM (scanning electron micrograph) is a photograph of a wool hair magnified about 2,000 times. The SEM illustrates the fragmentation of the cuticle (the exterior sheathing). *May Indoor Air Investigations LLC*

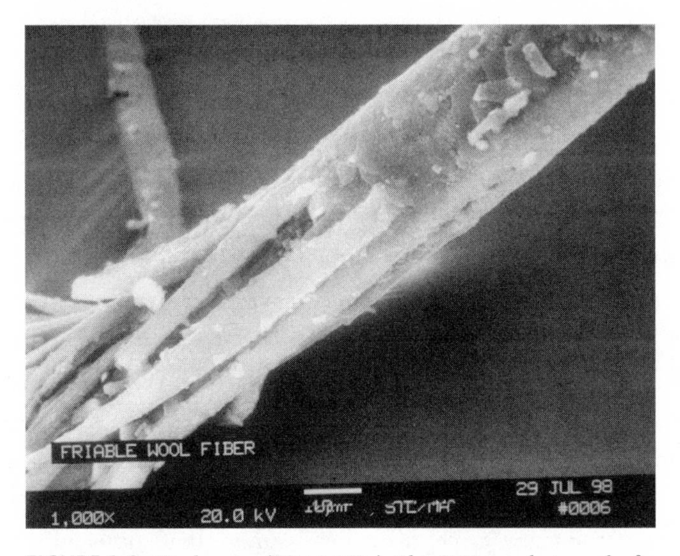

FIGURE 3.3. Wool cortex (SEM 1,000×). This SEM is a photograph of a wool hair magnified about 1,000 times. The intact cuticle is at the upper right. At the bottom left, the cuticle has disintegrated, and the individual cortex fibers (cable-like structures within the hair) are revealed. This is the wool-hair equivalent of a split end. *May Indoor Air Investigations LLC*

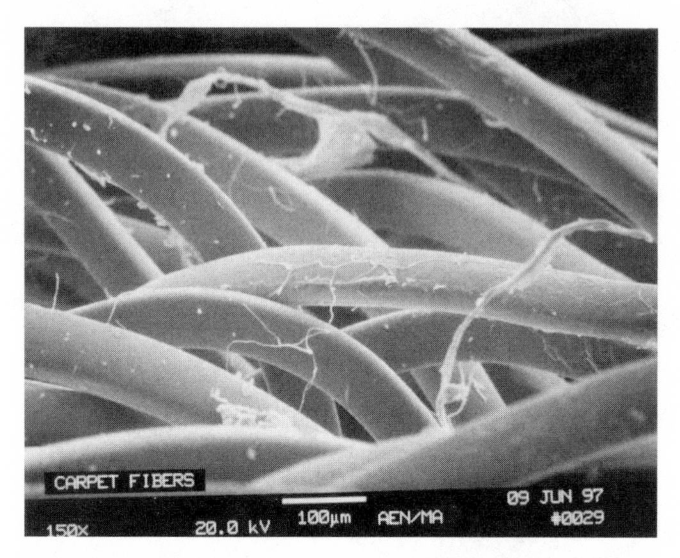

FIGURE 3.4. Mold hyphae on a carpet fiber (SEM 150×). The thick, curved, tube-like structures are loops of nylon from a sample of wall-to-wall carpet installed in a damp basement. Mold hyphae (the "roots" of fungi) are visible as fine threads, running across the smooth, nylon surfaces. The two coarser, thicker fibers are cellulose: paper or lint from settled dust. The mold hyphae were digesting the dust particles that had landed on the nylon. The carpet was so new (only two months old) that the settled dust and thus the mold hyphae were on top of the fibers, and not on top of the backing. *May Indoor Air Investigations LLC*

allergens, potentially stored in any carpet, can be aerosolized when the carpet fibers are disturbed by foot traffic.

The Carpet and Rug Institute claims that carpeting acts as a filter and can store dust until it is vacuumed away. Unfortunately, it is impossible to vacuum all the dust out of a carpet. A solid-surface floor (wood or vinyl) measuring 8 feet by 8 feet has the same dimensional area as a carpeted floor measuring 8 feet by 8 feet: 64 square feet. But the actual *surface* area of the carpet is more than fifty times greater than that of the vinyl or wood floor, because each of the many carpet fibers has a surface that contributes to the total surface area of the carpeting. Dust can be trapped on, between, and below the fibers and become nutrients for microbes. Add moisture, and microbial growth begins. Such dust and contaminants can become airborne when disturbed. One study found that dancing on carpeting as compared with dancing on a hardwood floor produced nine times as many aerosolized particulates.[2]

In general, I believe that permanently installed carpeting should not be placed in areas regularly subjected to wetting or soiling: near or at entrances to buildings, in bathrooms, and in kitchens. Some buildings have recessed metal grates in the vestibule area where people first enter from the outside, so that most of the tracked-in dirt, water, and snow falls through the grate and into a pan before people move into other parts of the building. A removable "walk-off mat" can be used to protect the carpet located beyond the grille.

Dampness in a carpet may come from a source not readily apparent. I investigated two offices in which occupants were experiencing asthma symptoms. In both cases I found mold growing in dust in the carpeting beneath vinyl/plastic chair mats. The buildings were slab-on-grade, and the carpeting was placed directly on the concrete slab. Moisture from the soil moved by capillary action through the concrete and carpeting, and from there it evaporated into each room. The moisture was not able to evaporate in places where the mats covered the carpeting, and the fibers remained damp. In some spots water even condensed on the bottom of a plastic mat. There were sufficient nutrients in the carpet dust, as well as moisture, for mold growth to occur. A similar situation can develop at upper-level floors when carpeting is washed and chair mats are put back before the carpeting has dried.

When the chairs were rolled across the plastic mats, spores were pushed out into the air from under the edges of the mats, as well as through holes that had been drilled into the plastic for "ventilation." There were many desks and chairs in this office, and so there were many islands of mold growth under numerous chair mats. I recommended that the carpeting be removed and that a moisture-impervious flooring be applied over the concrete before new carpeting was installed.

The Underpad

Carpeting may or may not have a pad underneath made of synthetic foam, rubber- or plastic-based materials, or a natural cellulose fiber such as jute. If made of a rubber-based material, the pad can off-gas an odor similar to the smell of a new tire. I know of one case in which a wool rug was placed on top of an odorous rubber pad. The pad was discarded, but the rug had to be washed and aired out for days before the odor that had adsorbed (collected) on the surface of the wool fibers dissipated.

Carpeting and carpet pads installed directly on cool concrete in below-grade spaces can also develop conditions of high humidity, resulting in microbial growth within. (I'll be discussing this further in the chapters that follow.) I was once asked to investigate a nursing home because one of the patients was experiencing respiratory problems in her room. The wall-to-wall carpet and padding were installed on concrete. When I lifted the carpet and pad, I found the concrete sprinkled with sawdust from construction. Intersecting black rings consisting of colonies of *Alternaria* mold covered the concrete. Apparently the carpet and pad had been laid down on the concrete before it had dried adequately (cured). The sawdust and other dust left on the concrete must have contained mold spores which then had the food (sawdust consists of wood fibers, mostly cellulose and other biodegradable components) and the moisture (evaporating from the concrete) that they needed to develop into colonies. Whenever people walked across the carpet, allergens were probably released into the air.

Adhesives

In public buildings carpeting is usually glued to the concrete, and vinyl composite tile is always glued down. To be applied to large surface areas, adhesive must be able to flow, and thus water or solvent is used in the adhesive mixture. In order for the adhesive to solidify, the solvent must diffuse through the tile or carpet and evaporate into the air, which can create irritating vapors. Water-based adhesives produce fewer volatile organic compounds, or VOCs, than solvent-based ones do. The Carpet and Rug Institute advises that after new carpeting has been installed, the space should be well ventilated and odors flushed out before occupancy, particularly if solvent-based adhesives are used.

FURNITURE AND EQUIPMENT

Many desks, bookcases, computer tables, and even room partitions are made of particle board laminates: pressed sawdust stuck together with urea-formaldehyde adhesive, which is then coated with or sandwiched between two thin layers of plastic. Formaldehyde by itself is a pungent gas that is irritating to the mucous membranes and that may cause chemical sensitization as well as an extremely rare occupational disease, nasopharyngeal cancer. When particle board first came into use, the emission rates of formaldehyde from the adhesive (from exposed surfaces) were high enough to create IAQ problems. (The emission from the laminated surfaces, however, was minimal.) These rates have been reduced by more careful manufacturing processes; however, some odor still remains and is particularly noticeable when such furniture is first unpacked.*

Copiers, laser printers, and specialized printing equipment such as blueprint machines and photographic processing devices also emit a mixture of chemicals that can have a significant negative effect on indoor air quality (see chapter 5).

Items made of vinyl (window screens, computer monitors, plastic cables, even vinyl-covered three-ring notebooks) can produce indoor air problems. Vinyl products may contain two common plasticizers: dioctyl phthalate (DOP) or diethylhexyl phthalate (DEHP). Both DOP and DEHP are made by combining phthalic acid with either the chemical 1-octanol, resulting in DOP, or the chemical 2-octanol, resulting in DEHP (see chapter 5). If present in the air, both octanols can potentially be irritating to inhale, or at least annoying

During the 1990s a process called *bake-out* was tested as a means of flushing out newly furnished or finished spaces. The process involved maintaining the heat in a new building at more than 90°F while diluting the indoor air with outdoor air. The idea was that the heat would cause a rapid off-gassing of solvent vapors, which could then be ventilated out of the building. The results were disappointing, however, because some of the solvent vapors diffused into and thus contaminated materials that didn't initially contain those chemicals. In addition, the high temperatures sometimes caused shrinkage and cracks in finished surfaces. The cost of heating the building and repairing the damage, as well as the work time lost while the building was vacant, led to the abandonment of bake-out. Nonetheless, whenever feasible it is always a good idea before occupancy to ventilate (flush out) a space that has new finishes or furnishings.

* The emission of formaldehyde from particle board adhesive depends on temperature and relative humidity. Below about 70°F and 50 percent relative humidity, emissions are low, even from problem materials (see chapter 4).

to smell. 1-octanol has a chemical odor, and 2-octanol has an unpleasant, mushroomy odor, which may lead some people to believe that mold growth is present. This moldy odor may become a problem with some computers that contain DEHP plasticizer in vinyl parts.

Dioctyl phthalate has been found in blood that has been stored in vinyl bags as well as in foods that have come into contact with vinyl packaging. Some people are concerned there may be health consequences to the buildup of DOP in the human body; others worry that DOP may act as a hormone mimic. (Chemicals that act as hormone mimics affect animal reproduction.)[3]

Floor mats under office chairs are made of vinyl. The flexible vinyl used in mats is only about 70 percent vinyl; the balance of the material is plasticizer. Solvent may be used in the processing. One of these solvents, xylene, emits the odor associated with vinyl products such as new shower curtains. Although some people find this odor irritating and even sickening, the odor usually dissipates in a few days.

Styrene butadiene plastic, from which computer monitors are made, is another source of an irritating chemical-like odor. Some monitors smell and others do not; some lose the smell with time and others continue to off-gas for months. In offices where all the computer monitors come from a single lot, if the computers off-gas, the odor can be quite strong.

MYSTERIOUS AND NOT-SO-MYSTERIOUS BUILDING ODORS

If there is a vase of flowers in a room, it is pretty easy to identify the source of the fragrance in the air. And the closer you get to the vase, the stronger the smell. On the other hand, if an entire ceiling, the carpet, or the walls in a room are producing small amounts of odor, it can be very difficult to locate the source, because the odor is spread out and diffuse, and other surfaces in the same space may acquire that smell (by adsorption). Something that generates an odor is called a *primary source,* and material that adsorbs that odor is called a *secondary source.* It is often easier to get rid of a secondary-source smell emanating from the wall than one emanating from the carpet, because the carpet has more surface area than the wall. (The greater the surface area, the greater the capacity for adsorption.)

Even when not in use, bathrooms can also be the source of odors. Hot- and cold-water supply pipes are always full of water under pressure, which is why water flows out of the pipe as soon as you turn a faucet handle. On the other hand, water flows through the waste pipes of a building by the force of gravity when people flush a toilet or drain a sink. (This is why drain pipes must always be sloped downward to drain water.) When fixtures are not in use, the drain pipes are full of air, not water, with one exception: sewer-line traps, which are U-shaped sections of pipe under sinks or in floor drains. The fixture side of the U contains room air. The drain side contains sewer gas: a mixture of gasses, some of which have unpleasant odors due to bacterial growth. In the middle of the U is water, which prevents the sewer gas from entering the fixture side of the U. If the water in the trap dries out, sewer gas is no longer "trapped" and can enter the room. If the bathroom exhaust is on, it will draw gas from the drain pipes that much faster. Then the bathroom can smell strongly of sewer gas, and airflows can carry that odor into adjacent rooms. People may experience nausea or headaches from exposure to even low concentrations of sewer gas.

In 2003 the virus that causes Severe Acute Respiratory Syndrome (SARS) raged among the residents of a high-rise apartment building in Hong Kong. People who were sick threw up or had diarrhea, and these waste products entered the drain piping of the building. All the bathrooms had floor drains; unfortunately, the traps were dry because the residents no longer cleaned the floors by inundating them with water from buckets. One theory for the spread of the disease was that aerosols containing the virus entered the bathrooms through the dry traps; three hundred people in the apartment block were infected, and thirty-five of them died.[4]

Sewer gas can also enter the bathroom through the gap between the floor and the base of the toilet if the wax ring (the seal between the toilet and the sewer pipe flange) is not airtight. Usually, though not always, a loose toilet is an indication of a bad wax seal. The ceramic base of a toilet should always be completely immobile.

THE THREE P'S: PAPER, PLANTS, AND PEOPLE

The chemicals in self-copy, pressure-sensitive *paper* forms (carbonless paper) are distributed on the paper surface in microscopic brittle packets *(microspheres)* that break under the pressure of the point of a pen or pencil. These chemicals then react with other chemicals in the paper to change color; thus the pattern of the crushed microspheres traces the path taken by the writing instrument. The chemicals in the microspheres include formaldehyde and solvents and can be irritating if touched or aerosolized and inhaled.

In most offices only a small number of self-copying forms are used, so those who use them may be the only ones who are exposed to the chemicals. In billing offices where high-speed equipment prints on rolls of perforated self-copying forms, however, more of the chemicals can become vaporized and cause more widespread eye and mucous membrane irritation. Inhalation of the chemicals from the microspheres can also cause hoarseness (due to laryngeal swelling) and cough.[5]

Green *plants* are not usually sources of indoor air quality problems, and some people believe that spider plants can remove contaminants such as formaldehyde.[6] One study showed that bacteria and moisture in the soil were responsible for the removal of the formaldehyde.[7] Still, excess moisture from overwatering the plant or from surfaces that are dampened because the flower pot is porous can lead to biological growth and to bioaerosol. And if leaves fall onto the soil and become moldy, and the plant and soil surfaces are disturbed by airflows from a heating or cooling system, mold spores may be aerosolized.

Pesticides in the soil or applied to the plant may occasionally cause a problem for someone who is sensitized. Finally, some plants produce allergen-containing aerosol such as pollen, though the pollen from most ornamentals is too large to remain airborne long enough to be much of an allergy issue. One popular indoor tree, a weeping fig (*Ficus benjamina*) can cause rhinitis (nasal irritation), urticaria (hives), swelling of the eyelids, and allergic asthma, if dust that has been in contact with the "latex" in the leaves is aerosolized and inhaled by sensitized individuals.[8]

People can spread illnesses in an indoor environment. In crowded spaces lacking fresh air (see the discussion on ventilation in chapter 7), there is a higher likelihood for the transmission of diseases spread by coughing and inhalation. People can also introduce irritants and contaminants into the building envelope. They may have residual chemicals from detergents or softeners in their clothing, or they may be wearing strong aftershave or perfume (I discuss fragrances in chapter 5). Most large office buildings don't allow pets, but in some cases employees may bring their pets to work, either literally or on their clothing in the form of pet dander. Have you ever noticed that you start to sneeze or cough every time some co-worker walks by? You may be reacting to mite allergens, or to cat or dog dander, on his or her clothing or even hair (especially if the person hasn't showered for a day or two).

I was once asked to investigate the air quality in a small office where one of the employees had threatened to contact the Occupational Safety and Health Administration because of asthma symptoms she experienced at work. I took air samples in her office and found that the air was extraordinarily free of particulates. The employee had taken the day off, so I had the opportunity to take a dust sample from the cushion of her chair. The sample contained feather particles and dust mite fecal pellets, which were not consistent with any of the particulates in the office air. The office manager told me that the employee normally sat on a down pillow she brought from home. Judging from the dust, the pillow was contaminated with dust mites (see chapter 6).

My samples from the woman's pillow also contained pet dander. Estimates of the numbers of Americans allergic to cats vary from 2 to 15 percent. Cat allergen, however, is common in all buildings, whether or not the animals are present, because the dander from cats is readily transported by and shed from the clothing of pet owners, and cat allergens accumulate in building dust (see chapter 14). One Swedish study found that 80 percent of children with cat allergies had never lived with a cat, suggesting that the levels of cat allergens in schools or other buildings were high enough to cause sensitization.[9]

Sometimes the animal products that cause problems do not come from domesticated animals. I just read a paper in the medical literature about someone who developed hypersensitivity pneumonitis as a result of exposure to droppings from Canada geese. The carpets in the individual's place of work

> Generally, dust mites colonize cushions that pick up warmth and moisture from frequent human contact. But even if a down cushion is free of dust mite allergens, air containing small fragments of feathers (and the numerous microorganisms often associated with feathers) is forced out of the cushions when compressed. Because these particles can cause lung irritation or allergy symptoms, I usually discourage the use of couches and chairs that have feather stuffing.

had probably become contaminated with goose droppings carried into the building on people's shoes, though the paper suggests that the droppings came in through the ventilation system because the antigens (allergens) were found on the office air filter.[10]

CLEANING DILEMMAS

Dust can be a source of allergens as well as nutrients for microbial growth, so it is important to remove dust. Ironically, the way we clean is often the source of indoor air quality problems. People who have concerns about IAQ should educate themselves about maintenance practices in the buildings in which they work or otherwise spend extended time, so that they can ask questions and convey their concerns to the appropriate individuals.

Hard Surfaces

Window cleaners and surface polishes are often sprayed onto the surfaces to be cleaned. Some of these chemicals then become airborne as small droplets, and when the water in the droplets evaporates, the cleaning compounds (detergents, fragrances, and other chemicals) may become potentially irritating vapor or airborne particles that can be inhaled. Pump sprays or squirt bottles are preferable to aerosol cans, because they produce larger droplets that are not so readily aerosolized. When working around sensitized individuals, maintenance staff should use cleaners that can be applied directly to a cloth for damp-wiping, rather than use sprays.

Hard-surface flooring has to be damp-wiped regularly, so in any building with wood or vinyl floors, there is usually a cleaning closet containing brooms, mops, and cleaning agents. If the mops are not rinsed thoroughly and allowed to dry after being used, they can develop sour or musty odors that can spread beyond the closet into the hallway or rooms nearby. The odor and microbes may also be spread during subsequent "cleaning," leaving a slime on the surface that dries to an invisible but frustrating source of foul odor.

Carpeting

Carpet maintenance is vital for indoor air hygiene, because collected dust and other contaminants that are in a carpet may become airborne. Carpeting in a high-traffic area of a building should be vacuumed daily.

All vacuum cleaners have powerful blowers that draw in air through the cleaning head, wand, and hose. Most vacuums contain a replaceable bag designed to capture (filter) the dirt and dust. Air passes through the bag and is then blown back into the room through the vacuum's exhaust. Unfortunately, the bag of an ordinary vacuum cleaner cannot capture smaller particles such as clay, some mold spores, and other allergens and microbes, and these particles are aerosolized as soon as they are emitted with the exhausted air. Many offices employ outside cleaning services. If these services use conventional or leaky vacuum cleaners, it is possible that contaminants from the carpeting in another building that the service cleans will be dispersed into the air. This is why I recommend that all vacuuming be done with machines equipped with *HEPA* (*high-efficiency particulate arrestance*) filters. A HEPA filter traps nearly all the particles in the airstream.

I was once giving a talk about indoor air quality at a respiratory hospital that had a carpeted hallway outside the auditorium. The doors to the room were open, and during my talk I could hear the distant roar of an approaching upright vacuum cleaner. As the vacuum drew nearer, people in the audience (including patients, some in wheelchairs and attached to oxygen tanks) began to cough. The machine had inefficient filtration and was exhausting allergens or irritants, and building airflows were carrying these particulates from the hallway into the auditorium.

When carpets are stained, they must be washed. Some carpet-washing systems (which can be either portable or truck-mounted) spray hot water into the carpet with a cleaning head. At the same time, a vacuum hose attached to the head extracts the water from the carpet. If the carpeting and pad dry out rapidly, this type of cleaning is not a problem, and it has been used successfully in hundreds of thousands of buildings all over the country. However, washing can never remove all the dust from a carpet, so if the carpet doesn't dry out quickly and if the temperature is sufficiently warm, microbial growth within the residual moist dust can begin within twenty-four to forty-eight hours. And if detergent or other chemicals are not properly rinsed from the carpet, residues can be left behind. These chemicals can then stick to dust particles remaining in the carpet after it dries and be aerosolized by foot traffic.

The chemicals used can create other indoor air problems as well. For example, when soiled water is drawn back into a carpet-cleaning machine, the soapy mixture has a great deal of air mixed in with it. To prevent this liquid from frothing and spewing out of the equipment, a defoaming chemical must be added. During an inspection of one sick school—a building experiencing IAQ problems as a result of contaminated dust in carpeting—I opened a bottle of defoamer from the supply closet. The bottle reeked of *MVOCs* (*microbial volatile organic compounds*) and was full of mold growth. I suspect that when exhaust air came out of the carpet-washing machine, some of this mold was aerosolized and settled into the carpet, to join the microbes already living there.

I always recommend that only certified and trained professionals undertake carpet cleaning, and that only chemicals approved by the carpet industry be used in the cleaning process. The Institute of Inspection, Cleaning and Restoration Certification trains and certifies professional carpet cleaners and is a good resource. Though I do not agree with some of the statements on its website, the Carpet and Rug Institute is another source of information (see the Resource Guide).

Sometimes we dampen carpets unintentionally when we spill beverages. A small amount of water can be soaked up with paper towels and the carpet simply be allowed to dry, but when beverages other than water (such as coffee or soft drinks) are spilled, the liquid should be blotted up and the area spot-cleaned. You can never remove every trace of the spill, but clean as much of it out of the carpet as you can, to minimize nutrients for mold and bacteria. This is particularly important if the carpet is on concrete that is resting on soil (slab on grade; see chapter 2) or is below grade, because even after the carpet has dried, conditions of high humidity and residual sugars remaining in the carpet from the spill may fuel microbial growth (see chapter 4). In carpeting in below-grade spaces, I have seen colonies of mold that delineated long-forgotten food spills!

Bathrooms

Because bathrooms may have bacterial contamination, powerful disinfectants are used for cleaning. Some of these cleaners may be chemically incompatible with each other and produce toxic fumes when mixed. Diluted bleach (hypochlorite) may be used to clean some bathroom surfaces, but bleach should never be mixed with either acids (such as hydrochloric acid, also called *muriatic acid*, sometimes used to clean toilets) or ammonia. When bleach is mixed with acid, toxic chlorine gas is produced; when bleach and ammonia are mixed, toxic choloramine gas is produced. Exposure to mixtures of bleach fumes, chloramine, and chlorine are a source of occupational asthma among cleaning workers.[11]

Microbial growth is likely to occur in any room where water is routinely present, so bathroom surfaces must be kept as clean and dry as possible. Leaks should be repaired promptly. In cases where leaks have continued for a long time, any mold-damaged materials should be cleaned or professionally removed and replaced, depending on the extent of the damage.

Perfumed Restrooms

Strong fragrances are often used to mask bathroom odors. A potpourri sachet treated with chemical fragrances such as vanillin and raspberry ketone is propped in a vase or hung on the wall. Occasionally an aerosol can of fragrance is left on a bathroom shelf. Sometimes a block of paradichlorobenzene (a toxic pesticide also known as mothballs) is placed in the men's urinal. Even though the block is a solid, the chemical *sublimes* (goes directly from a solid to a vapor) at room temperature.

Fragrance is a masking agent, not a cleaning agent. A properly maintained, cleaned, and ventilated bathroom should not need to be doused in "perfumes." Fragranced bathrooms are particularly problematic for individuals with chemical sensitivities.

Air Purifiers

When occupants are dissatisfied with the air quality in a building, they sometimes purchase portable air purifiers for their individual spaces. The simplest type of air purifier, which comes in a variety of sizes and capacities, has a blower to move air through the equipment and a HEPA filter to remove particulates. Such a device does clean the air, but unfortunately it does not remove contaminants within the carpet or mechanical system; these contaminants can become airborne faster than the HEPA filter can remove them. One type of portable HEPA air purifier has a large gooseneck supply that can be directed toward the user's face and therefore toward the person's breathing zone. If the diameter of the supply is at least 4 to 6 inches, this type of air purifier is likely to significantly reduce the number of allergens that an occupant will inhale (see the Resource Guide for *IQAir*). More sophisticated air purifiers contain charcoal filters to remove VOCs as well as HEPA filters to remove particles.

Another type of purifier, called an *ionizer*, produces electric fields that charge (ionize) the air to create airflows. Unfortunately, in this process, minute sparks occur and irritating ozone gas is formed. Most of the manufacturers of this kind of equipment claim that the ozone produced in a typical-sized room does not exceed the Food and Drug Administration's (FDA's) concentration guideline, but in small rooms the ozone produced can exceed the guideline. There are many manufacturers selling air purifiers that produce ozone, because we associate the smell of this gas with clean outdoor air. Though ozone gas can be useful in high concentrations to eliminate certain odors, even low concentrations can cause problems for people with asthma (see chapter 5). A building's occupants should not risk unnecessary exposure by being present when ozone is being used to eliminate odors; and I believe that this is the *only* purpose for which ozone should be produced in occupied spaces, particularly spaces where people with asthma work or live.

In the end, no matter how many individual room air purifiers are in use, there is no substitute for first getting rid of the *sources* of contaminants within the building envelope.

SOME PRACTICAL STEPS

- Consider using a leather-covered rather than a fabric-covered office chair. Fabric-covered cushions allow dust and moisture to build up in the cushioning, supporting the growth of dust mites.
- To determine if a vinyl product such as an insect screen is off-gassing an irritating smell, remove the item and ventilate the room to see if the odor goes away.
- If a carpet is wet, the room should be dehumidified or ventilated (with dry, not humid air).
- Carpeting should dry within twelve to twenty-four hours after it has been washed. If the carpet in your building has been washed

and stays wet for more than twenty-four hours, and a musty or sour smell develops, there is a good chance that microbial growth has occurred. The carpet should then be evaluated by an IAQ professional. The carpet may have to be removed.

- If you suspect that irritants in a carpet are being aerosolized by foot traffic and the carpet cannot be removed immediately (under containment conditions, to prevent allergens and irritants from contaminating adjacent spaces), cover high-traffic *dry* areas of the carpet with a nonslip heavy-duty plastic runner or adhesive-backed plastic film (see the Resource Guide). Don't put a runner over a damp carpet.
- If new wall-to-wall carpet is to be installed in your workspace and you are sensitized to the chemicals, ask if you can "sniff-test" a carpet sample before the carpeting is installed.
- If carpeting or new furnishings are brought into a space and a strong odor develops, the area should be well ventilated until the odor disappears. Individuals who are sensitized to the odor may have to move to another space if such a space is available.
- To find out if a surface area is emitting an odor, you can conduct what I call the foil test. Lay a piece of paper toweling, folded into quarters, over an area on a floor or wall, cover the exposed side of the paper towel with a flat piece of aluminum foil, and tape the edges of the foil to the surface (being careful to use tape that will not damage the surface or covering). Leave the covered paper towel on the surface for twenty-four to forty-eight hours. When you remove the assembly, fold the paper towel into the aluminum foil so that the towel is completely covered on both sides and sealed within the foil. Take the wrapped towel outside and, without unwrapping it, loosen an edge of the foil and cautiously take a small sniff. If the surface on which the towel rested is off-gassing, the towel should have adsorbed some of the VOCs.
- Avoid using spray pesticides indoors.
- Encourage cleaning personnel in your building to use unscented products and a HEPA-filtered vacuum.
- Avoid using ozone-generating air purifiers.

CHAPTER

4

A Sea of Air

A woman was renting an apartment on an upper floor of a four-story building with a commercial cleaning company on the first floor. When she entered the building stairwell, she could smell the chemical fumes arising from solvents stored in the basement. She would rush upstairs holding her breath, unlock her front door, and run in to open a window in her bedroom. This didn't help much in the winter when the heat was on, because more warm air flowed out the apartment window than cold exterior air flowed in. As a result, more air flowed from the stairwell through the gap under her closed door and into her kitchen, bringing the chemical fumes into her apartment.

Like water, air is a fluid that flows. We cannot see clean air because it is colorless and transparent, but outdoors we can tell that it moves because we feel wind against our bodies. We usually aren't aware of air movements inside a building, though, unless the flow is so strong that we can feel it on our skin. But the fact that most of the air movement indoors is imperceptible does not mean that the air is still.

Air carries invisible vapors and gases in its currents: fumes from solvents, combustion gases entering from heating systems, emissions from furniture, and fragrances from perfumes and cleaning products. Airflows also carry particulates. In the air inside a building, particularly in a beam of light from the sun or a projector, we may see cigarette haze or suspended dust particles called *motes,* which consist mostly of skin scales: microscopic cells that we all con-

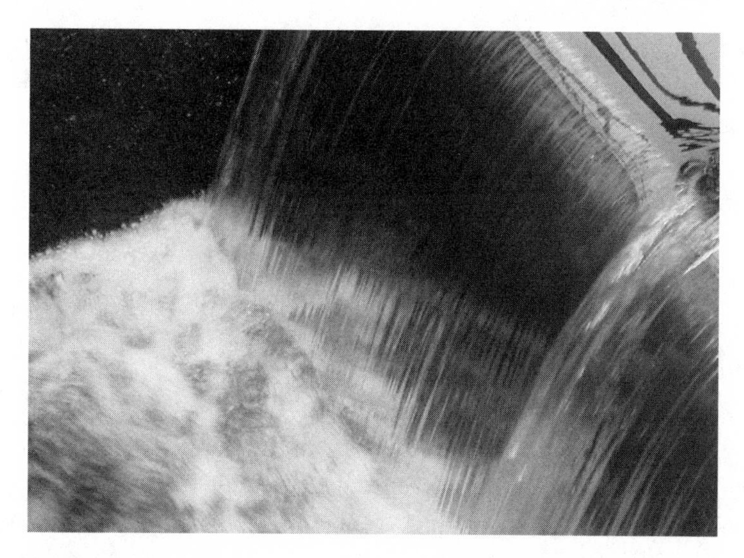

FIGURE 4.1. Fluid flows. Captivating to watch, flowing water has been a source of energy for centuries. The flow of air can also be harnessed (by windmills) for energy. *Jeffrey C. May*

stantly shed (about 30 grams per month) from our bodies. Clothing lint, paper fibers, soot, rust, mold spores, and minute insect body parts are also part of the mote mix. Some of the gases and particulates mixed in air are benign; others may be irritating, allergenic, or even toxic.

If enough fresh air enters and stale air exits a building, many irritants and contaminants are diluted and even flushed out. In older buildings, windows can be opened in the warmer months, and air will also infiltrate and exfiltrate (leak in from the outside and vice versa) through construction gaps and uninsulated wall cavities. But most newer buildings are tightly constructed and lack operable windows, so fresh air must be provided by mechanical systems. These complex systems are often inadequately designed, installed, or maintained (or intentionally shut down, as at the University of Massachusetts Boston; see chapter 1). As a result, fresh air distribution may be poor, compounding any indoor air quality problems that may be present.

In the chapters that follow I will be discussing vapors, gases, and particulates as well as heating, ventilation, and air-conditioning (HVAC) systems. In this chapter I discuss how air moves, which has an effect on what the airflows may contain and thus a potential impact on the health of building occupants. To understand the movement of fluids such as air, we must first understand a bit about the composition of matter and how it behaves.

MARBLES OF MATTER

Matter is made up of atoms and molecules. Just about every atom in your body was once part of either another living organism or an inanimate object. Some of the calcium in your bones probably came from milk produced by a cow that ate grass growing in soil that contained calcium that came from rocks. In a pregnant woman's womb, the fetus is formed from nutrients in the mother's blood that came from the food she ate, and so on. Just as the twenty-six letters in the English alphabet can be arranged and rearranged into thousands of words and the same words rearranged into gossip magazines or even Shakespearean plays, atoms are combined and recombined in myriad ways to make up the food we eat, the clothes we wear, and even the family members we love. The "stuff" of life is constant but shared and recycled.

Atoms combine in various ways to make up molecules. Some molecules are small and simple, some large and complex, but all are too small to see. (The number of air molecules that would fit on just the surface of the period at the end of the last sentence is greater than 100,000,000,000,000,000!)

Infinitely small though molecules are, imagine that they looked and behaved like many tiny marbles. In a solid, the marbles would be packed together, much as they would be in a box filled to the brim, and each marble would be attached to its immediate neighbors by an imaginary string called a *bond.* (Bonds in matter result from the attraction of opposite charges, like the opposite poles of a magnet.) The marbles can neither move freely about nor rotate, but at every temperature other than absolute zero (the theoretical coldest temperature measurable), the marbles are vibrating back and forth a minute distance, as if tethered together by tight springs. In a liquid, the marbles are still held close together but are more weakly bonded than in a solid, with the strength of the bond depending on the particular liquid. Nonetheless, the molecules can rotate and move. In a gas, such as air at sea level, the marbles are not bonded to each other and are thus free to rotate and move more

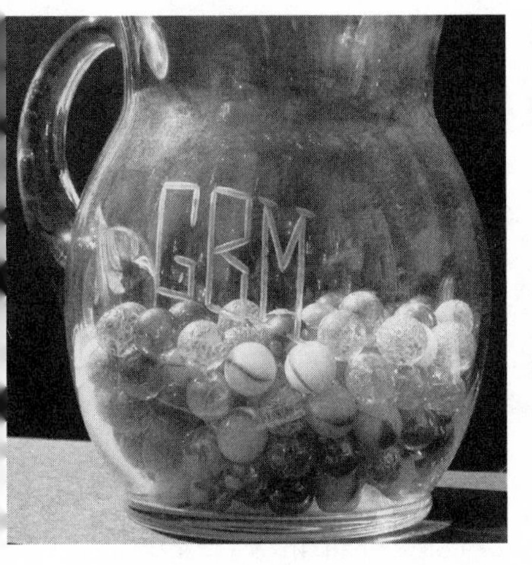

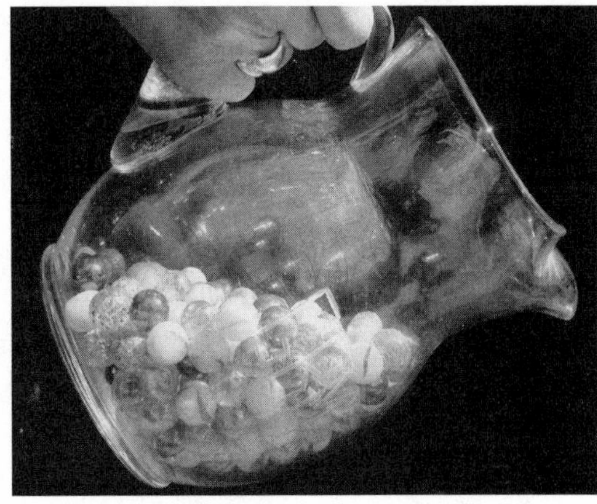

FIGURE 4.2. The marble theory of matter. The molecules in a liquid, here represented by marbles, are pulled by the force of gravity. At rest, the surface of a liquid is flat and level. If you tip the vessel, the molecules (marbles) roll and move until the surface becomes level again. *Jeffrey C. May*

than in a liquid. In addition, at sea level the molecules in air are about ten times as far apart as those in a liquid; there is more space between the marbles.

Temperature is a measure of how fast the marbles are vibrating if they are in a solid, or vibrating, rotating, and moving if they are in a liquid or a gas. Inside a vessel containing a gas at any temperature above absolute zero, the marbles are constantly in motion, colliding with one another and with the walls of the container. The hotter the gas, the faster the marbles are moving and rotating. The colder the gas, the slower the marbles are moving and rotating. The fact that the marbles move gives a gas its pressure and substance. Think of it this way: If a few hundred flies start buzzing around inside an open garbage bag, the bag will appear to inflate. If the insects stop flying and settle down to feed, the bag will appear to deflate.

As the marbles in a contained gas move faster, they exert more force when they collide with the walls of the vessel, and therefore the pressure within increases. As the marbles slow down, they exert less force, and therefore the pressure within decreases. This is why manufacturers recommend that you measure air pressure in a car tire when the tire is cool, after the car has been sitting still for a while, rather than when the tire is warm from driving. If you measure tire pressure after you've driven a while, you may get a falsely high reading. Then if you let out some of the air to correct the overpressure, the tire will be at too low a pressure when it cools.

The pressure of a gas is related to volume (the amount of space a three-dimensional object occupies) as well as to temperature. Reducing the volume of a gas-filled container like a syringe or an air pump crowds the marbles of matter so that the number of their collisions with each other and with the container's walls increases, and the pressure within rises.

When I was a high school science teacher I liked to use a basketball to illustrate the relationships among the volume, temperature, and pressure differences of gases. The more air you pump into a basketball, the greater the internal pressure. If you sit on the ball, decreasing the volume slightly, the pressure within will likewise increase. If you heat the ball, it will expand slightly as the molecules move faster and the internal pressure rises. If you cool the ball, it will shrink slightly as the internal pressure decreases. And if there is a small hole in the ball or if the valve leaks, air will leak out, and the pressure within will again decrease because air at a higher pressure flows toward air at a lower pressure.

Elevator Shafts and Mold

When an elevator descends, it compresses the air beneath it and rarefies (thins) the air above it. Since the pressure is then greater below the elevator than above, air will flow upward in the narrow space between the elevator and the walls of the shaft. When the elevator is ascending, it rarefies the air beneath and compresses the air above. Air will then flow downward in the space between the elevator and the walls of the shaft. Where the air pressure in the shaft is higher than the pressure in an adjacent hallway, air will flow out of the shaft into the hallway through gaps in the doors.

In one interesting case of a high-rise office building with mold problems, the source of the mold was the drywall (acting as a fire separation wall) lining the interior of the elevator shafts. The drywall was installed at the lower levels of the building, including the basement, before the upper levels had been made weather-tight. When it rained, rainwater blew across the exposed floors and into the open elevator shafts, puddling at the bottom and soaking the drywall, which was soon overgrown with mold. Once the building was completed, the mold growth was disturbed as the elevator ascended and descended, and spores and allergens became airborne and spread through the shaft and into the building hallways on airflows.

Wall and Ceiling Cavities

A wall consists of vertical studs (the framing) to which the surface material, such as drywall, is fastened. The vertical studs (made of wood or metal) give the wall strength and are usually spaced 16 inches apart. The space between the studs is called the *bay* or *wall cavity.* Similarly, a *ceiling cavity* is a space between two floor joists, enclosed at the top by the floor and at the bottom by a drywall or plaster ceiling (not a suspended ceiling).

You may not think of wall and ceiling cavities as parts of the rooms you occupy, but particulates or gases in these spaces can affect a building's indoor air quality. Sometimes rodents nest in wall cavities, and then odors from their droppings or from the decaying bodies of dead animals may enter the habitable space. Insulation is also installed in wall cavities, particularly in the cavities of exterior walls, because the insulation blocks air flowing from the exterior of the building through the cavity into the interior. Insulation also slows down the rate at which water can evaporate. If there have been any leaks resulting in water in a wall or ceiling cavity and the insulation remains wet long enough (over twenty-four to forty-eight hours), mold can grow on the paper at the backside of the drywall, or even on the wood framing. Then odors from the fungi (MVOCs; see chapter 3) can diffuse through the wall, even if the cavity is packed with insulation, resulting in a low-level musty odor in the room.

The spread of contaminants from a ceiling or wall cavity into the habitable space depends on differences in air pressure as well as on the size and nature of openings (construction gaps, electrical outlets, openings for pipes) leading from the cavities into rooms. The pressure of the air in a building with many bathroom and kitchen exhausts may be lower than the pressure of the air outside, leading to a flow of exterior air into wall cavities and, from there, into the interior. Air can flow from a pressurized ceiling cavity around ceiling light fixtures or from a pressurized wall cavity through electrical outlets into the room. And some buildings with mechanical ventilation systems have powerful fans that blow fresh air in, which might make the pressure in the building greater than the pressure of the outdoor air, resulting in airflows from the interior into ceiling and wall cavities and, from there, to the exterior.

Pressure differences also drive airflows from one interior space to another. (When air flows in this way from one space to another, the spaces are said to be *in communication* with each other.) In many buildings the interior drywall along the exterior perimeter does not extend beyond the drop ceiling, and the exterior wall cavities may thus be open at the top to a ceiling plenum. Air can then flow from the room into the wall cavity and from the wall cavity up into the ceiling plenum. This air is then drawn back into the fan coil and distributed to the spaces served by the building's heating or air-conditioning system (see chapter 7).

Most building occupants can't measure or adjust pressure differences, but knowing how and why air is flowing will help you understand potential pathways for the spread of contaminants within the building envelope.

Sinking and Floating

Understanding air quality means understanding how fluids behave when mixed together; this in turn means understanding density.

Weight is a measure of the relationship between mass and gravity, or how much matter you put on a scale. *Density* is a measure of the *mass* (the quantity) that a given volume of matter contains. Different volumes of the same pure substance at room temperature may have different masses, but they always have the same density (as the amount of the substance is increased, both the volume and mass increase in the same proportion). The density of water in a cup will be the same as the density of water in a bathtub or water in a reservoir, as long as the temperatures of the water in the cup, tub, and reservoir are the same.

Cooling a liquid, however, can increase its density as the marbles of matter move closer together (the same amount of matter takes up less space as the liquid approaches the solid state, so the matter is more dense). And heating a liquid can decrease its density as the marbles of matter move farther apart (the same amount of matter takes up more space as the liquid approaches the gaseous state, so the matter is less dense). If the water in the tub is warmer than the water in the reservoir, the tub water will be less dense than the reservoir water.

Substances that are less dense float on substances that are more dense. Warmer water will float above cooler water, as many of us have experienced when we are swimming in a fresh-water lake and notice that the water at our toes is cooler than the water at our shoulders.(Solids are usually more dense than the liquids from which they form. Ice is an exception: ice is less dense than liquid water, so it floats on the surface of a pond or lake.) Cool air is denser than warm air, so cooler air sinks and warmer air rises in a room—a very important concept in understanding air quality.

In the winter in a heated building, the warmer air will rise to the upper levels and exfiltrate through any openings or construction gaps. Cooler outdoor air will then infiltrate through doors and gaps at the lower levels. In multistory buildings, the movement of air from the lower stories to the upper stories is called the *stack effect,* because it approximates what happens in a chimney stack. The stack effect can spread contaminants. For example, in a building with an elevator shaft, air leaks out of the shaft at the upper levels and leaks in at the lower levels, carrying carbon monoxide and diluted fuel vapors from an underground garage, if present.

Some gases, such as pure carbon dioxide, are denser than air and will sink toward the floor. Sewer gas is a mixture of carbon dioxide, water vapor, and other gases, and the mixture is denser than air. Utility workers can suffocate if they descend into a manhole that is filled with sewer gas. The space looks as if it were filled with air (though it may have an odor), but there is insufficient oxygen for breathing, because the sewer gas has displaced the oxygen-containing air. To prevent such disasters, utility workers use blowers to introduce fresh air into a manhole.

When ice is heated sufficiently, it turns to liquid water. When water is heated sufficiently, it turns to water vapor (a gas). *Solids, liquids,* and *gases* are the *states* or *phases of matter.* When solids become liquids and liquids become gases, and vice versa, these changes are called *phase changes.*

Filling stations provide another illustration of how dangerous dense vapors can be. As you pump gasoline into your car, the liquid fuel displaces the air and the fuel vapors in the gas tank. Sometimes you can even see the vapors spilling out of the fill pipe and flowing down the side of the car; the light passing through the vapors shimmers as it is refracted (bent). Because the vapors are denser than air, they collect on the ground. If ignited by a spark, these fumes can burst into flames. This is one reason why people are warned not to smoke while filling their cars with gasoline. As you walk from your car to the cashier to pay for the gas, you are probably stepping through fuel vapors; this movement (as well as any wind present) mixes the concentrated vapors into the air, diluting the vapors.

The vapors from solvents in paint strippers are also denser than air, which is why manufacturers of paint strippers recommend that people use these products in well-ventilated spaces. I recall reading one newspaper story about a man who was stripping paint at the bottom of a narrow stairwell where there were no open doors or windows. The solvent evaporated into the space around the worker and displaced most of the air. He might just as well have been under water. Unfortunately, the fumes from methylene chloride (the same paint stripper used on the University of Massachusetts Boston campus) are narcotic at high concentrations. In the end, the man suffocated; no doubt he became drowsy and disoriented before lapsing into unconsciousness. It is doubtful that he would have recognized the threat when he first started stripping the paint, because the solvent fumes are not visible.

Density is a physical property of matter. Other physical properties of matter may include color or luster as well as electrical or heat conductivity. The physical properties of glass include transparency, brittleness, and a relatively low softening point. Some types of substances, such as metals, have many physical properties in common: most metals conduct electricity, are shiny, and are denser than water.

Construction materials are chosen because of their physical properties. Steel has great tensile and compressive strength; that is, it resists stretching as well as crushing. Masonry materials such as brick, concrete, and stone (which consist of minerals) also have great compressive strength, but concrete must be reinforced with steel because it does not have much tensile strength. (It breaks when it is under tension, or stretched.)

BUILDING DISCOMFORT

If a room is comfortable, people working in it under normal conditions are neither hot nor cold, sweaty nor dry, and the temperature and humidity of the air are not generally noticed. But because there will always be some people who are dissatisfied, *thermal comfort* is defined by the American Society of Heating, Refrigerating, and Air-Conditioning Engineers (ASHRAE) as a building condition in which 80 percent of the occupants are comfortable at that temperature. (You cannot satisfy all the people all the time!)

Whether consciously perceived or not, changes in our environment—fluctuations in temperature, pressure, movement, sound, and light—can be unsettling. A room that is too hot or too cold can be an uncomfortable workspace. A very tall skyscraper can sway back and forth in a strong wind (up to several inches or more, I've heard), and the motion can cause feelings of uneasiness or disorientation. Too much noise, regular and systematic changes of pitch in background sound, too much light or glare, or even too little light can affect one's work performance and job satisfaction.

Temperature

Temperature is a physical variable that can have a major impact on comfort; it is hard to concentrate on your computer screen when your feet are freezing. In the winter in a northern climate, the outside air is much colder than the inside air, and there may be large temperature differences in various areas of a building. A wall facing the sun will be warmer than a wall not facing the sun. The entry level of the building may be cooler than the floors above. We may not notice slight temperature differences as we move from room to room, but large temperature differences can lead to complaints that some rooms seem too hot and others too cold.

Whether someone is comfortable at any given temperature also depends on a person's individual metabolism. Under the same conditions, some people feel warm and others feel chilled. And individual comfort can also depend on the level of activity and the type of clothing worn. Someone sitting at a computer who is lightly dressed might feel comfortable while a nearby coworker who is wearing a long-sleeved shirt and a tie and is moving files may find the room too hot.

Humidity

People complain about sore throats and eye and skin irritations when the air is dry, particularly in the winter. In the summer, if the air is too humid, people may find it hard to concentrate, especially if they naturally sweat a lot. It's not very pleasant to try to work when your clothing is pasted to your back and the papers on the desk stick to your palm!

The humidity of the air also affects our perception of what constitutes an "acceptable" temperature. If the air is very dry in the winter, a temperature of 67°F might feel cold. Add a little moisture to the air, and that temperature might be more comfortable, because the rate of evaporation of moisture from the skin will be lowered (evaporation of moisture from the skin cools the body). In the summer, humid air at 78°F will be uncomfortable, but dry the air a little and it can be acceptable.

The amount of water vapor in the air inside a building envelope can have an enormous impact on indoor air quality, because humid conditions can lead to microbial growth. It is therefore important to understand how and why water vapor concentrations can vary.

There are several ways to talk about the amount of water vapor in the air. One simple measure is the percentage moisture content. We can readily sense the difference between air containing 0.1 percent water vapor (desert conditions) and air containing 3 percent water vapor (tropical conditions). The most meaningful way, however, to express how much vapor is in the air is to talk about *relative humidity (RH)*, a measure of how much water vapor the air at a given temperature holds versus the total water vapor that air at that given temperature *can* hold. If air at 70°F is at 70 percent RH, it can still hold 30 percent more water vapor before it reaches the point at which it can hold no more: 100 percent RH, the *saturation* point.

As air is heated, its ability to hold water increases. If air that is 80°F and saturated is heated to 85°F, it will no longer be at 100 percent RH, because its ability to hold water vapor will increase. Conversely, as the temperature of air decreases, its ability to hold water vapor decreases. If we have air in a container that is 70°F with 50 percent RH and we lower the temperature to 60°F, the air will then be at 70 percent RH—an increase, but not yet reaching the saturation point. At both temperatures the *amount* of water vapor present (the

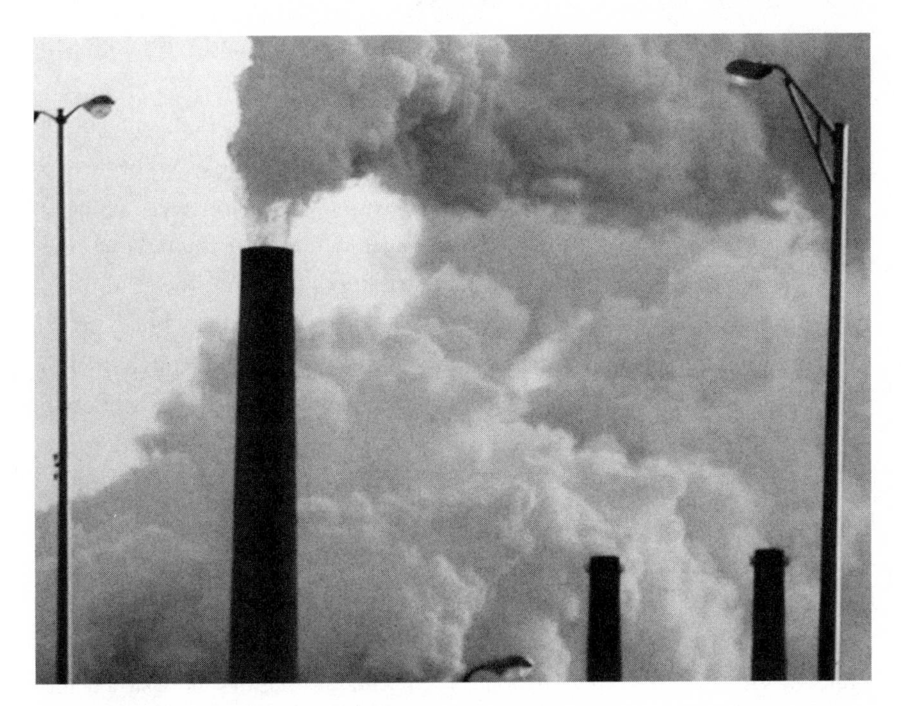

FIGURE 4.3. Man-made clouds. This view of a power-plant smokestack was taken on a bitterly cold winter day. The plant burns natural gas, so the combustion products consist mostly of hot water vapor. A colorless gas, the water vapor can't be seen just above the smokestack, but after the vapor mixes with the air and cools, it condenses to liquid droplets, and billowing white clouds appear. *Jeffrey C. May*

percentage content) will remain the same, but the air's capacity to hold more water vapor will increase or decrease. In other words, the RH of air with the same percentage moisture content varies, depending on the temperature.

Relative humidity is not an obscure scientific concept but a condition that constantly impacts our comfort. As I write this sentence, I am in Vermont, and it is a beautiful sunny day with fair-weather clouds floating by in a deep-blue sky. A hint of the autumn to come is carried in the crisp air coming in through my partially open window. A thermo-hygrometer, which measures temperature and relative humidity (and which I take with me everywhere), tells me that the temperature is 71°F and the relative humidity is 57 percent. I feel great, and words are flowing onto the page. Today seems miraculous compared with yesterday, when I was in Boston and it was 94°F at noon with a relative humidity of 85 percent. The air was like syrup, and every step—indeed, every breath—was an effort.

Halfway on my drive to Vermont yesterday afternoon, the sky turned black, with flashes of lightning on all sides. Within moments, large drops of rain began to thud against my windshield. I could see a dark curtain ahead, beneath which the pavement was drenched with splashing rain. As I entered the thunderstorm, I could hear nothing but rain striking the car, and the road disappeared from view. I rolled up my window to keep the rain out, but even the small gap at the top was wide enough to let a spray of rain through. Within minutes, the windshield fogged with condensed moisture. Ironically enough, since my car's air conditioner was broken, I was forced to turn on the defroster (on heat mode!) to clear the windshield. The rain soon stopped, and I opened my window to enjoy the cooler air. By the time I arrived in Vermont, the RH had dropped 20 percent and the temperature was 80°F. Heaven.

Now let's look as scientists at some of the changes that occurred during that trip. Whether or not we are aware that we are sweating, water is always evaporating from our skin. When the RH is high, water evaporates more slowly into the air, and liquid water (sweat) accumulates on our skin. Air movements can speed up evaporation, because drier air displacing the humid air near the skin surface can take away more moisture. This is why fans make us feel cooler. In hot and very humid air, however, a fan is nearly useless. I was sweating while I was loading up the car and leaving the city in fairly dense traffic, and the open car window didn't bring me much relief until I could go fast enough to get a strong cross-wind going, which carried away my body's moisture.

The thunderstorm occurred because cool dense air from Canada flowing across northern New England encountered the sweltering moist air that was settled over southern New England. Turbulence and even violent air flows occurred where the two air masses collided (the *weather front*). The denser colder air slipped under the less dense warmer air, forcing the humid warmer air upward. The warmer air was cooled as it rose into the colder layers of atmosphere above the Earth. The air's RH increased, and water vapor within condensed into rain.

Some people think that the process of raining "dries" the air, but the reverse is often true. Rain first forms high in the atmosphere, and as the drops fall they may pass through a drier air mass. Some drops may evaporate into water vapor before hitting the ground, thus increasing the relative humidity of the air (sometimes, if the air is dry enough, the rain never reaches the ground). Rain can also increase the RH by evaporating from surfaces after it falls. (Because rain is formed high above us, it doesn't have to be 100 percent RH at the Earth's surface for rain to occur.)

When the thunderstorm started and I closed my window, the air inside the car remained humid because of the evaporation of the rainwater that had come in through the partially open window as well as the evaporation of moisture from my body. The windshield, on the other hand, was drenched on the outside with cooler rainwater, thus lowering the temperature of the glass on the inside. Air in contact with the windshield was cooled, lowering its ability to hold water vapor and raising its RH, and the air eventually reached the *dew point*. Water vapor then condensed onto the inside of the windshield, which is why I had to turn the defroster on. (Dew point conditions exist when the air is saturated—is at 100 percent RH—at any given temperature, and water then condenses onto surfaces that are cooler than the temperature of the air. The more water vapor there is in the air, the higher the dew point temperature. In other words, air containing more water vapor will reach the dew point at a higher temperature than air containing less water vapor will.)

I stated earlier that high RH can lead to microbial growth. It is generally accepted that in occupied buildings with nonoperable windows, the RH should be limited to a maximum of around 60 percent. When the RH is over 75 percent, the moisture content of a surface can be sufficient for mold to grow. Carpeting laid over concrete can develop mold problems, particularly in below-grade spaces, because a concrete surface is often cooler than the room air. Air near or within the carpet fibers is thus cooled and its RH rises, increasing the moisture content of the carpet dust and fostering mold growth.

Pressure

Air pressure differences can be another source of building discomfort. The higher you go, the fewer the molecules and the less dense the air. When an elevator moves from the first to the fiftieth floor of a building, the air pressure within the shaft drops, because the air pressure is lower at the top of the shaft than at the bottom, despite the fact that the elevator is compressing the air above as it ascends. We can feel the pressure differences in our ears, as we of-

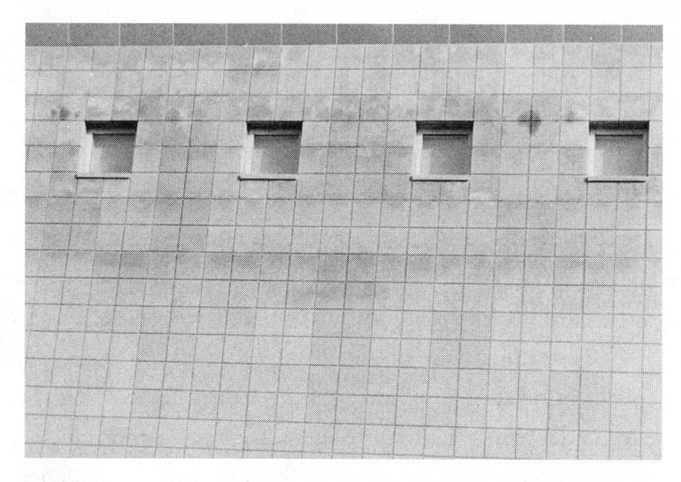

FIGURE 4.4. Indoor moisture finds its way out. This building has a masonry panel exterior, and during the winter the relative humidity indoors was high: 50 percent. Because of pressure differences between the interior and exterior of the building envelope, warm, moist air was exfiltrating into the wall cavities behind the masonry. The water vapor condensed on the cool backside of the masonry and moved through the panel joints to the exterior. There it evaporated, leaving behind stains and crystals of efflorescence. Buildings must have a continuous air barrier (usually consisting of plastic film) somewhere in the wall to prevent indoor air from exfiltrating into wall cavities. Either this building lacked air barriers or the air barriers were improperly installed. *May Indoor Air Investigations LLC*

ten do when we are in an airplane and the air pressure changes during takeoff (a reduction of pressure) and landing (an increase of pressure). It can be painful if the pressure difference is great enough across the eardrum (a taut membrane like the skin of a drum); swallowing, yawning, or chewing gum equalizes the pressures and relieves the discomfort.

We expect pressure differences when we are riding in an elevator in a tall building or traveling in an airplane, but other pressure differences we are not as aware of can exist within the building envelope. The air pressure can vary according to the operation of the ventilation equipment, for example. Just as a poorly balanced spinning tire can shake a moving car, the vibrations of an improperly balanced fan can create small pressure fluctuations that can be disconcerting to those who unconsciously sense them.

Noise and Sound

We live and work with a background hum of computers, printers, copiers, telephones, fax machines, and air-conditioning systems. Fluorescent light fixtures can flicker or hum. Outside we are surrounded by the sounds of traffic moving through the streets and jet planes flying overhead. Excessive noise either indoors or outdoors can be a problem for some people.

What is noise, and how it is different from music? A child thumping on piano keys makes noise, and yet when the child learns to play the instrument, what comes out of the piano is music (we hope). Music is the *organized* occurrences of sounds (notes) sequenced in time. Noise is the *disorganized* mixture of many notes.

Sound consists of small fluctuations in pressure that travel through the air. Think of a tuning fork or a loudspeaker. When the surface generating the sound is moving forward, the air in front of the surface is compressed and its

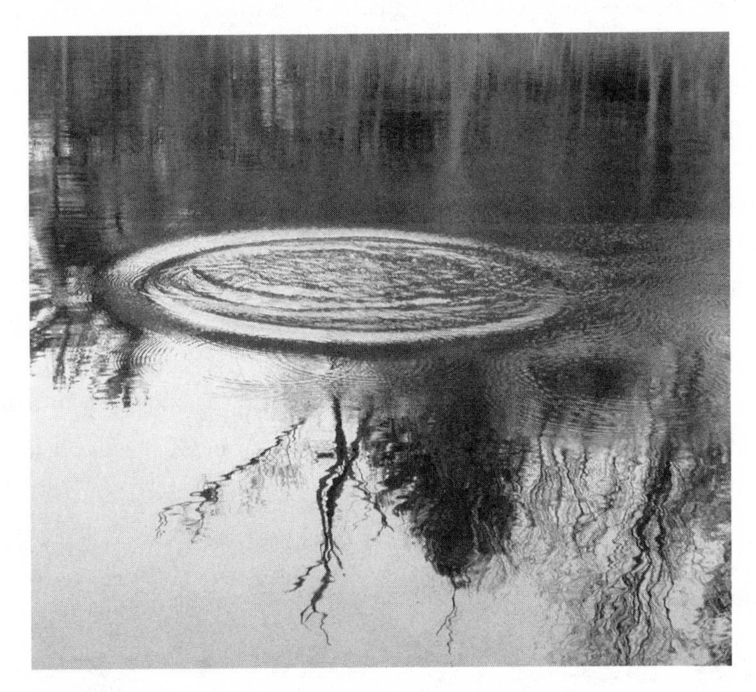

FIGURE 4.5. Waves in a pond. A stone dropped into a quiet pond creates circular disturbances on the water's surface. The rings travel until they reach the shore. *Jeffrey C. May*

pressure is increased; when the surface is moving backward, the air in front of the surface is rarefied (thinned) and its pressure is decreased. These pressure changes travel out in waves, just the way swells appear to roll away in concentric circles from a stone dropped into a quiet pond of water: the crest of a wave is analogous to the elevated pressure, and the trough to the reduced pressure. When these sound waves (periodic pressure variations) arrive at the eardrum, it too starts to vibrate "sympathetically," and the brain translates these vibrations into what we perceive as sound.

Whether we hear sound depends on *loudness* and *pitch*. Loudness is a measure of the *energy* associated with sound and determines how far the eardrum—a membrane—will move in and out. A very loud sound can be painful, because its amplitude (sound intensity) stretches the eardrum, while another sound may be so feeble that the vibration of the eardrum cannot be detected. The pitch characterizes the *frequency* of a note, which determines how rapidly the eardrum moves in and out. Inaudible sounds of higher frequency are called *ultrasound* (used in imaging fetuses). Dogs can hear ultrasound that humans cannot. Inaudible sounds of lower frequency are called *infrasound*. Infrasound at great amplitude can cause mild stress reactions and strange pulsating auditory sensations, reported by some people to cause fatigue and nausea (two of the symptoms associated with sick-building syndrome; see chapter 1), but the amplitude of infrasound in most buildings is not great enough to be a significant cause of such symptoms.

Some animals can detect infrasound that human beings cannot. On the morning of December 26, 2004, one of the worst tsunamis in recorded history struck villages and cities on the Indian Ocean coasts, following an earthquake off the island of Sumatra. Over 150,000 people perished in the flooding, but many animals, including elephants, fled from beach areas before the

> Because sound consists of particles moving and vibrating, sound waves can only travel through matter: solids, liquids, and gases. In the vacuum of space there are almost no particles, and therefore space is silent. Light consists of waves or packets (photons) of energy and therefore does not need the presence of matter for transmission. If sound could travel through a vacuum the way light can, we would be able to hear the violence of nuclear explosions on the sun and even perhaps more distant stellar events, and life on Earth would be a lot noisier than it already is.

giant waves struck. On the Khao Lak beach in southern Thailand, one group of elephants, their handler reported, cried out about the time the earthquake occurred. Approximately an hour later, just before the tsunamis came ashore, the elephants fled inland, scooping up some tourists and carrying them to safety as they rushed to higher ground. Scientists know that elephants communicate with infrasound, which would have been "broadcast" by the earthquake and incoming ocean waves, providing the warnings these animals detected.

Sound waves from one or more sources can interact in surprising ways. Perhaps the most familiar is when two notes with nearly identical pitches are played simultaneously, and you hear *beats:* not the plural of *beat,* which refers to rhythm, but a periodic change in amplitude that can be disconcerting and even stressful. When musical instruments are tuned, they are adjusted so that the notes do not produce any beats.

One common significant source of indoor noise can be the mechanical (heating and cooling) system. In a larger building the system may contain one fan (blower) for supplying air and a second fan for removing air from the conditioned (heated or cooled) space. The operation of each fan is associated with sound—mostly noise, but nonetheless containing pure pitches. If the frequencies of some of the louder pitches are close enough (when fans are operating at nearly the same speed), they may interact to produce beats.

Even a relatively pure pitch from a single source can create significant disorientation. Because we have two ears, the brain deduces our position with respect to the source of a particular pitch from the loudness in each ear. If a sound seems louder in the right ear, then the sound appears to be originating from the right. If louder in the left ear, the sound appears to be coming from

> For human hearing, the range of audible pitches spans the frequency range of about 20 cycles per second (cps) of pressure changes to 20,000 cps. The human ear is most sensitive to sounds in the range of about 600 cps to 3,000 cps, the range of the human voice. Loudness of sounds can be measured in watts per unit of area, and in decibels (dB). The lowest level of audible sound is about 15 dB. Levels above 120 dB are painful. The noise from a typical rock concert can be as loud as 100 to 230 dB, and musicians, as well as members of the audience, can experience hearing loss when exposed to this level of sound.

the left. But sometimes when sound is reflecting off surfaces, the source of the sound can appear to change location with even the slightest head movements.

I first became aware of this phenomenon while riding a bus. I was just sitting quietly in my seat, looking at the people and reading the ads, when suddenly I became aware of a high-pitched engine whine that seemed to fill the bus. Although I had not been aware of the sound before, now that I was hearing it, I couldn't ignore it. One moment the sound was louder in my left ear and the next moment louder in my right ear. As I moved my head, the loudness switched from one ear to the other, and it felt as if the sound were coming from everywhere. The effect, like a ringing in the ears, was disorienting.

Such variations in loudness are caused by the interaction of a sound wave with itself. Remember that beats are produced by two pitches interacting, but a single pitch can be reflected from a surface, and when reflected waves meet they can interact like two pitches. This is why it can be nearly impossible to locate chirping smoke detectors or misplaced pagers, because the high-pitched sounds they make are being reflected throughout the spaces they occupy.

SOME PRACTICAL STEPS

- If you think that mold growth or pest infestation in a wall or ceiling cavity is creating odors indoors, you might ask building maintenance personnel to put an exhaust fan in one of the doorways or windows while closing the other doors or windows in the room. Air will then flow from the cavities into the room through construction gaps, electrical outlets, light fixtures, and other openings in the wall or ceiling. This is one way to find the general location of an odor source, because the strongest smell will emanate from the openings nearest the mold growth or pest infestation. I would recommend that you vacate the room while this "treasure hunt" is going on!
- If you suspect that the light or sound of a fluorescent fixture in your office is causing you discomfort, turn the fixture off and use a plug-in desk lamp with an incandescent bulb for a few days, to see if this makes a difference. If you are not able to switch the lighting in this way, try wearing dark glasses.

- If your office seems cold, find out if it is possible to use an *oil-filled* portable heater (or some other heater that does not get red hot) to make the space more comfortable for you.
- If the air is dry where you work, consider using a portable warm-mist humidifier with a built-in humidistat. (Ultrasonic and evaporative humidifiers can become contaminated with microbial growth.) To minimize the chances of mildew growth in the room, monitor the relative humidity with a hygrometer to ensure that the RH doesn't rise above about 40 percent in winter. For comfort in summer, the RH should not be greater than 60 to 65 percent.
- If background noise in the office might be a problem, try wearing ear plugs as an experiment. To isolate possible sources of the noise, turn off printers, computers, copiers, speakers, and even fans or blowers, and then turn them back on one at a time. Once you have identified the source of the problem, you can consider erecting a hanging (made of fire-retardant material) between you and the sound source to muffle the sound, or, if appropriate, you can request that noncombustible sound-proofing be added to enclosures containing mechanical equipment. Blowers may have to be balanced, just as car tires have to be.
- To determine if physical factors are a source of building discomfort, an expert who measures levels of sound and light, such as an industrial hygienist, can be hired.

CHAPTER

5

Gases in the Sea of Air

A sea of air—the atmosphere—envelopes the Earth. Our atmosphere is a mixture of gases that contains about 21 percent oxygen and 78 percent nitrogen. The remaining 1 percent consists of helium, hydrogen, carbon dioxide, among others, and varying amounts of water vapor. The air we breathe indoors comes from the atmosphere but may contain other gases and vapors that can cause health problems. In the preceding chapters I described the sources of some of these contaminants: carpeting that off-gasses chemicals and ceiling tiles that smell like vomit, for example. In this chapter and the chapter that follows I concentrate on the contaminants themselves: what they are and how they can affect health.

ORGANIC VERSUS CHEMICAL

In common usage, the word *organic* often has a positive connotation and the word *chemical* a pejorative connotation. Yet water is a chemical; blood, sugar, and even hamburgers and apples are all made of chemicals. Flour, whether "organic" and stone ground or white and processed, is still a mixture of different chemicals: atoms variously arranged or combined together into molecules. I am an "organic" chemist, which means that I was trained in the chemistry of carbon-containing substances.

Not all man-made chemicals are harmful, and not all "organic" and naturally occurring substances are beneficial. Mad cow disease, also called *BSE,* or *bovine spongiform encephalopathy,* is caused by a naturally occurring molecule

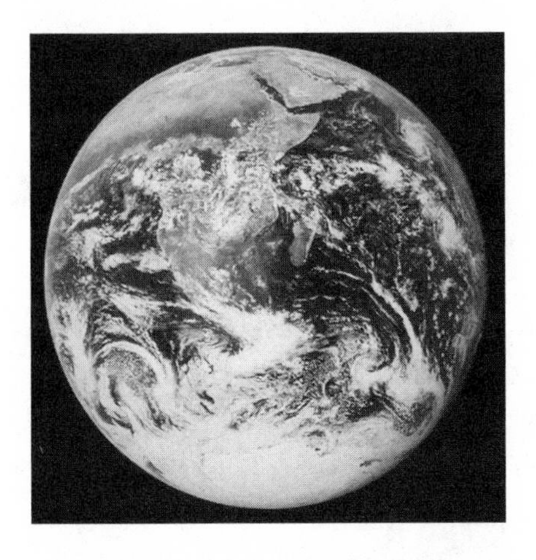

FIGURE 5.1. Earth from space. This view of Earth shows Africa and Antarctica. The diameter of the Earth is about 8,000 miles; most of Earth's atmosphere is less than 20 miles thick. In this photograph, the atmosphere is visible (barely) as a thin white line (most obvious at the top and left) around the Earth's circumference. *NASA*

called a *prion*. Another type of prion is believed to be the cause of a similar human brain disease, Creutzfeldt-Jakob disease, in which the protein molecules in the brain merely change shape. This minute shift leads to the destruction of tissue and eventually to death.

One woman who had an unknown debilitating disease saw scores of physicians and had hundreds of X-rays. In the end, through her own research, she figured out that her symptoms were consistent with lead poisoning. Unfortunately she had never told any of her physicians that she was consuming large amounts of "organic" bone meal, derived from horses that had grazed on grass contaminated with lead from automobile exhaust (this occurred when gasoline still contained the antiknock compound tetraethyl lead, which is now banned). That the bone meal was organic did not prevent the lead from poisoning her. And the X-rays used in the effort to determine what was wrong with her eventually led to cancer.

When I see the word *organic* on a food label, I still read the ingredients. When someone calls me to say he is worried about "chemicals" in his indoor environment, I ask him to report in greater detail the difficulties he is having and where he is having them, because the word *chemicals* alone doesn't necessarily describe a problem.

As you read the rest of this chapter, I hope you will free yourself of any preconceived notions you have about the connotations of words like *chemicals* and *organic*. View the world objectively, and you will be able to make informed decisions about what might be injurious and what might be beneficial to your health.

THE LANGUAGE OF CHEMISTRY

If you want to talk about the effects that vapors and gases can have on indoor air quality, you must learn a few phrases from the language of chemistry (particularly if you want to understand IAQ test reports, which I discuss in part III).

Single letters or pairs of letters are used to name the elements that constitute matter: the solids, liquids, and gases that surround us. H is hydrogen, O is oxygen, N is nitrogen, Na is sodium, Ca is calcium, and Cl is chlorine. Since there are 110 identified elements (more will be identified in the future), there are 110 letters or pairs of letters to name these elements. These letters and pairs of letters make up the chemical alphabet.

Hydrogen gas consists of two hydrogen atoms bonded together (H_2), and oxygen gas consists of two oxygen atoms bonded together (O_2). Atoms combine with different kinds of atoms to create *compounds*; for example, two

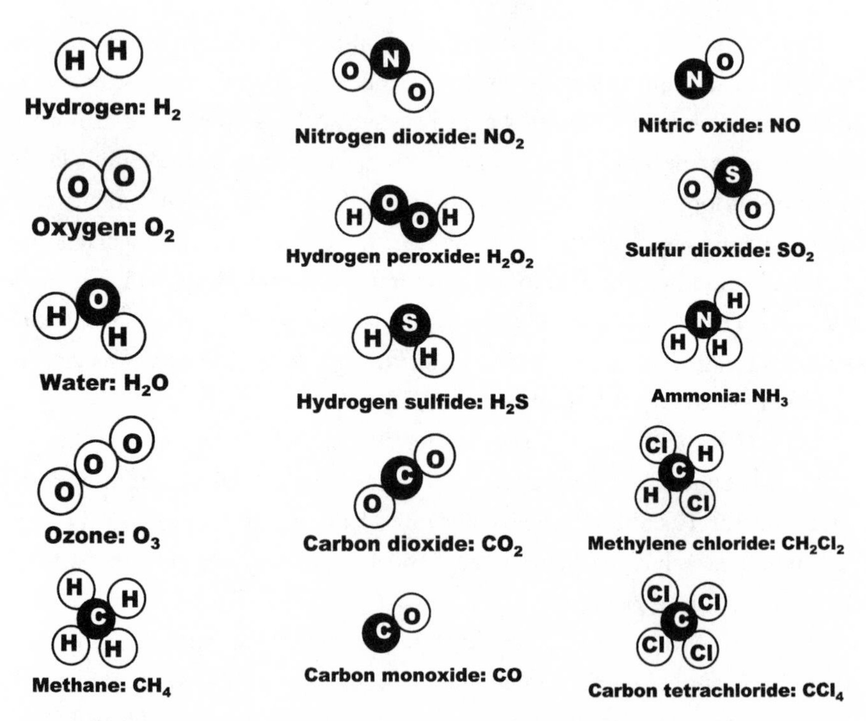

FIGURE 5.2. Some molecules. Here are the formulas and structures of the molecules of some of the chemicals discussed in this chapter.

atoms of hydrogen combine (are bonded) with one atom of oxygen to create water, H_2O. Hydrogen peroxide, H_2O_2, used in hair bleach and as a disinfectant, is also made from a combination of hydrogen and oxygen—again, two hydrogen atoms, but this time two oxygen atoms rather than one. Hydrogen sulfide (H_2S) differs from water: between the two hydrogen atoms there is a sulfur atom instead of an oxygen atom, and the substitution of this one atom creates a foul-smelling gas that in low concentrations is associated with the odor of rotten eggs and sewer gas, and that in high concentrations is toxic. (The *chemical formulas* H_2O and H_2O_2 are chemical "words" that define the type and number of atoms in each water or hydrogen peroxide molecule.)

Now let's take a look at some of the irritating, toxic, or carcinogenic gases that can be present in the air we breathe.

OZONE

The molecules of ozone gas, O_3, are made up of three oxygen atoms—only one oxygen atom more than in the oxygen molecule (O_2). Ozone is formed when ultraviolet energy from sunlight, or energy from the electrical discharges of lightning or sparks, passes through air and breaks molecules of O_2 (oxygen gas) into separate atoms. Each of the two separated oxygen atoms then combines with another molecule of O_2 to produce O_3. (When atoms separate and recombine in this way, it is called a *chemical reaction*. Those separated and recombined atoms have gone through a *chemical change*.) After lightning strikes, you can smell ozone gas, but even on a sunny day there is a small amount of ozone (a *background level*) in the outdoor air.

Ozone gas reacts with many substances in both living and nonliving things. Latex rubber that is exposed to ozone becomes brittle and falls apart. In our

> Ozone at the fringe of the Earth's atmosphere protects us from the sun's ultraviolet light, which can cause skin cancer. There is a widely accepted scientific theory that chlorine atoms (Cl) released by the degradation of chemicals from air-conditioning refrigerants formerly used around the globe are destroying portions of the ozone layer above the South Pole. The resulting thinning of the ozone layer is allowing increased levels of ultraviolet light to strike the Earth, which some people fear is increasing skin cancer rates in the Southern Hemisphere.

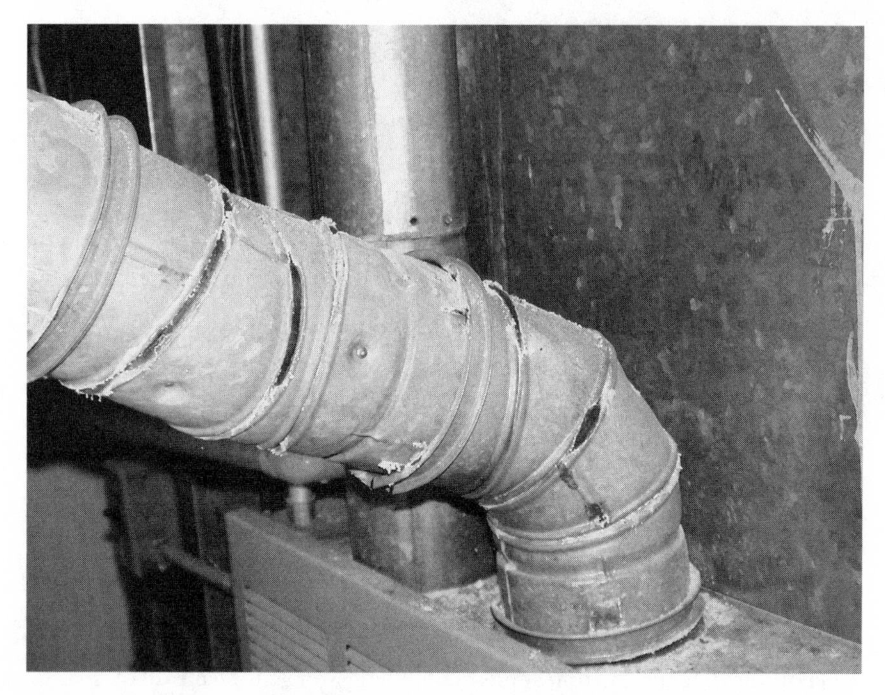

FIGURE 5.3. Corroded vent pipe. This pipe carries toxic combustion gases from a furnace into a chimney. The pipe is made of galvanized iron (iron coated with zinc metal). Metals corrode and form oxides when they combine chemically with the oxygen in air. There are two types of corrosion visible in the joints of this pipe. The white fluffy material is zinc oxide; the darker material is iron oxide (rust). Eventually, holes will develop in the pipe and combustion gases will leak out. *May Indoor Air Investigations LLC*

lungs, ozone gas can kill cells, cause inflammation, and lead to symptoms in people with asthma. As I discussed in chapter 3, ozone gas is produced by certain types of air purifiers and office equipment, including photocopiers and laser printers. Even the small amounts of irritants released from copiers can be a problem for people with chemical sensitivity (see chapter 1).

Automobiles emit chemicals (hydrocarbons, discussed later in this chapter) that enhance the formation of ozone. On a clear dry day in the country when there is no automobile traffic, there might not be more than a background level of ozone. Yet in the middle of a traffic jam in the city, the ozone level can be unhealthy for some people. Ozone levels outdoors are a problem for many inhabitants of cities that regularly have pollution alerts, because ozone is one of the very irritating components of smog. In Los Angeles, a

"Stage 1 Smog Alert" is declared whenever the ozone concentration reaches 0.2 part per million (ppm).[1] (One part per million of ozone gas, or any kind of gas for that matter, means 1 part of the gas and 999,999 parts of air.) A study published in 2002 claimed that young athletes in cities had more asthma than young athletes in the country, because of increased exposures to ozone.[2]

The Occupational Safety and Health Administration (OSHA) limits the workplace concentration of ozone to 0.1 ppm, and the FDA guideline for ozone production by medical devices is 0.05 ppm. (The odor threshold of ozone—the level detectable by sniffing or breathing—is reported to be in the range of 0.0076 to 0.036 ppm,[3] though some hypersensitive individuals can detect the odor at even lower concentrations.)

CARBON DIOXIDE

Carbon dioxide (CO_2) is a gas consisting of molecules that contain one carbon atom and two oxygen atoms, each oxygen bonded to the carbon. General recommendations for CO_2 levels indoors vary from about 600 ppm to 1,000 ppm.

If present in high enough concentrations (above 1,000 ppm), CO_2 can make the air in a room seem "stale" or even cause drowsiness. In a bedroom in which two people are asleep with doors and windows closed, the concentrations of CO_2 overnight can rise to about 2,000 to 2,500 ppm, or 0.25 percent of the inside air, depending on the tightness of the house. In some poorly ventilated schools, the CO_2 levels in classrooms may be as high as 3,000 ppm or more. While high levels like these are not much of a problem in a bedroom when people are sleeping, these levels can affect students' and teachers' abilities to focus. Monitoring the levels of CO_2 can therefore provide a measure

> In the 1960s, a popular song used the phrase "one in a million" to describe a lover. The song wouldn't have been as romantic if it had referred to Romeo as "one part per million," but the idea is the same: one "part" out of one million "parts" (or 1 Romeo and 999,999 other men). If the lyrics had said "one in a billion," then the person (or part) would be one of a billion, rather than a million. When talking about concentrations of gases and vapors, *parts per million (ppm)* and *parts per billion (ppb)* describe how much of a substance is present in air. So if room air contains 600 ppm of CO_2, it means that there are 600 molecules of CO_2 and 999,400 molecules of other gases and vapors (600 ppm is the same as 0.06 part per hundred, or 0.06 percent).

of the efficiency of the ventilation system (which introduces fresh air into the building; see chapter 7).

Plants take in carbon dioxide and use the carbon for growth; they release the oxygen into the air that animals then breathe. Animals breathe in oxygen and combine it in cells with carbon from food to form carbon dioxide, CO_2, which is then exhaled. Carbon dioxide is also produced during the combustion process (I discuss the combustion process in greater detail later in this chapter). If there were no animals (including human beings) or combustion sources of CO_2 inside a building, the CO_2 levels would be the same indoors as outdoors: about 360 ppm. Because people are exhaling inside, however, the indoor levels of CO_2 rise.

Compared with the amount of nitrogen and oxygen in air, the amount of carbon dioxide in air is small, about 0.036 percent, yet the concentration of carbon dioxide in the atmosphere has been increasing slowly as a result of the burning of carbon-containing fossil fuels such as natural gas, gasoline, oil, and coal. Scientists think this increase is responsible for global warming.

Carbon dioxide is called a *greenhouse gas*. Much of the energy from the sun enters Earth's atmosphere as light. Some of the light is ultraviolet, a shorter wavelength than visible light, and some is infrared, a longer wavelength than visible light. When visible light and infrared light hit the earth, the energy is absorbed and surfaces heat up like a car in the sun. Much of the energy from sunlight heats the oceans, evaporating water and creating weather. Some of the light energy is used by plants, both in the oceans and on land, in the process of photosynthesis. Some of the energy is radiated out in all directions (like the heat from pavement after the sun sets) through the atmosphere back into space, in the form of infrared.

Carbon dioxide molecules in the atmosphere absorb infrared and re-emit it in all directions, including back toward the Earth—in a sense, reflecting and re-reflecting the heat back to the planet's surface.

CARBON MONOXIDE

A molecule of carbon monoxide gas (CO) has one carbon atom and only one oxygen atom, rather than the two oxygen atoms in carbon dioxide; CO is potentially deadly because it reduces the capacity of the blood to carry oxygen.

Oxygen by itself is only slightly soluble (dissolvable) in water, so if the blood in our veins and arteries consisted of nothing but water, it couldn't carry enough oxygen from the lungs to the cells. Red blood cells are full of an iron-containing substance called *hemoglobin;* every hemoglobin molecule bonds reversibly with one oxygen molecule and then releases the oxygen to the cells where it is needed. Thus hemoglobin makes it possible for blood to supply oxygen from the lungs to the rest of the body—a major reason why iron is so important in the diet.

Carbon monoxide also bonds *reversibly* with hemoglobin, but the bond is about 250 times stronger than the bond between oxygen and hemoglobin, so CO reduces the ability of the blood to carry oxygen. Chronic low-level exposures to carbon monoxide may cause heart problems, depression, or even psychosis. (Some people suspect that the author Edgar Allan Poe was not a drug addict but rather a victim of low-level CO poisoning, though of course he may have been both.) Inhaling 3,200 ppm of CO will cause headache, dizziness, and nausea within ten minutes and unconsciousness and death in less than half an hour. Because carbon monoxide bonds *reversibly* with hemoglobin, however, most people can recover within a few hours from a nonlethal exposure as oxygen in fresh air replaces CO in their blood, though around five hundred people in the United States die annually because of involuntary, non-fire-related carbon monoxide poisoning, and others suffer permanent brain damage due to lack of oxygen.[4]

Our bodies produce a small amount of carbon monoxide, so there is less than 1 percent of carboxyhemoglobin (hemoglobin with carbon monoxide) in most people's blood. In a heavy smoker's blood, however, the level of carboxyhemoglobin can be more than 5 percent, because cigarette smoke contains carbon monoxide. (A heavy smoker's breath can contain a CO concentration of from 20 to 100 ppm.) Cigarette smoking is bad for all of us, but it is particularly bad for people with heart problems, since carbon monoxide reduces the oxygen-carrying capacity of the blood. When people quit smoking, the amount of carboxyhemoglobin in their blood decreases.

ASHRAE follows the EPA's National Ambient Air Quality Standards for the indoor exposure limits for carbon monoxide: 9 ppm for eight hours or more, or 35 ppm for one hour or more.[5] The permissible exposure limit (PEL) set by OSHA for the industrial workplace is 50 ppm. (PELs are generally based on time-weighted averages of concentration measurements, rather than on single measurements.) In my opinion, carbon monoxide concentrations indoors should be close to zero. I recommend that all buildings have CO detectors. Because the gas is colorless and odorless, a detector is the only way, short of illness or death, to tell if there is an elevated level of CO indoors.

Automobile engines produce carbon monoxide, so CO concentrations inside tunnels during traffic jams can reach 150 ppm. And in buildings in which there is incomplete combustion (defined below) of fuel in the heating or hot-water systems and not all the combustion products exit the building, there can be elevated levels of CO indoors.

COMBUSTION PRODUCTS

More than 50 percent of residential and commercial buildings burn natural gas in their heating systems. Over 90 percent of natural gas consists of methane molecules: one central carbon atom bonded to four hydrogen atoms (CH_4). Methane gas and oxygen gas can exist in the same mixture without burning; some source of high temperature is required to start the combustion process. To burn methane in air, oxygen from the air is first mixed with the methane, and the mixture is ignited by heat from a match or spark. Atoms and molecules then collide with each other and separate and recombine in various ways. Heat is produced when something burns, and the heat energy from the combustion process itself, once started, supplies the energy needed to continue the chemical reactions taking place.

If *complete combustion* occurs, a CH_4 (methane) molecule collides with O_2 (oxygen) molecules, and after a series of steps, the hydrogen atoms combine with oxygen atoms to form water, and the carbon atom bonds with two oxygen atoms, resulting in CO_2 (carbon dioxide). In *incomplete combustion* (occurring when the flame is disturbed, or when there is not enough oxygen), the carbon atom ends up with one oxygen atom to form CO (carbon monoxide). Soot, formaldehyde gas, and other chemical vapors may also be produced as end products of incomplete combustion.

Even in a gas stove or heating system with complete combustion, formaldehyde is produced when the flame first ignites. If a heating system is properly vented, all the combustion gases, including formaldehyde, go up the chimney. Unfortunately, most kitchen exhausts do not vent to the exterior, so formaldehyde (as well as carbon monoxide) produced by a gas stove or oven usually enters the kitchen air. Unless there is incomplete combustion, however, the amount of formaldehyde produced is minimal (though some people find even this small amount of the gas irritating).

Nitric Oxide and Nitrogen Dioxide

When something burns, atoms from the combustible material are combining with oxygen. But only 21 percent of the air is oxygen. In every flame, all the air (which consists primarily of nitrogen) is heated. At high temperatures, a rapidly moving nitrogen molecule (N_2) may collide with an oxygen molecule (O_2) with sufficient energy to break bonds. The molecules "trade partners," and two molecules of nitric oxide (NO) are formed.

Because of its ability to combine (reversibly) with hemoglobin and reduce the ability of the blood to carry oxygen, colorless nitric oxide is toxic and, like carbon monoxide, can cause asphyxiation. (The concentration NIOSH considers to be "immediately dangerous to life or health," or IDLH, is 100 ppm.) And because it is fat soluble, NO can be absorbed through the skin. This gas can also be an eye irritant, because in the presence of moisture and oxygen, NO reacts to form acids.

Nitric oxide was not considered much more than a pollutant until the 1980s, when researchers discovered dozens of life processes for which the presence of NO is vital. In 1992, *Science* magazine named nitric oxide "Molecule of the Year" (whatever that means). The most significant process involving NO as a "messenger molecule" was discovered accidentally. According to one physician's anecdote, when the drug sildenafil citrate, which affects nitric oxide concentrations, was being tested by the pharmaceutical company Pfizer as treatment for high blood pressure and angina, some male participants refused to give up their unused portion of the drug at the end of a trial. Dr. Ian Osterloh, one of the researchers, asked why, and the rest is history.

The drug, christened Viagra and approved as a cure for male impotence, became the fastest selling drug in history; some people estimate that over forty thousand prescriptions were written per day during the first weeks of sale. Viagra slows the rate of removal of NO in cells, which in turn enhances the relaxing effect that NO has on the constriction of blood vessels. This can increase the blood flow to the penis, thus improving erectile function. (Fireflies utilize NO to control their flashing, used to communicate with and select mates. We are *all* truly part of the world of nature!)

Nitric oxide is not very stable in the presence of oxygen; even at room temperature, when a nitric oxide molecule and an oxygen molecule collide, if the NO bonds to one of the oxygen atoms, nitrogen dioxide (NO_2) is formed. Thus there will always be some nitrogen dioxide in air containing nitric oxide.

Nitrogen dioxide is a brown gas responsible for the haze that hugs large urban areas during smog alerts. (Stack gases from power plants contain nitrogen dioxide as well as carbon monoxide.) Both NO_2 and NO are toxic by-products of all internal combustion engines. When an automobile is being driven outside, combustion products exit the tailpipe and are diluted by the air around the car. When an engine is running indoors, however, in a parking garage or a warehouse, combustion products can build up if the space is not ventilated adequately, and these products can be carried on airflows to other parts of the building. Nitrogen dioxide and nitric oxide can also be produced in gas stoves, heating systems, and heating appliances such as kerosene heaters, most of which are unvented, so the gases enter the indoor air. Cigarettes also produce nitrogen dioxide.

Exposure to NO_2 above 300 parts per billion (ppb) can exacerbate asthma symptoms.[6] Exposure for ten minutes to 4 parts per million of NO_2 can cause a loss of the sense of smell, increasing the likelihood that continued exposure to other contaminants may go unnoticed. If NO_2 is present in high enough concentrations, a slightly fishy odor can result. Inhalation of air containing over 100 ppm of NO_2 can cause swelling of lung tissues (pulmonary edema) and death. Nonetheless, compared with most other indoor contaminants, nitrogen dioxide does not appear to pose a significant health hazard in typical buildings.

Passive monitors are available to measure nitrogen dioxide concentrations (see chapter 13), but testing is not required under most circumstances. It is wiser to determine and eliminate the sources of combustion products than to spend money on testing. (For example, exhaust vents for kitchen stoves can be installed, and water heaters and fireplaces can be vented to the exterior.)

Sulfur Dioxide and Sulfurous Acid

Solid and liquid fuels like coal and oil usually contain a small percentage of sulfur. At high temperatures in a flame, a sulfur atom bonds with two oxygen atoms from O_2 in air to produce sulfur dioxide (SO_2) molecules. SO_2 is a very irritating toxic gas. At low levels, it causes a peculiar taste sensation, described as metallic by people who experience it. A level of 0.25 ppm can cause bronchoconstriction (narrowing of the airways) in some asthma sufferers when they are exercising.[7] SO_2 is used as a preservative in dried fruits, wines, and other food products and can also cause breathing difficulties for people with asthma who consume them.

Sulfur dioxide may be present indoors when sulfur-containing fossil fuels are burned in unvented kerosene heaters. This gas can also be present in the outdoor air, near where sulfur-containing compounds such as copper or lead sulfide are processed in smelters or where sulfur-containing fuels are burned in power plants. The SO_2 may then infiltrate buildings located nearby.

Sulfur dioxide gas is soluble in water (H_2O) and combines chemically with H_2O to form sulfurous acid ($SO_2 + H_2O = H_2SO_3$), an irritating liquid. Because the mucous membranes in the eyes, nose, and respiratory system are wet, exposure to sulfur dioxide at about 10 ppm produces H_2SO_3, which can irritate the tissues.

HYDROCARBONS

The fuel gases methane, ethane, propane, and butane are called *hydrocarbons* because they consist of molecules that are combinations of hydrogen and carbon atoms. Gasoline, kerosene, and fuel oil are mixtures of liquid hydrocarbons.

Solvents

Many of the solvents found in paints and caulks are liquid hydrocarbon mixtures. Residues of solvents can be found in carpets, plastics, and furniture. As discussed in chapter 3, construction materials, furniture, carpeting, and plastics in computer equipment and in cables have the potential of slowly releasing residual vapors (off-gassing) from solvents that might have been used in the manufacturing process or application. If present in the air in high enough concentrations, any of these hydrocarbons, either alone or in combination, can cause eye and mucous membrane irritation or even a sensation of burning on the lips.

A solvent is not just something used in the dry-cleaning process. Solvents get their name from one of their physical properties: they cause other things to dissolve. When a solid dissolves in a liquid, the molecules merely separate and spread out through the liquid (like sugar in water, for example). Hydrocarbons mix with each other but not with water or with most things that dissolve in water. Hydrocarbons also mix with other organic compounds, including fats and vegetable oils. (The phrase *organic compounds* originally referred to the fact that these substances were associated with living organisms. Today, most organic compounds in plastics, furniture, and paints are synthetic.)

One reason why solvents can affect the body is that they have an affinity for fats. A very high percentage of the brain and nervous system consists of fat that acts as an insulator around the neurons, the "wires" that conduct the electrical impulses of the nervous system. When solvent vapors are inhaled, they enter the blood in the lungs and are distributed by the blood into the body's fat, where they have an immediate effect on the nervous system. People can feel disoriented, tingly, nauseated, and even inebriated. The vapors of some solvents, like ether and chloroform, can act as anesthetics when inhaled, presumably because of their impact on the fat that insulates nerves. Very high inhaled doses of solvent vapor or ingested doses of solvent liquid can be narcotic and even lethal.

Chlorinated Hydrocarbons

Another class of compounds, called *chlorinated hydrocarbons,* are solvents in which one or more of the hydrogen atoms in a molecule have been replaced by an atom of the element chlorine. Methylene chloride (CH_2Cl_2), for example, is the solvent used in many paint strippers, including the one used by the employee of the University of Massachusetts Boston whom we encountered in chapter 1. Carbon tetrachloride (CCl_4), a carcinogen, was formerly used to remove spots on clothing. (The dry-cleaning process today uses another chlorinated hydrocarbon solvent, tetrachloroethylene, to dissolve grease or fats in fabric.) Carbon tetrachloride can't burn, because the molecule CCl_4 has no hydrogen to combine with oxygen, and so it was also formerly used in fire extinguishers. When sprayed into a fire, CCl_4 changes state to vapor, pushing away the air and thus the oxygen needed for the combustion process to continue. The CCl_4 in fire extinguishers has now been replaced by less toxic chemicals.

Many chlorinated hydrocarbons are used as pesticides, such as DDT, dieldrin, and eldrin, which can be toxic to people as well as to insects.

HYDROGEN SULFIDE AND HYDROGEN CYANIDE

Two lethal gases with characteristic smells are hydrogen sulfide (H_2S), which gives sewer gas its rotten-egg odor, and hydrogen cyanide (HCN), which has the odor of almonds. A hydrogen sulfide molecule consists of two hydrogen atoms and one sulfur atom. A hydrogen cyanide molecule consists of three different atoms: a hydrogen attached to a carbon atom that is attached to a nitrogen atom. Cyanide and sulfide from these gases bind *irreversibly* with the iron in hemoglobin (as well as with other components of the cells in the body). When present in high enough levels, these gases can be deadly after only a few minutes of inhalation. In December 2003, H_2S gas was accidentally released from an underground well in China, killing over two hundred villagers and sending thousands more fleeing from their homes. HCN has been used in gas chambers to execute death-row prisoners. HCN is not normally present in buildings except during fires, when acrylic plastic (used in paints, caulk, fabrics, and carpets, among other building materials) is decomposing (burning).

AMMONIA AND AMINES

An ammonia molecule (NH_3) consists of three hydrogen atoms, each attached to the same nitrogen atom. We all are familiar with the odor of ammonia gas, which is commonly dissolved in water for use as a cleaning agent. Pure ammonia gas is extremely irritating and toxic. Ammonia gas is used as a refrigerant in commercial coolers, and if the ammonia leaks out, toxic exposures to the gas can occur.

When nitrogen atoms are bonded to hydrogen atoms (as well as to carbon atoms), compounds called *amines* are produced. Many amines have ammonia-like odors. Compounds called *diamines* contain two amines. Many diamines produce downright disgusting odors.

"Nylon 66," one of the first man-made fibers ever synthesized, is found in plastics as well as in clothing and is made by mixing two reactive chemicals

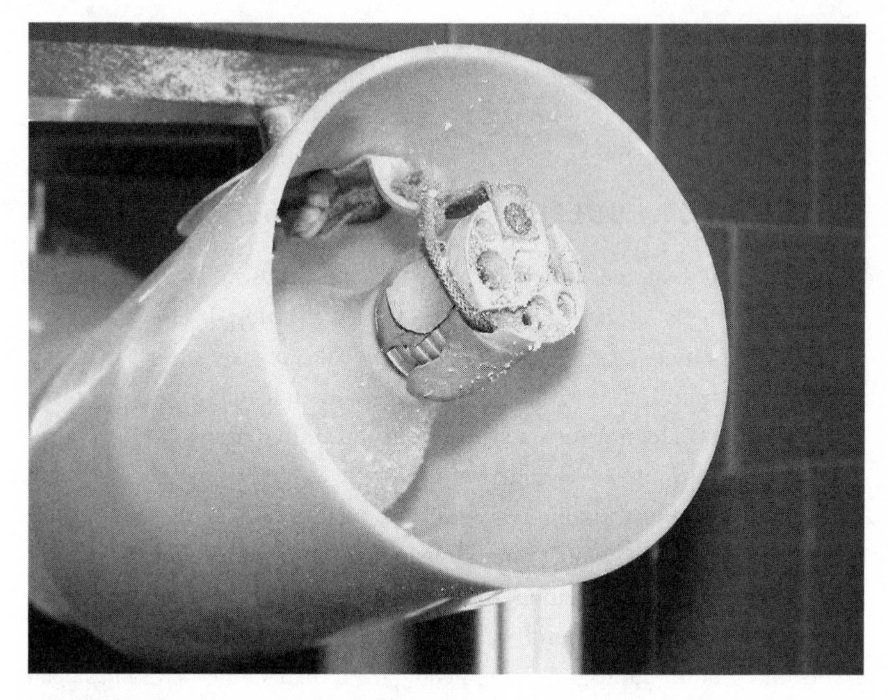

FIGURE 5.4. A putrid light fixture. This fixture caused a foul, dead-fish odor in a bathroom. You are looking at the fixture from the back; the light bulb is partially visible at the left. The plastic base is burned and broken. *May Indoor Air Investigations LLC*

together. One of these chemicals is a diamine consisting of a short chain of carbon atoms in the middle, each with two hydrogen atoms attached, and a nitrogen atom at each end, each with two hydrogen atoms attached. Each carbon atom with two hydrogen atoms attached (CH_2) is called a *methylene* group, and the nitrogen at each end with two hydrogen atoms attached (NH_2) is called an *amine* group.

Nylon is made from hexamethylene diamine, $NH_2(CH_2)_6(NH_2)$: six methylene groups and two amine groups. The diamine series also includes the compounds cadaverine (pentamethylene diamine, or five methylene groups and two amine groups) and putriscene (tetramethylene diamine, or four methylene groups and two amine groups). Both cadaverine and putriscene are present in decaying fish. When organic compounds differ by only one CH_2 group, the compounds are said to be in a chemical series called a *homologous series,* and the compounds in a homologous series can produce similar odors. This is why heated nylon plastic in some light fixtures and lamps can produce a sickening odor.

One day we received a call from a woman who worked in a building in which one bathroom had an irritating fishy odor, so strong that people had avoided using that facility for weeks. The building owner had hired a contractor, a plumber, and even an industrial hygienist to investigate, but no one had been able to find the source of the smell. The owner was so frustrated that she was about to have the entire bathroom demolished and rebuilt.

I had asked that all the ventilation be shut down before I arrived at the site. I soon regretted this request; the smell was so disgusting that I could hardly stand to remain in the room. I quickly opened the bathroom door and window and turned the exhaust back on. By sniffing various surfaces, I found the source of the smell: a multisocket light fixture with cracked and melted plastic bases, located above the sink. Removing the fixture eliminated the primary source of the odor, but the walls and ceiling near the fixture had become secondary sources. Rinsing the surfaces with diluted vinegar a few times eliminated the smell and saved the bathroom from demolition. (Because vinegar is an acid and a diamine is a base, or alkaline, the vinegar neutralized the smell of the diamine.)

RADON GAS

Radon gas is an invisible airborne carcinogen (see chapter 1). Air containing radon enters basements and other below-grade spaces through gaps or cracks in the foundation floor and walls when the air pressure in such spaces is less than the air pressure in the surrounding soil.

In general, the air pressure in a building is slightly different from the air pressure outside; infiltration and exfiltration occur in the presence of very small pressure differences. The air pressure in a basement is often less than the pressure in the soil, particularly in winter, because of the stack effect (see chapter 4). When a storm approaches, the barometric pressure (the air pressure outside) falls, and the pressure *above* the surface of the soil becomes less than the air pressure *in* the soil. Exfiltration will cause the air pressure inside a building to drop. Air from the soil will then flow not only into the atmosphere above the soil surface but also into the building, potentially carrying radon in air into below-grade spaces.

Levels of radon in air are naturally higher in some parts of the country than in others. While radon in air is more of an issue in residential spaces than in commercial spaces, I still recommend that radon levels be measured whenever people are spending extended periods of time in a below-grade space. The most common way to measure the amount of radon in air is to place a container full of activated charcoal in a space for a fixed period of time, usually around two days. The charcoal adsorbs the radon gas, and the container is then covered and sent to a lab for analysis. One way to express radon levels is in picocuries/liter of air, or pCi/L of air (a picocurie is a measure of radioactivity). A level of radon in air greater than 4 pCi/L is considered to be above the EPA's action level, and further testing or remediation is needed. (Refer to the Resource Guide for information on obtaining the EPA's "A Citizen's Guide to Radon.") Although testing for radon in air is important, typical levels of radon in air can *never* produce the symptoms associated with sick-building syndrome. Nonetheless, air with radon can be carcinogenic if inhaled at elevated levels over a prolonged period of time.

A radon mitigation system uses a fan to remove air from the soil beneath the basement floor, thus ensuring that the air pressure in the basement will be greater than the air pressure in the surrounding soil. The air that is removed is exhausted via a pipe to the outside above the roof, to prevent that air (which contains radon) from entering the basement.

FRAGRANCES

Men and women alike use perfumes, colognes, or fragranced body products such as shampoos and skin creams. They wash their clothes with perfumed detergents and put scented softener sheets in their dryers. Some people plug in heated fragrance-emitters and use sprays that "freshen" the air with scents. Scented candles are everywhere, magazines come with perfumed inserts, and there are even "scratch and sniff" stickers for children. Advertisements make strong connections among scents, Nature, cleanliness, and health. There is even an alternative health practice called *aroma therapy,* involving the use of so-called natural fragrances for mood adjustment.

Some of the chemicals in fragrances can cause symptoms in people with asthma. I consider myself physically intolerant of fragrances. Some scented products make me cough, and others make my wife wheeze. My home and office are fragrance-free. My wife and I don't use scented detergents, soaps, deodorants, or garbage bags. I can detect when someone has used fragrance, just, I suppose, as many nonsmokers can identify a smoker by the odor clinging to his or her clothing.

I wasn't always like this. At one point in my career I worked as a product-development chemist. One of my projects involved formulating a milky-white silver polish. Most polishes have an unpleasant odor. I wanted to create a polish with a familiar, pleasing odor, so I chose the scent of almond oil so that people would associate the cleaner with a popular hand lotion that had the same scent. The odor of almond is produced by the chemical benzaldehyde (C_7H_6O), which belongs to a class of oxygen-containing compounds called *aldehydes*. Aldehydes generally have strong and often pleasing (though sometimes irritating) odors. Despite the fact that in very low concentrations benzaldehyde is "generally regarded as safe" (GRAS) by the FDA for use as a fragrance in lotions, perfumes, and cleaning products and as a natural flavor in foods, the chemical in its pure form can cause rashes if applied directly to the skin.

Pinene (a liquid hydrocarbon responsible for pine odor) and limonene (a liquid hydrocarbon responsible for lemon odor) are two irritating volatile organic compounds (VOCs) found in paint thinners, solvents, plug-in air-fresheners, and cleaning compounds. (Turpentine—one type of paint thinner—is nearly pure pinene.) Both limonene and pinene can react with oxygen or ozone from air. When limonene reacts with oxygen, it produces a chemical that causes skin sensitization and dermatitis.[8] Both limonene and pinene vapors in the air react with ozone gas to produce irritating chemicals,[9] which can then be inhaled—another reason to avoid ozone-producing devices (see chapter 3).

TOTAL VOLATILE ORGANIC COMPOUNDS

Fragrances add to the load of total volatile organic compounds (TVOCs) that people must tolerate indoors. When VOC levels are elevated, the tear film in the eyes can become thinner, causing people to blink more in order to renew the film. Some building researchers have actually proposed using blinking rate as an indication of air quality.[10] However, staring at a video terminal may suppress the blinking rate, so exposure to VOCs might not cause someone looking at a computer monitor to blink more.

Based on studies of buildings in which people were not complaining about indoor air quality, a mixture of common VOCs called M-22 was formulated to simulate the TVOC mix typically found indoors.[11] Several investigators exposed groups of subjects to air contaminated with various levels of M-22. The subjects then filled out questionnaires regarding their symptoms at the different concentrations tested. TVOC concentrations of less than 1 milligram per cubic meter (mg/m^3) were generally not a problem for the subjects (though hypersensitive individuals might have disagreed). Symptoms started to appear when M-22 was in the range of 1 to 10 mg/m^3 and became common when M-22 was above 25 mg/m^3.[12] The symptoms experienced were typical of sick-building syndrome and included irritation or dryness of mucous membranes of the eyes, nose, and throat as well as headaches, sleepiness, and fatigue.

TVOC levels considered normal range from 0.2 to 0.5 mg/m^3.[13] If the TVOC concentration indoors is much over 0.5 mg/m^3, there is probably either a VOC source in the building or inadequate ventilation. The identities and concentrations of all the VOCs in any given building can fluctuate hourly, daily, or weekly, depending on the sources. Some offices contain specialized printing equipment, such as blueprint machines and photographic processing devices, each of which emits its own particular mixtures of chemicals.

Most offices contain photocopiers, which produce VOCs in a range of between 1 and 20 milligrams per hour of use.[14] Photocopiers use ink called *toner,* a dry powder consisting of black pigment (carbon) in microscopic plastic beads (composed of plastics such as polystyrene, polybutylacrylate, and polyethylene, and also containing some residual solvent). Inside a photocopier, a high-voltage wire helps to transfer the light image from a text page to a rotating drum. As the paper rolls over the drum, the image is applied to the paper by means of the toner. Then the paper passes under a light tube (a *fuser*) containing a very hot filament that heats and melts the plastic beads onto the paper surface. The high temperature of the fuser also thermally decomposes some of the plastic, and the residual solvents are flashed off (evaporated), producing irritating odors. In addition, depending on the temperature and humidity of the air as well as on the condition of the copier, the high-voltage wire can produce ozone gas.

Laser printers (not ink-jet printers) produce VOCs in a range of between 1 and 8 milligrams per hour of use.[15] Laser printers operate on principles similar to copiers and also contain a fuser that melts the toner onto the page, which is why the paper is hot when it comes out of the printer. Laser printers can therefore also produce VOCs from the heated plastic in the toner powder.

In a worst-case scenario, imagine a printer located in a small room (10 cubic meters, or about 6 by 6 by 9 feet in size) and producing VOCs at the top of the range (20 milligrams per hour of use). If there is very little ventilation, after an hour of copier use the TVOC concentration could be 2 mg/m^3 (20 milligrams divided by the volume of the room, or 10 cubic meters): high enough to produce sick-building symptoms in sensitized individuals. It is not uncommon in schools and offices for copiers to be used in small, poorly ventilated rooms just like this.

Any type of printer that uses powdered toner may also produce pigment aerosol. I was once looking for mold spores in an air sample I had taken in an office, when I noticed several particles that resembled spores but were too brightly colored: yellow, magenta, and cyan (blue-green)—the primary colors of printing inks. I was mystified until I remembered that someone had been operating a color laser printer in the office while I was sampling. I then realized that these were not spores at all but rather microscopic spheres of plastic toner containing pigment that had become airborne. But I'm not aware of any studies connecting inhalation of toner particles with health symptoms.

SOME PRACTICAL STEPS

- If the air in your office seems stuffy, the simplest thing to do is to be sure that there is a supply of fresh air.
- If your heat is supplied by a gas- or oil-fired appliance, it is a good idea to have a plug-in carbon monoxide detector (see chapter 13). Be sure to install it where you can hear it if it goes off. Such detectors are available at most hardware stores.
- In my opinion, equipment that emits chemicals, including printers and copiers, should be housed in rooms that have exhaust ventilation and partition walls that extend from floor to ceiling deck (the bottom of the floor above), so that emissions cannot flow with air from one ceiling plenum to another and thus enter other spaces in the building.

- If a bathroom in your building has an unpleasant, fishy odor, it may be caused by nylon heated in a light fixture. Turn off the lights one by one to see if the smell abates.
- To filter out vapors, you can buy a single-use charcoal mask, available in most hardware stores. You can also purchase a reusable half-face respirator with charcoal filters that remove VOCs.

CHAPTER

6

Particles in the Sea of Air

Air flowing inside buildings carries particles as well as gases and vapors. For years, one of the major sources of air quality problems indoors was smoke from cigarettes. Cigarette smoke, formed by combustion of dried tobacco leaves, is a contaminant that consists of particulates (solids such as ash as well as aerosolized droplets containing nicotine and tars), gases (hydrogen cyanide, carbon monoxide, and carbon dioxide, among others), and vapors (including acrolein, acetone, and methyl ethyl ketone). (Vapors are gases that have evaporated from substances that are liquid at room temperature.) In many cities in the United States, smoking is banned in most public buildings, including restaurants. While smoking in public places is still common in many other countries, in January 2005 Italy followed Ireland and Norway in enacting a smoking ban in enclosed public spaces (except restaurants and bars with ventilated smoking rooms).

Even when cigarette smoking is banned in a building, people can still be exposed to the smoke. Time and time again I have seen smoking areas located right outside a building entrance, and people were forced to move through clouds of cigarette smoke as they walked in and out of the building. Secondhand smoke or ETS (environmental tobacco smoke) is considered by the EPA to be a carcinogen. Children are susceptible to ETS, particularly those with asthma, so I think infants and children should not be taken into buildings where people are allowed to smoke. I also do not think susceptible children should live in houses where people smoke, but unfortunately many parents smoke.

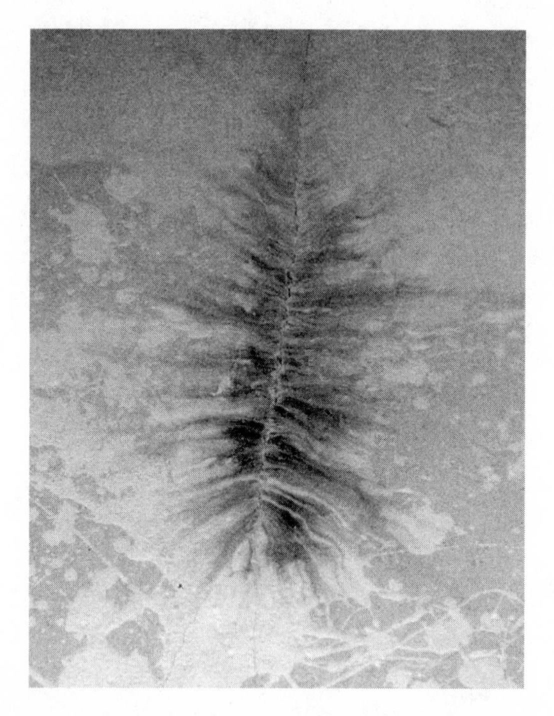

FIGURE 6.1. Soot reveals airflows. This 1-inch-thick concrete floor (resting on plywood) was covered by wall-to-wall carpet that was removed after a serious building fire. The fire started in the level below at the other end of the building. During the fire, hot gases carrying soot moved more than a hundred feet through a ceiling plenum (see chapter 7) and penetrated through cracks in plywood and concrete. The feather-like soot deposits in this photograph delineate the pattern of air flowing through the crack. (The white paint splatters were present from the time of construction of the building.) *May Indoor Air Investigations LLC*

INDOOR FOG

I investigated an air quality problem in an office, part of a manufacturing facility. A very large, open storage room inside the building had a floor area of about 30,000 square feet and a ceiling height of about 30 feet. The air outside was extremely humid and hazy. Indoors I noticed that the most distant ceiling mercury lights in the storage area looked blurry, whereas lights in the smaller rooms were shining perfectly clearly. I asked the owner if something inside the building was producing smoke, and he said no. There was, however, a strong exhaust fan drawing in thousands of cubic feet of air per minute from the exterior into the storage area. The air in that space, therefore, was not much different from the hazy air outside.

Atmospheric haze, like fog, often consists of small droplets of suspended water. Remember that on a very humid day, the air is holding water vapor close to its capacity to do so (see chapter 4). On that particular day the relative humidity was 85 percent, so the air could have held only 15 percent more water vapor before reaching its saturation point. Water vapor molecules are attracted to surfaces, and when they collide with these surfaces, some stick. Cotton clothing, for example, can feel "heavy" on humid days because cotton can adsorb more than 25 percent of its (dry) weight in water from vapor in air. Aerosolized particulates also offer water vapor a surface on which to collect, so on humid days water vapor molecules can adsorb on airborne particles and combine and grow into small microscopic droplets.

I measured the number of aerosol particulates inside the storage area using a laser particle counter, which counts the number of particles in different size ranges. The concentration of particulates greater than 0.5 micron in size was 5 million per cubic foot (177 per cubic centimeter) of air. On a clear, dry day outside there might not be more than 200,000/ft^3, or 7/cm^3. I also collected some of these particulates on a glass slide with an air-sampling instru-

The terms *percent* and *rate* both express concentrations and are ratios: comparing the quantity of one thing with the quantity of another thing. With percentages, the "things" are the same: ten oranges out of one hundred oranges, or 10 percent. Rate, on the other hand, compares the *number* of something with the *amount* of something different: four tires per car, or ten fingers per person. The same rate can be expressed in a number of ways, which can make understanding a rate confusing. For example, if you are earning $10/hour, you are earning $5 / half hour, $80 / eight hours, or if you work a 40 hour week, $400/week. If you work 50 weeks a year, your salary could also be expressed as $20,000/year or even 20k/year. These are all the same rate, conveyed in different ways. Similarly, 100 parts per billion is the same rate as 0.1 part per million (100 ppb = 0.1 ppm), and 100,000 particles per cubic foot of air is the same rate as 3.53 particles per cubic centimeter of air (100,000 particles/ft^3 of air = 3.53 particles/cm^3 of air).

ment and looked at the slide with a microscope. Nearly every particle on the slide was a tiny water droplet with a speck of dust within.

The light fixtures in the storage room appeared to be blurry because I was peering at them through a mist of these droplets. In the smaller rooms of the building, the lights were not as far away from me as they were in the cavernous storage room. In addition, there wasn't as much exterior air in those smaller rooms, because there wasn't as much ventilation, so there were not as many droplets between the light bulbs and my eyes to reflect (scatter) light.

THE LONELY ORANGUTAN

A particle counter saved the life of Minyak, a very rare orangutan caged in the Los Angeles zoo. The twenty-three-year-old male had suffered for years from breathing problems and respiratory infections, and had even endured lung surgery. His problems often landed him in the zoo's health center, where he was isolated from other orangutans. He was so weak and unhappy that his keepers administered him antidepressants along with his antibiotics.

The zoo turned to an IAQ investigator for help. Using a particle counter, the investigator measured the concentration of aerosol outdoors, in other zoo facilities, and in Minyak's "bedroom," where she found elevated levels of particulates—more than 10 million per cubic foot of air that were 0.3 micron or larger, rather than the average of 950,000 measured in six other locations at the zoo. She then measured the particles in the air coming from the supply vent in the room, to find 12 million per cubic foot of air.[1]

The investigator hypothesized that the source of the particles was dirty, deteriorating fiberglass lining material in the heating system (see chapter 7). The next day the fiberglass was sealed, the air-handling system was cleaned, and efficient filtration was installed. Minyak's health improved so drastically over the next few months that he went off his meds and was soon courting a mate.

PARTICLES FROM LIVING AND NONLIVING THINGS

In some of the samples I took from the factory storage room, the specks of dust within the water droplets consisted of particles of soil. Other specks were mold spores or bits of rubber from tires. Particles that come from living things, like spores from mold growth, are called *biogenic,* and particles that come from nonliving things, like the dust from weathered rocks, are called *nonbiogenic.*

Biogenic Particles

The air we breathe may contain a whole host of biogenic particles that can potentially cause disease. Viruses and bacteria are transiently in the air in droplets expelled by people sneezing and coughing. Bacteria, yeast, and mold require moist conditions such as those found in air-conditioning equipment or in carpeting that has been chronically damp.

According to a 2004 report commissioned by the CDC and undertaken by the Institute of Medicine, there is no evidence that exposures to "toxic" molds lead to cancer, fatigue, or neurological problems, a conclusion that attracted a great deal of media attention. Unfortunately, in consequence, a very important aspect of the report was downplayed: that exposure to microbial growth in damp buildings is associated with respiratory symptoms.[2] In a more recent (2005) study of major importance, researchers looked at respiratory symptoms experienced by people working in a twenty-story office building in the northeastern United States. There had been long-term roof and exterior water leaks, as well as plumbing leaks, in this building, and extensive mold growth as a result (especially on the upper levels). The building occupants

Bacteria are microscopic organisms consisting of single cells, each surrounded by a cell membrane made up of a variety of components, including fats, proteins, and other substances. Depending on how the bacteria are affected by Gram stain (a mixture of a blue dye and a red dye), they can be classified into one of two groups. Those that adsorb both dyes in the stain and turn purple or blue are called Gram-positive bacteria (GPB). Those that adsorb only the red dye in the stain and turn pink are called Gram-negative bacteria (GNB). Many of the common bacteria that cause infections are GNB. GNB are dangerous for another reason: their cell membranes contain a substance called *endotoxin,* a toxin that can cause inflammation of lung cells, chest tightness, and fever.

If water from a reservoir contaminated with GNB is aerosolized, or if the reservoir dries out and the desiccated (dried out) membranes are aerosolized, the endotoxin may be inhaled. Endotoxin may be found outdoors at low levels and in homes and offices at moderate levels, particularly if GNB-contaminated humidifiers are present. In industries where organic dusts are present (such as in the cotton or grain industry) or where water-based lubricants are used (such as in metal-cutting), concentrations of the toxin indoors can be thousands of times higher than concentrations outdoors (see chapter 14).

suffered from wheezing and asthma symptoms up to two and a half times the rate found in workers in healthy buildings, and adult-onset asthma at over three times the rate found in workers in healthy buildings (two-thirds of these new asthma cases occurred after people began to work in the building). One-third of time lost for sick days was blamed on respiratory symptoms, and "abnormal lung function and/or breathing medication use was found in 67 percent of the respiratory cases."[3]

Despite this report and others like it, mold and the by-products of its growth continue to be underestimated and misunderstood indoor health threats in buildings. In order for mold to grow, spores (microscopic "seeds"), moisture (either from humidity or from liquid water), oxygen from air, the right temperature conditions, and a food source must be present. There are myriad nutrition sources for mold, including paper, food crumbs, wood and wood products, and human skin scales in dust. Since oxygen and sustenance for mold exist everywhere inside a building, the limiting growth factor for mold is *moisture*.

If flooding or leaks have occurred in a building, or if there are conditions of high relative humidity (consistently greater than 75 percent), there is a strong chance that mold growth is present. Do not ignore a moldy smell, for although some plastics off-gas a smell reminiscent of mold growth (see chapter 3), a musty smell most likely signals the presence of mold. Do not be complacent if you see mold growth or mildew. While mold is part of the natural world, that doesn't mean that people should live or work in its midst in indoor environments. In fact, I do not think that there should be any visible mold growth indoors.

Mold is at the bottom of a food chain the components of which can be both microscopic and macroscopic (visible without a microscope). In New England I often find a variety of mite species foraging on mold, particularly in below-grade spaces. Sometimes I find that a sample of what I thought was only mold growth on a wall is actually fecal pellets full of partially digested mold spores. When disturbed, this biological fuzz can become aerosolized, and people breathing the "dust" are exposed to mold as well as to insect allergens. In some highly infested locations I even find predator mites, such as *Cheyleus eruditis* mites, that feed only on other mites. A storage mite called *Tyrophagus putrescentiae* is common on farms, and a majority of farmers have serum IgE (immunoglobulin E) antibodies to it.[4] The same mite can cause dermatitis in dogs; almost 90 percent of dogs have IgE antibodies to this mite.[5]

There are two species of mites, *Dermatophagoides pteronyssinus* and *D. farinae,* that are referred to as house dust mites (HDMs) because they feed on human skin scales in dust. (*Blomia tropicalis* is another indoor dust mite common in warmer climates.) Dust mite allergens are a major trigger for asthma symptoms. HDMs live in cushioned materials such as couches, mattresses, and pillows and are thus more likely to be present in homes than in office spaces. But HDMs can be found in constantly used cushioned desk chairs (see chapter 3) as well as in school carpeting, particularly if the carpeting is laid on concrete, either at or below grade. And frequently worn, rarely washed clothing (such as a down parka or a wool sports coat) can become infested with HDMs and become a source of allergens, either for the wearer or for others who are exposed to dust from the item.

Dust mites are fragile and defenseless and thus live hidden from predators, like spiders, in fleecy or fibrous materials (such as beds and couches) in which the relative humidity is elevated as a result of body moisture from human beings. (Mites take moisture directly from the air, but they can do this only if the relative humidity is above 70 percent.)

Allergy to house dust mites is one of the major triggers of asthma symptoms, and HDMs are the species for which allergists test. To determine if someone is allergic to HDMs, physicians use extracts of the principal HDM allergens: enzymes (chemicals that digest food) present in the mite gut as well as fecal pellets. Despite a negative HDM allergy test, though, you can still be highly allergic to mites, because there are probably over a dozen species of mites common in buildings that can cause sensitization, and you may react to allergens from one kind of mite but not another.

Silverfish feed on mites, and booklice feed on mold. Spiders are often at the top of this vast food chain. If you see a lot of spiders or spiderwebs in a building, you know that you have a micro-ecology in place. Cockroaches, booklice, silverfish, and various larvae (such as those from wool moths) all produce digestive enzymes and eject fecal pellets (containing bits of what was ingested) that can be allergenic if aerosolized and inhaled.

Other biogenic particulates present in interior environments may include fragments of wool fibers emitted from rugs and wall-to-wall carpet (see chap-

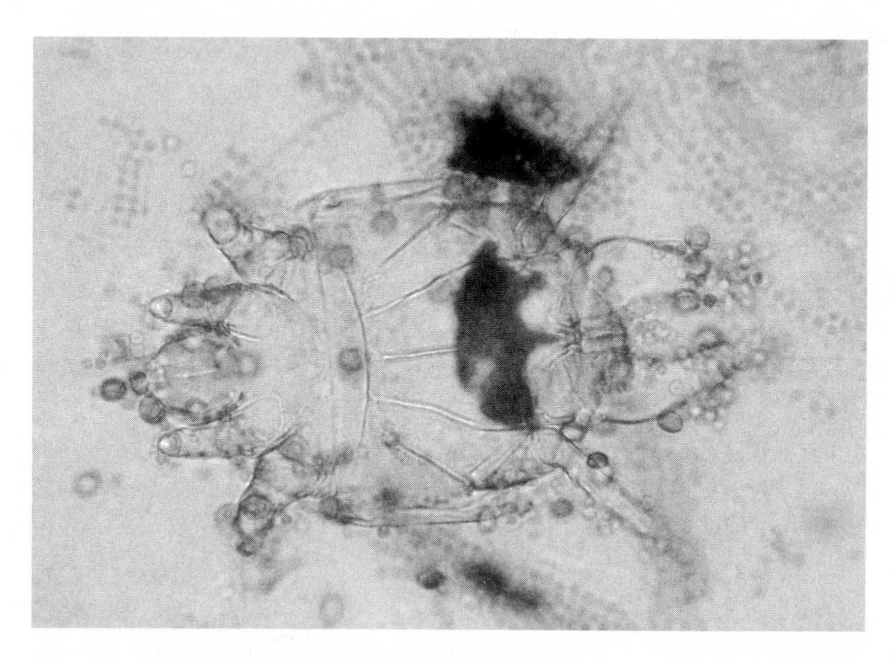

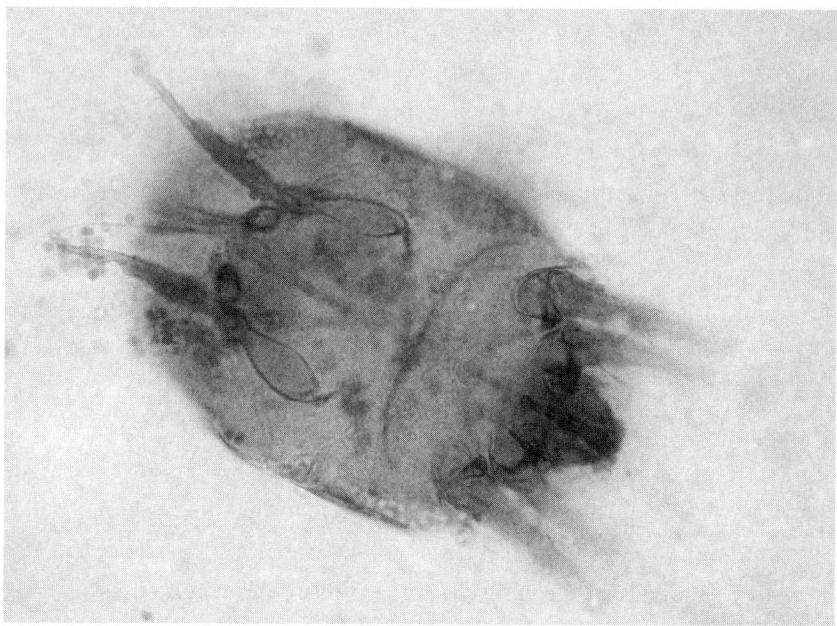

FIGURE 6.2. Mold-eating mites. These two mites, each just over three-hundredths of an inch long (125 microns, slightly greater than the thickness of a hair), were found foraging on *Aspergillus* mold growing in a damp basement. The small spheres are the mold spores.
May Indoor Air Investigations LLC

ter 3). In environments where a great deal of paper is being processed (mail sorting, printing, and photocopying), cellulose fibers may be present in concentrations high enough to cause irritation. In buildings where many latex rubber gloves are used, such as hospitals, allergens from the latex (carried on starch granules that become aerosolized) have caused allergic responses. Latex allergy, most often caused by skin contact with latex products, can be a life-threatening condition and is discussed in greater detail in chapter 10.

Pollen can sometimes enter a building with airflows. Pollen is not much of an issue in bigger buildings where the mechanical system filters and supplies most of the air, but in smaller buildings where exterior doors open and close frequently and where the windows can be opened, infiltrating pollen can cause allergy symptoms. Obviously, pollen is hard to avoid during certain times of the year.

Nonbiogenic Particles

The soil in which we grow our crops and on which we construct our buildings consists of many small particles of clay, silica, limestone, and granite dust (nonbiogenic particles) mixed with humus (decaying plant and animal material: biogenic material). Soil can be tracked into a building on shoes and end up in carpets, from which particulates can be aerosolized by foot traffic. Lead paint dust, made up of nonbiogenic particles from exterior paint, can also become mixed with soil and find its way into buildings. Pesticides can make the same trip, because these chemicals adhere to soil particles.

SINKERS: PARTICLES THAT SETTLE

Some particulates remain airborne longer than others. In quiescent (quiet) air, the rate at which a particle falls depends upon its size and shape. In general, smaller particles stay afloat longer than larger particles do. Flat particles will float longer than spherical ones, and light spherical ones will float longer than heavy spherical ones (assuming the same breeze conditions).

The *settling rate of particles* (how quickly they settle onto surfaces in quiescent conditions) is extremely important in determining the exposures that people may have to the particles. Dust mite allergen is mostly contained on 25-micron spherical particles that settle out of the air in less than a minute. In a typical workplace setting, fiberglass fibers do not pose much of a health

TABLE 6.1. Approximate time for a particle to settle from a ceiling height of eight feet

Particle size	Time
100 microns	3 seconds
50 microns	12 seconds
30 microns	34 seconds
15 microns	2.25 minutes
10 microns	5 minutes
5 microns	20 minutes
1 micron	8.5 hours
Smaller than 1 micron	Permanently suspended

Source: Adapted from "Particle Settling Rate" (Memphis, Tenn.: National Safety Associates, 1989).

Note: One micron is one-millionth of a meter; a human hair is about 100 microns thick. These times are for spherically shaped particles.

risk via inhalation if they are removed with regular, thorough maintenance, because the fibers are large (mostly bigger than 20 microns) and tend to settle out of the air fairly quickly. (Contact with fibers that are not removed and that thus settle and collect on surfaces can cause skin irritation, however.) Pollen particles are also relatively large (over 10 microns) and settle out of the air within seconds to minutes, so indoor spaces should be vacuumed more frequently during pollen season.

Mold spores that are about 3 microns in size can remain suspended in air for half an hour or more. Particles less than 1 micron in size remain permanently suspended because the molecules in air are in constant motion, and even in "still" air there is enough molecular energy to keep these very small particulates afloat. (Asbestos fibers can be 0.1 to 10 microns in length, and most are less than 1 micron in thickness, so those fibers can remain suspended in air for hours.) Of course, any settled dust containing irritants, allergens, or toxins can be disturbed and then inhaled, but the level of exposure to particles that settle quickly depends on the level of activity rather than on the settle rates of the particles themselves.

BREATHING IT IN

Aerosolized particulates are characterized according to how deep they penetrate into the respiratory system. Particulate matter (PM) with an *aerodynamic diameter* (the diameter the particulate appears to have as it moves through air) larger than 10 microns and up to about 100 microns in size is trapped in the nose and throat and is referred to as *inhalable*. People eliminate inhalable PM

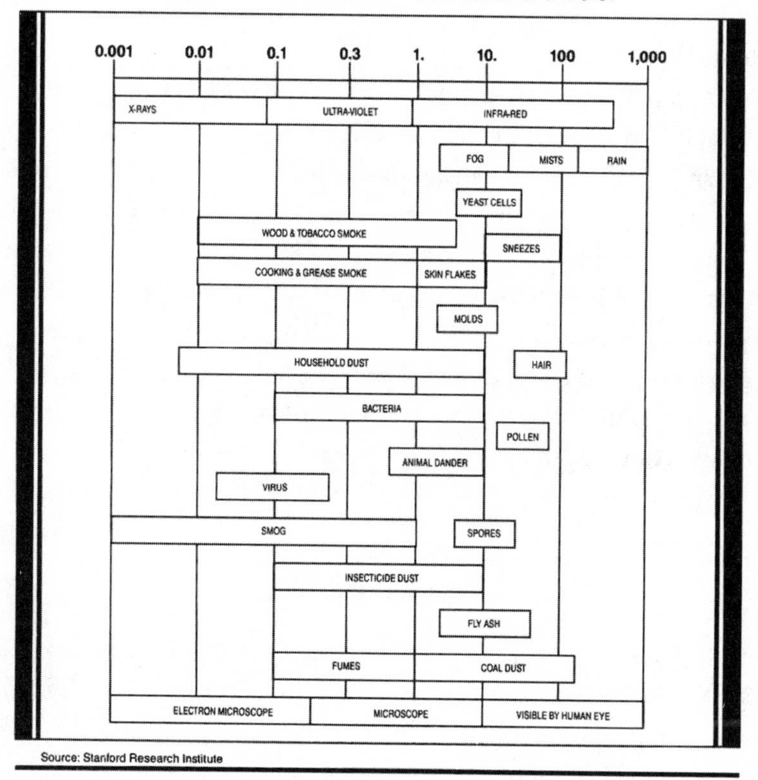

FIGURE 6.3. Particle sizes. This chart indicates the range in sizes of aerosols. At the top, the chart shows the size ranges for different wavelengths of light, included for size comparisons. The bottom row indicates how the particles can be observed. *Courtesy of SRI International*

by swallowing, sneezing, or coughing. PM less than 10 microns in size is referred to as PM_{10} and is divided into three fractions (types): coarse (between 2.5 and 10 microns), fine (from 0.1 micron to 2.5 microns), and ultrafine (less than 0.1 micron). The coarse fraction of PM is called *thoracic* and penetrates into the upper part of the respiratory system, beyond the nose and throat. The fine and ultrafine PM (smaller than 2.5 microns in size) is designated $PM_{2.5}$ and is called *respirable*. $PM_{2.5}$ can penetrate deep into the lung and deposit on the delicate membranes of the lung's air sacs and smallest passageways. Most outdoor $PM_{2.5}$ is generated by processes that take place when fuel is burned in power plants, cars, trucks, wood stoves, and so on. Indoors, cooking and cigarette smoking also generate $PM_{2.5}$. The concentrations of ambient (outdoor) PM are significant, because in most buildings much of the $PM_{2.5}$ may infiltrate from outdoors.

Spores produced by the mold *Stachybotrys chartarum* (the so-called toxic black mold) are about 8 microns in size, so they are not respirable. On the other hand, the spores from many species of other fungi such as *Penicillium* and *Aspergillus* (commonly found in damp, "sick" buildings) are respirable, and many also contain mycotoxins.

A study of the dust emissions from ceiling tiles contaminated with *Stachybotrys chartarum* demonstrated that many dust particulates were coated with mycotoxins from the mold growth.[6] The particulates, which consisted of fungal and ceiling tile fragments, were less than 1 micron in size and were thus respirable. Although this study only determined the presence of mycotoxins, it is likely that other allergenic, fungal by-products were also present on the particulates.

CATASTROPHE

At the beginning of the attack on the World Trade Center on September 11, 2001, the intense heat from the burning jet fuel set fire to all of the combustible contents of several floors. Because the initial explosion had stripped much of the insulation from the steel supporting the floors, the horizontal steel was softened by the heat, ultimately leading to the collapse of a few of the concrete floors. As soon as the falling concrete hit an intact floor below,

Epidemiological studies have shown a strong relationship between exposures to ambient (outdoor) air containing elevated concentrations of particulate matter and increased mortality from cardiovascular and respiratory diseases as well as increased hospitalizations for asthma. In 1987 the EPA created the National Ambient Air Quality Standards (NAAQS) for particulate matter. To protect public health, the NAAQS sets limits for the quantity of PM_{10} in the outdoor air. Because most of the health effects of PM are due to the fine and ultrafine fractions of PM_{10}, however, in 1997 the EPA issued a $PM_{2.5}$ standard for outdoor air.

the horizontal steel support beams snapped at the vertical supports under the impact of the excessive load. One after another, each level crashed down onto the one below. Each successive failure contained a greater weight of concrete, so that the building accordioned on itself, and the concrete and building materials were pulverized (turned to dust) as they fell.

Immediately after the Twin Towers collapsed, over a million tons of dust spread out in a thick blanket over nearby sidewalks, streets, cars, and buildings, not to mention survivors, and entered apartments and businesses.[7] Most of the dust consisted of solid particles that came from building materials, including the concrete in the floors, gypsum in the drywall, and glass fibers in the ceiling tiles. Asbestos fibers were also in the dust; most of these fibers settled within a half-block of ground zero.[8] The billowing clouds of smoke from the fire as well as the dust from the collapse of the buildings obscured the entire lower end of Manhattan Island, and the growing cloud could be seen by satellites in space.

The liquid droplets in the smoke included the combustion products not only from burning jet fuel but also from burning plastics (computers, wires and cables, pipes, furniture) and burning paper and oils from the electrical power transformers. These combustion products contained many organic compounds, including chlorinated hydrocarbons such as PCB (polychlorinated biphenyl, a carcinogenic oil used in transformers), as well as other highly toxic products of combustion such as dioxin (a carbon-based, chlorinated, carcinogenic compound). Most of these liquid droplets weren't volatile and therefore did not evaporate; rather, they settled with and stuck to other solid particles and mingled with the dust.

Ninety-five percent of the dust was larger than 10 microns and 50 percent was larger than 53 microns.[9] Still, Dr. Philip J. Landrigan, principal author of a study funded in part by the National Institute of Environmental Health Sciences, said that "the collapse of the towers generated thousands of tons of particulate matter comprised of cement dust, glass fibers, asbestos, lead, aromatic hydrocarbons, and organochlorine compounds, many of which significantly increased the subjects' susceptibility to bronchial spasms and asthma." Landrigan also noted, "Our results indicate that the environmental exposures following the WTC disaster were associated with profound adverse effects on respiratory health." For example, over three hundred of the ten thousand firefighters who were exposed long-term to the particulates developed the chronic "World Trade Center cough."[10]

It took nearly a year to clean up the actual building site. The dust problem in the vicinity of ground zero took even longer to eradicate. Hundreds of workers were brought in from all over the country to clean up the dust that had crept into heating and cooling systems, carpets, and wall cavities in nearby buildings. The dust had also spread into underground garages in the area.

After the cleanup, the EPA did extensive testing and assured residents of lower Manhattan that the dust and smoke were at safe enough levels for the area to be reoccupied.[11] But a group of residents and workers disagreed and filed suit against the EPA for making "misleading statements about air quality" after 9/11.[12]

DEMOLITION AND RENOVATION PROJECTS

The destruction of the World Trade Center produced catastrophic amounts of dust, but even the dust generated by the ordinary demolition of buildings or the destruction of building materials indoors can have a negative impact on health.

Tearing down drywall and sawing, sanding, and grinding other building materials can produce large numbers of aerosolized particulates. If ceiling tiles are replaced, bits of the tile material can become aerosolized and then settle into carpeting and onto surfaces. If there is fiberglass in the dust, people may get rashes. During the construction phase of a renovation project, new walls or partitions are erected, new carpeting is installed, and walls are painted. Paint aerosol may be produced, and new carpeting and furnishings, caulks, adhesives, and paints may off-gas (see chapter 3).

My wife once had an appointment in a doctor's office in a large commercial complex that was being renovated. The space had been cut in two by a temporary wall so that patients could still enter without interrupting the renovation work. Workers had opened the windows to ventilate the work area while the walls were being painted; unfortunately, wind was blowing into the windows, increasing the air pressure within the workspace. Air containing paint fumes and construction dust flowed around gaps in the temporary wall into the patient waiting room, where the air pressure was lower. The fumes and dust were irritating for patients who came and went, but the receptionist had the greatest exposure and had a headache all day long. If the workers had put a window fan on exhaust and closed the other windows in the space undergoing renovation, the pressure in the work area would have been lower than the pressure in the occupied office area. Air would then have flowed from the office area to the work area, reducing or even eliminating the spread of contaminants.

It is essential during all phases of renovation to minimize the spread of irritants and contaminants from the work area into adjoining spaces, and to prevent the contamination of the HVAC (heating, ventilation, and air-conditioning) system with biodegradable dust. Registers and grilles in the HVAC system should be covered with filter material, and the highest level of filtration should be used at the fan coil while work is in progress. If possible, during very dusty operations the HVAC system should be shut off. If the system must be operated, steps should be taken to isolate the zones under construction from the rest of the space so that contaminants are not spread to other zones.

The work area should be completely contained (isolated from the rest of the building) and the air pressure reduced (the air pressure in the work area should be less than the air pressure in adjacent areas). Workers should come and go through areas that are also isolated, so that dust and debris on their clothing will not spread to occupied spaces of the building. And occupants should not have to walk through the work area to reach their offices or classrooms.

If you work or live in a building in which renovation work is being undertaken, the risk is minimal if the correct procedures are followed and the utmost precaution taken.

SOME PRACTICAL STEPS

- If smoking is allowed in a building, it should be confined to an isolated space that is ventilated to the exterior.
- In a building with operable windows, carpets can be HEPA-vacuumed more frequently than usual during the height of the pollen season.
- During renovation, a work area should be isolated to prevent the spread of vapors and particulates. Highly sensitized individuals may have to relocate temporarily.

- *IAQ Guidelines for Occupied Buildings under Construction* is an excellent resource for the type of planning and control that should be exercised during renovation work in occupied buildings (see the Resource Guide).
- A mask with a NIOSH rating of N95 can filter out airborne particulates. If wearing a NIOSH N95 mask is not an option, you can purchase a portable HEPA air purifier with a gooseneck discharge so that you can direct the flow of purified air toward your breathing zone (see the Resource Guide).

CHAPTER

7

Menace in the Mechanicals

One memorable hot summer evening, my extended family and I took my seventy-five-year-old aunt to dinner at a Chinese restaurant. There were eight of us, and our reserved table was in a corner where there was not much air circulating. By the time the drinks were served, my aunt was feeling hot and asked if we could be reseated. The waiters set up another large round table in the middle of the restaurant and moved the beer, wine, and water glasses. Soon after we resettled at the new table, my aunt complained of feeling chilly and pointed to a ceiling air-conditioning diffuser (register) that was blasting her with "arctic" air. She wanted to switch tables again, but the rest of us were too embarrassed to ask. After a few minutes she draped a heavy cloth napkin over her head to try to keep warm.

My brother offered to switch seats with her. As he rose from his chair, he pushed against the table. Unfortunately, a set of collapsible legs at the opposite side of the table had not been set properly, and that end of the table started sinking. All the drinks tipped over. Frothing liquids ran down the sloped surface of the table, flowed over the laps of those unfortunate enough to be sitting at the lower end, and dripped onto the floor. After we stopped gasping, we could see that all the conversation in the restaurant had stopped and every head was turned toward us. My horrified teenaged son dropped his head to the table and hid under his arms.

This incident would not have happened if my aunt hadn't first been too hot and then too cold. When the mechanical system in a building keeps us comfortable, we take the conditions of the indoor environment for granted. If not properly designed or maintained, however, any mechanical system can create thermal, environmental, or air quality problems. How does a building's mechanical system operate? If you are concerned about air quality, it's important for you to know.

WHAT DOES IT DO?

The purpose of the mechanical system is to keep the temperature and the relative humidity comfortable and, in buildings without operable windows, to remove stale air from and introduce fresh air into the building envelope—in other words, to ventilate the building. For most of us, the only "communication" we have with a mechanical system in the building where we live or work is through the thermostat. At the other end of the wires or tubes leading from a thermostat is a complex system that is supposed to provide us with the comfort we need.

On dry days when the outdoor temperature is mild, a heating, ventilation, and air-conditioning (HVAC) system can just draw outdoor air into the building and circulate both this air and the indoor air, sometimes without any change other than filtration. More often, though, this mixture of indoor and outdoor air must be cooled or heated. On a cold day, a building is similar to a hot oven in a kitchen. In both, energy is supplied to heat the air within and to replace the heat that is lost to the surroundings. If you are baking a cake at 350°F, you set the thermostat for that temperature, and the oven remains on until that set point (350°F) is achieved. Because the air in the oven is much hotter than the kitchen air, heat flows into the room from the inside of the oven (heat moves spontaneously only from higher temperatures to lower temperatures). As the oven cools, the thermostat within senses the temperature drop and turns the gas or electricity back on to raise the temperature. Similarly, components of the mechanical system in a building will turn on and off (cycle) to maintain the set points in the spaces within the building envelope.

FORCED HOT-WATER AND STEAM HEAT SYSTEMS

Many offices, classrooms, and homes contain hot-water or steam radiators or hot-water convectors—all *heat emitters.* (Steam and hot-water heating systems operate with *boilers,* which heat water; *furnaces* heat air.) Convectors are

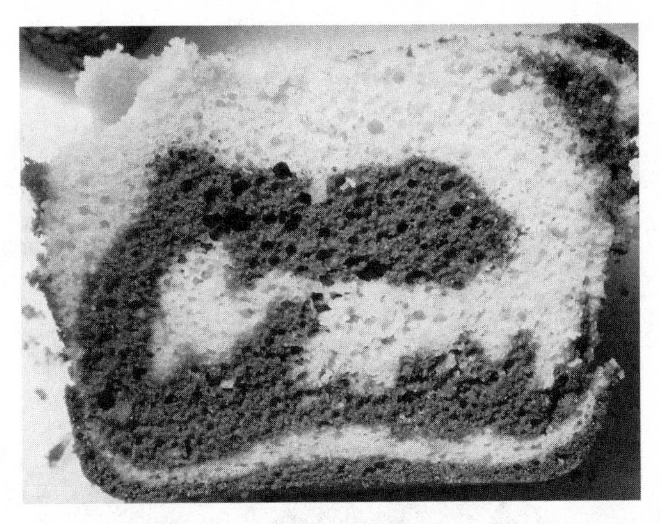

FIGURE 7.1. Marble cake. In making this cake, about half an inch of chocolate batter was placed in the bottom of a greased glass pan. White batter was then carefully layered on top and covered with another, quarter-inch layer of chocolate batter. The layers were not mixed prior to baking. In the oven, the chocolate batter at the bottom was warmed first, became less dense than the batter above, and rose, moving in a circular pattern. Thus the movement of heat and matter by convection caused the marbling in the cake. *Jeffrey C. May*

usually located along the bottom of the wall, hence the name *baseboard convector.*

In the simplest kind of system, either hot water or hot water vapor flows through pipes and heats the metal emitter. Air that is close to the hot surface is heated, becomes less dense, and floats upward. Cooler air at the bottom of the radiator or convector then moves upward to replace the air that floated out, and that air in turn is heated and rises. On an *exterior wall* (a wall facing the exterior), heated air cools as it comes into contact with the colder surfaces of the upper walls, and then the air sinks toward the floor. This circular pattern of airflow—the movement imparted by differences in density generated by the heat transfer—is called a *convection cycle.* Assuming that no windows or doors are open and that the emitter remains on, mixing due to convection raises the temperature of all the air within the room.

Heat can also move by *conduction*, a process by which heat is transferred through solids or fluids by collisions among particles of matter such as atoms

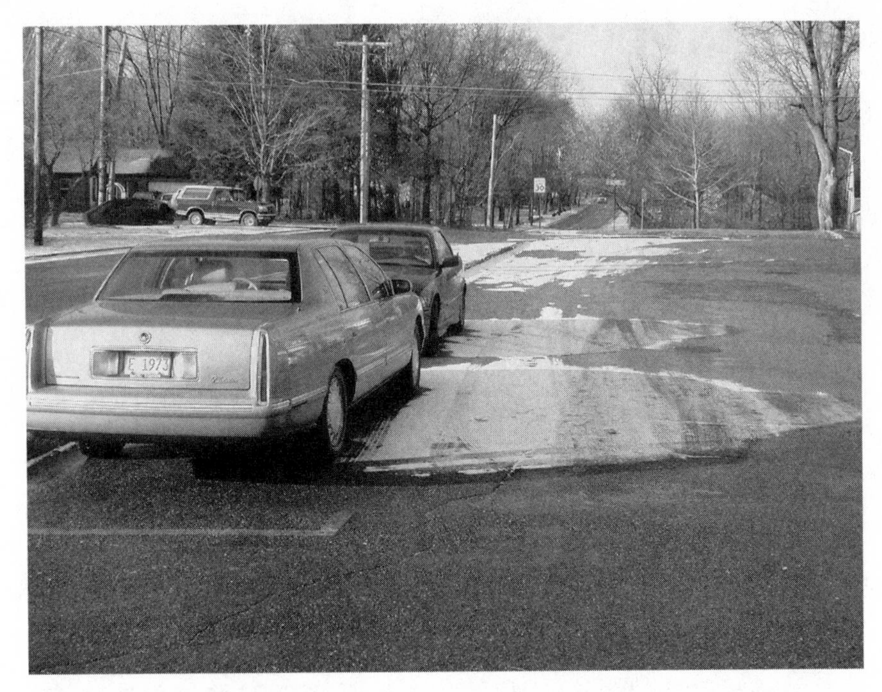

FIGURE 7.2. Cold car shadows. In the early morning, light snow fell on the asphalt in this parking lot. The rising sun cast long shadows. Radiant heat from the sun melted the snow, except where the cars' shadows fell on the ground, blocking the sunlight. *Jeffrey C. May*

and molecules. If you stir boiling water with a metal spoon, heat moves by conduction from the higher temperature (the water) to the lower temperature (the spoon). To avoid burning your hand, you should use a wooden rather than a metal spoon to stir hot liquids, because metal conducts heat much faster than wood does. In a hot-water or steam system, heat from the fluid within the pipes is transferred by conduction to the metal of the pipes. The

> One type of steam heating system, called a *vacuum system,* contains only water vapor and no air. Another type of steam heating system, called an *atmospheric pressure system,* when it is not operating contains air and water vapor, much of which condenses to liquid as the pipes cool. When the atmospheric pressure system is operating, however, the pipes are full of hot water vapor rather than air or the aerosolized droplets of liquid that most people call *steam.* Nonetheless, the hot water vapor in the pipes of a heating system and the mist that forms above a pot of boiling water are both referred to as steam.

In a microwave oven, microwave radiation (which is lower in energy than either light or heat) makes some water molecules spin faster than others. If a slow-moving water molecule collides with a more rapidly spinning water molecule, both molecules bounce away from the collision, now moving at much higher speeds and thus increasing in temperature. (Remember that temperature is a measure of how fast molecules are moving, so greater speeds mean higher temperatures.) Dry foods don't heat up very well in a microwave oven, because they lack the water molecules required for the process to work.

air trapped between the fins in a baseboard convector is heated by conduction (collision with the surface area of the fins), expands, becomes less dense, and then rises because of its increased buoyancy.

Piping in a steam or hot-water system also radiates heat out, hence the name *radiator.* In *radiation,* heat is lost (radiated) in the form of infrared energy. Convection requires the presence of a fluid, and conduction requires the presence of a fluid or solid, because convection and conduction can only take place when particles of matter move or vibrate. Heat radiation does not require the presence of a solid, liquid, or gas, because radiation is a form of energy that travels in waves through either matter or a vacuum. (The energy from our sun travels by radiation through 93 million miles of space vacuum to reach the Earth.) When heat in the form of radiation travels through matter, however, the energy in the waves causes the particles of matter to vibrate, and the matter heats up.

In radiant heating systems, piping that carries hot water is usually placed in the floor. The heat travels by conduction from the pipes into the floor material (usually concrete). The floor material, warmer than the air and the surrounding walls and ceiling, radiates heat to the other surfaces. They in turn absorb the heat and warm up. Air that comes into contact with the warm floor will be heated by conduction and convection, but most of the heat loss from the floor occurs through radiation. Radiant systems provide a very even and comfortable heat, because instead of one or two heat emitters warming a room, the entire floor surface emits heat.

PROBLEMS WITH HOT-WATER AND STEAM SYSTEMS

Room air containing particulates flows around or through the emitting components of a hot-water or steam system. As these particles collide with the components, some particles stick to the surfaces and accumulate over time. This dirt or dust usually contains biodegradable material; baseboard convectors can also accumulate pet dander if dogs, cats, or birds have spent time in the space. If the relative humidity is high enough (over 75 percent), mold may grow in the dust, and in the winter allergens can be released into the convective airflows. *Any type of heat emitter should therefore be kept free of dust.*

In older buildings with big cast-iron radiators, heat distribution can be uneven. When convection drives airflows in a room, heat tends to stratify, so that air near the ceiling is hot and air near the floor is cool, or one area of the room may be too hot and another area too cold. One room may have too large a radiator and be hot, while another room may have too small a radiator and be cool. And in many steam boilers the water is treated with chemicals to prevent excessive scaling (rusting) of the interior. These chemicals can be present in the steam and can occasionally enter the building air through air vents on radiators (or via a steam humidification system, if present; I discuss such systems later in this chapter), causing odors or irritation.

Any system containing water is prone to leakage. Wherever there are leaks, mold and bacteria can grow. I investigated an odor problem in the office of a senior editor of a newspaper. He claimed that there was a musty smell in the room, but everyone except his wife thought he was addled. The office was heated by hot-water convectors fed from vertical supply pipes in a corner chase (a walled shaft). I opened the small access door to the chase, which had been stuck shut for years, and found water dripping from a leaky valve. The water had soaked into the concrete and moved by capillary action into the carpet in a corner of the office, and mold was growing in the carpet dust.

AIR-CONVEYANCE SYSTEMS

Rather than having radiators or baseboard convectors in individual rooms, many buildings have air-conveyance systems in which air is drawn into a mechanical system (at a *return*), heated or cooled in a nearby or remote location, and then sent back to the room (at a *supply*). The warmed or cooled air travels through ductwork and enters the room through ceiling diffusers (or, in many residential buildings, through floor diffusers). Dampers, usually consisting of a set of movable louvers that can be opened, closed, or left in some position in between, may regulate the flow of the conditioned (heated or cooled) air. In modern mechanical systems, the louvers are controlled by a series of mechanical links or levers that in turn are moved either by pneumatic pistons (controlled by air pressure) or by electric motors.

The Furnace

In smaller office buildings the furnace may be in the basement, in which case the combustion gases must be vented from the furnace through a chimney or vent pipe to the outside of the building envelope. Some low-rise (one- to three-story) commercial and residential buildings may even have several furnaces on the roof (each called a rooftop unit, or RTU); these units are vented directly into the outside air. (Most RTUs contain a furnace for heating and air-conditioning equipment to supply cooling.) In some larger apartment or residential buildings each residential unit has its own furnace located in a mechanical closet accessible from an outside balcony, and each furnace vents directly to the exterior through a grille in the closet wall.

Fan Coils and Heat Pumps

Some bigger buildings have *fan coils,* each of which contains a blower (fan), a filter, and one or two coils (fluid-filled convectors). Other buildings have *heat pumps,* each of which contains a blower, a filter, a coil, and a compressor with a second coil (fan coils do not have compressors). In other words, a fan coil is not a heat pump, but a heat pump contains a fan coil (the blower, the filter, the coil). Heat pumps and fan coils provide heat and cooling, depending on the season.

Fan coils are usually located in the ceiling plenum (see chapter 3), though one kind of fan coil, called a *unit ventilator* or *univent,* sits against the inside of the exterior wall. (Univents are common in schools, and I discuss them in chapter 8.) In most nonresidential buildings with heat pumps, the coils and compressors are combined in a single unit, also suspended in the plenum. In a residential building, a heat pump (or a split air-conditioning system, if the

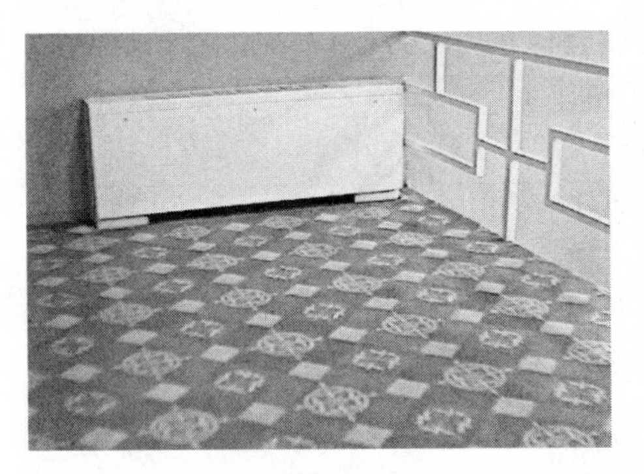

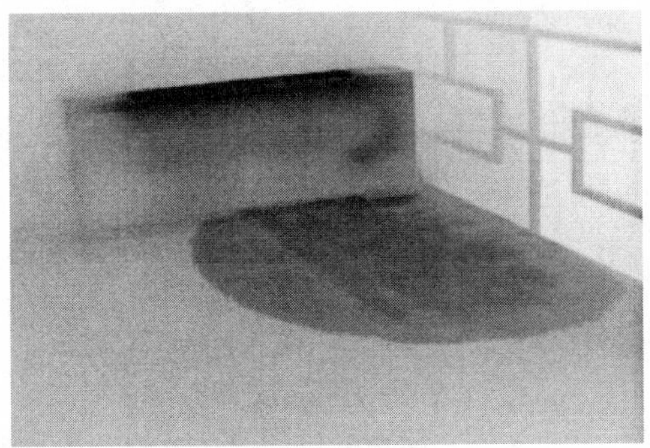

FIGURE 7.3. A leaking fan coil. A musty smell was noted in the vicinity of this fan coil. An investigator with an infrared camera was hired to locate the source of the odor. The photograph on the left was taken using visible light; the photograph on the right was taken with the infrared camera, which records temperature differences of surfaces. A darker color indicates a lower temperature. The area where the carpet was damp as the result of a leak from the fan coil was cooler than the dry area of the carpet, because water was evaporating (evaporation results in a reduction of surface temperature). Mold was growing on the dust in the dampened carpet. *Lew Harriman, moistureDM.com*

system only supplies cool air) consists of an indoor unit with one coil and an outdoor unit with the compressor and the second coil.

The coils in fan coils and heat pumps are called *heat exchangers,* because they either impart heat to the air in the heating season or remove heat from the air in the cooling season. In a fan coil that is cooling air, the heat is transferred to water that is circulated to a *chiller* (a large heat exchanger with a compressor) located in the basement or on the roof. The chiller removes the heat and transfers it to another "loop" of water where it is pumped to a *cooling tower.* Cooling towers are also used to dissipate the heat removed by heat pumps.

Cooling towers (not necessarily tall!) are located outside the building envelope, either on the roof or in an adjacent space at grade such as a parking area. A cooling tower gets rid of heat energy that has been removed from the inside of the building by spraying the warm water over an assembly, such as a series of louvers with a large surface area. A fan at the top of the cooling tower draws large volumes of air over the warm water, some of which then evaporates. The fan blows this warm moist air away and up into the atmosphere. Often the vapor condenses as it cools, creating clouds in the air that appear to be smoke. The remaining water on the assembly collects in a basin, where it is strained before being returned to the chiller.

Some large buildings contain so many heat-generating pieces of computer and other electronic equipment that air conditioning is required, even in the winter, so the "clouds" above a cooling tower can occur in any season. (Cooling towers are ugly; because of the large fans they contain, they are also noisy, as many of you have no doubt noticed.)

The Fatal Cooling Tower

In 1976 the fifty-eighth annual convention of the Philadelphia Chapter of the American Legion was held at the city's Bellevue-Stratford Hotel. One hundred and eighty-two of the attendees developed pneumonia; some fell ill while they were at the hotel, and others became sick after returning home. Ultimately, twenty-nine people who had been at the convention died.

The CDC in Atlanta discovered the culprit: bacteria, subsequently named *Legionella pneumophila,* growing in the water in the cooling tower. Clouds of water droplets containing the bacteria were blown around as air moved through the towers. Some of the droplets entered the hotel, and others were circulated at the exterior near the hotel.

One of the first recognized outbreaks of building-related illness, Legionnaires' disease brought about a shift in people's thinking. We know that people can disseminate pathogens, but this was the first time we realized that a component of an air-conditioning system can also spread a deadly disease. The water in most cooling towers is now treated and tested for *Legionella* bacteria.

The Ducts

Buildings may contain hundreds and hundreds of feet of ductwork, supplying warm or cool air to inside spaces and returning air to the coils.

Ducts come in a variety of sizes and shapes. Some are 6 inches in diameter; others are 6 feet in diameter. Some are round, others rectangular. Ducts are made of different materials. Some ducts, made of a material called *duct board,* have a thin aluminum foil exterior and consist of either rigid fiberglass cylinders or fiberglass boards about an inch thick. (Duct board can be folded into rectangular shapes.) Other ducts, called *flexible ducts,* are made of plastic on the inside and outside, with fiberglass sandwiched in between and a stiff metal spiral (like a stretched-out spring) embedded in the inner plastic layer to give the ducts shape.

I think the best kind of ductwork is metal, because metal ducts retain their shape and are more easily cleaned than other kinds of ducts (I discuss duct cleaning later in this chapter). But metal ducts can be noisy, because the hard metal interior surfaces reflect the sounds of the blower and the air movement through the ducts. Most metal ducts are therefore lined on the inside with fiberglass insulation (which if uncoated and damaged can represent a source of airborne fiberglass fibers) or with synthetic foam, or wrapped on the outside with fiberglass insulation.

Insulation prevents the ducts from losing or gaining heat, thus decreasing energy usage and cost by increasing the efficiency of the system. Whenever air flows through a metal duct, the duct surface will eventually reach the same temperature as the air within. If the outside metal surface of the duct is warm (during the heating season), heat will be lost to the plenum. If the outside metal surface of the duct is cool (during the cooling system), the duct will absorb heat from the air around it. If the outside of the duct remains cool enough, water may even condense on the metal surface and drip onto the backside of the ceiling below, which can sometimes lead to microbial growth.

A British architect faced manslaughter charges because she canceled a maintenance contract for the air-conditioning system at an arts complex and then negotiated a new contract, one that did not include measures to clean the water in the rooftop cooling towers. For two months, air contaminated with *Legionella* bacteria sprayed into a busy alleyway between a market and a bus stop, and then spread on prevailing winds toward the town center. Over 170 people became infected with Legionnaires' disease, and 7 of them died.[1]

1. N. Bunyan, "Council Architect Denies Legion Deaths," *Telegraph,* 26 February 2005, www.telegraph-co.uk.

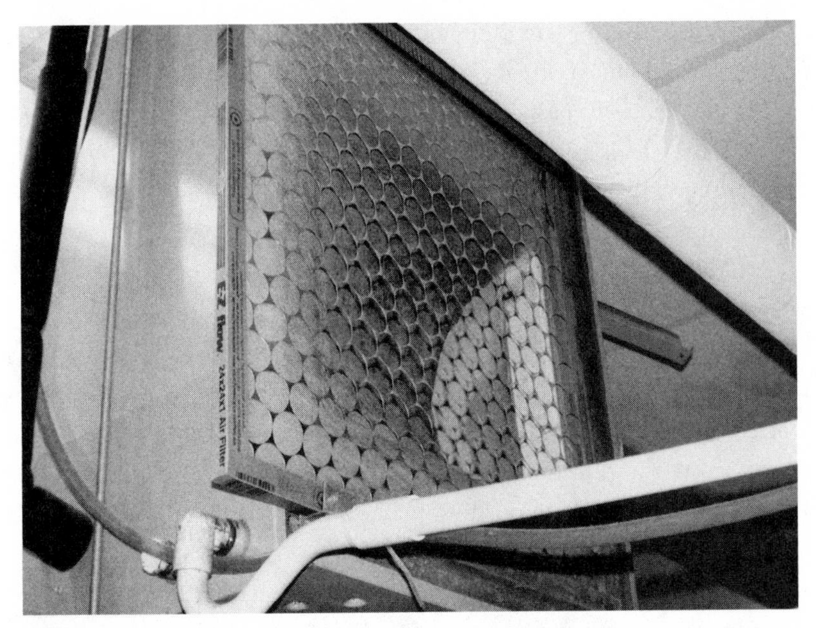

FIGURE 7.4. Clogged, damaged air-conditioning filter. The filter on this ceiling-mounted AC unit had not been changed for a very long time. The filter was so clogged and soiled that air couldn't pass through it. Thus the airflow forced the right side of the filter backward, out of its frame (at the lighter, U-shaped area) and into the unit, leaving a gap in the filter. *May Indoor Air Investigations LLC*

The Ceiling Plenum as a Return

In larger office buildings it is common for supply ductwork to be located in the ceiling plenum. Sometimes return ducts are present, but in general the space within the ceiling plenum itself is used as the return path back to a fan coil or heat pump suspended in the plenum, or back to a furnace in a mechanical closet that is open to the plenum. This air comes from the rooms below the drop ceiling, either through ceiling openings (one or more ceiling tiles replaced by plastic grilles) or through narrow gaps at the perimeter of fluorescent light fixtures designed to act as returns.

Filtration

Any mechanical equipment that has a blower and that moves indoor air must have filtration. Many people think that filtration cleans the room air—

and it *can* clean the air—but from an indoor air quality perspective, *the critical function of filtration is to trap biodegradable particulates that might otherwise build up on components of the air-conveyance system: blower, cooling or heating coil, ducts, and condensate pan* (the pan that holds water that has condensed on the cooling coil). Fan coils, heat pumps, and unit ventilators must all have adequate filtration to prevent soiling of the coil.

Why is cleanliness essential? A layer of dust on an air-conditioning coil can be dampened by condensed moisture. Some of the dust may also accumulate in the condensate pan and block the drain. If the drain overflows, water will soak into the soiled fiberglass lining material. Sometimes the water leaks out of the condensate pan and drips onto a floor or onto ceiling tiles. This entire progression can lead to the proliferation of mold, yeast, and bacteria in the condensate pan as well as on dust in the system or on adjacent surfaces. (When a contaminated air-conditioning system is first turned on, the air can have a sweat-sock odor, signaling the growth of bacteria and/or yeast, or a musty odor, signaling the presence of mold.) The purpose of filtration is to prevent this progression from occurring.

The filtration in most of the mechanical systems I have seen is inadequate, such as the flimsy, paper-framed, coarse blue, yellow, or green filters installed on home furnaces and often used in smaller offices, schools, commercial buildings, and rooftop units in midsized buildings. Some buildings have costly electronic filters. Larger buildings generally have pleated (accordion-like) filters or bag filters (so called because they look like cloth bags), which are usually more efficient than electronic filters. I think pleated media filters are ideal, because they trap nearly all of the biodegradable matter that can enter the mechanical system with airflows, and they can be easily replaced when soiled.

Until recently there were three different systems used to rate the efficiency of a filter. Because each of these was based on different criteria, the same coarse fiberglass filter could be described as having either 80 percent, 40 percent, or zero percent efficiency. There is now a more reliable fourth rating system called MERV (minimum efficiency reporting value). In my opinion, no mechanical system should be operated with a filter rated less than MERV 6 or 8 (MERV 12 is even better). (ASHRAE Standard 62, "Ventilation for Acceptable Indoor Air Quality," now recommends that new AC installations in commercial buildings have a minimum of MERV 6 filtration.) Unfortunately, even in systems

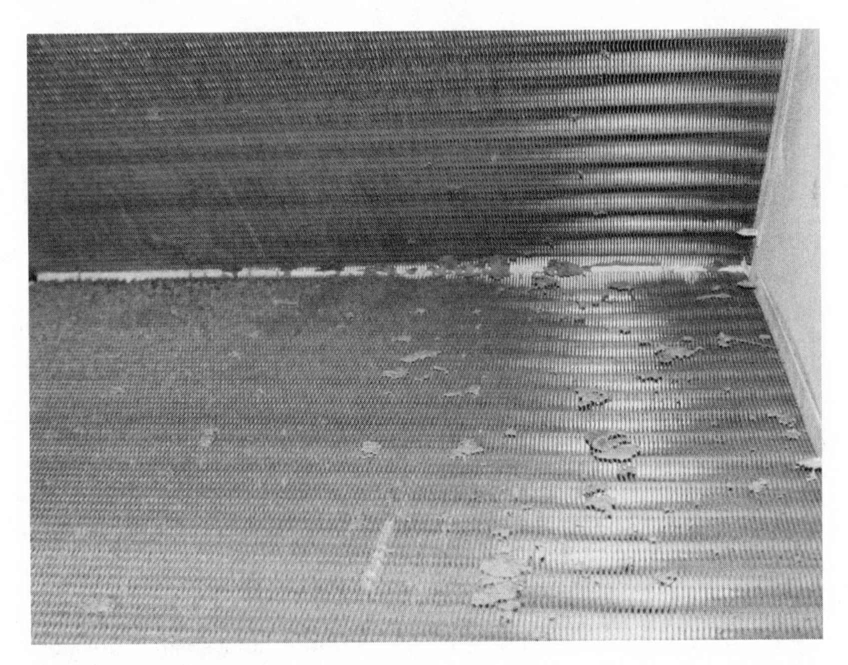

FIGURE 7.5. Clumps of dust on an air-conditioning coil. Because of the gap in the filter (see figure 7.4), unfiltered air flowed over the AC coil. Dust accumulated on the coil, and mold grew in the damp dust. *May Indoor Air Investigations LLC*

that have adequate filtration, the filters usually aren't changed frequently enough. And sometimes an improperly sized filter is installed, allowing air to bypass the filter and dust to soil the coil, or the slot that holds the filter is open to the air so that even if the filter is the proper size, unfiltered air can still enter the system through the gaps. In other words, a filter has to be efficient and of the proper size, and it must be placed in a secure holder that does not allow any air to flow from the mechanical room around the filter through gaps.

Dehumidification

Ironically, air conditioning reduces the amount of moisture in the room air but creates cooler air with higher relative humidity within the supply side of the mechanical system. If the air reaches its dew point (see chapter 4), moisture will condense on the system's coil and drip into the condensate pan below the coil. If the speed of the air moving across the coil is too great, some of the water may be caught up into the airflow and carried onto the surfaces immediately downwind from the coil, saturating the material lining the ducts and leading to microbial growth.

Many HVAC technicians swear by the capacity of air conditioners to dehumidify air, but unfortunately most AC systems are only operated by a thermostat, which controls temperature alone and *not* relative humidity (RH). If the temperature is 75°F and the RH 60 percent, then the inside air would be much more comfortable than if the temperature were 75°F and the RH 75 percent. There is no way to reduce the RH with a thermostat alone, so the temperature has to be lowered. Ordinarily, when the temperature of air is lowered and the amount of moisture in the air remains the same, the RH rises. In this case, however, the air conditioner removes more moisture from the air as the air is cooled further.

With a modified AC system containing a separate component for dehumidification, and with the addition of a dehumidistat, the equipment could continue to remove moisture without having to lower the room temperature. In the end, this would not only create drier conditions but also allow for higher air temperatures, which would save energy.

Air conditioning has become a necessity in modern office buildings. Years ago, cooling equipment contained electric heating coils to warm the saturated, cold air coming off the evaporator coil. The air's RH was lowered, thus reducing the potential for microbial growth in dust within the supply ducts. During the energy crisis of the 1970s, however, regulators thought that heating coils were a waste of energy, so engineers eliminated the coils. After all, why cool air and then expend energy to warm it?

Humidification

In New England, where I live, exterior winter air can be cold yet still have a high relative humidity, sometimes even 100 percent. That same air, when heated inside a building envelope, has a vastly increased capacity to hold water vapor, and thus its RH will decrease as long as the air's vapor content remains the same. This is why heated inside air in a cold climate can feel uncomfortably dry, particularly in a leaky building. In a building that is more airtight, moisture from human activities can be kept within the envelope and the vapor content can rise within.

In some buildings moisture is added by the mechanical system, sometimes in the form of steam blowing into the airflow. The steam can come from a separate steam-generating unit or directly from a steam boiler to which chemicals may have been added to reduce rusting within the system. These organic chemicals, called *amines*, contain nitrogen, and they can have a fishy smell and can irritate mucous membranes (see chapter 5). The steam in a humidification system should not come from a boiler treated with volatile chemicals; any water used for humidification purposes should be of drinking quality. In another type of humidification system, a metal mesh pad is placed in the airstream, and water trickles down the mesh and evaporates into the airflow. As long as there are no puddles of warm water that can sustain microbial growth, this type of humidification system is safe if properly maintained.

Regardless of the humidification system used, if the relative humidity within the mechanical system is excessive (over 75 percent), microbial growth can occur in any biodegradable dust present, whether there is condensation or not.

OTHER PROBLEMS WITH AIR-CONVEYANCE SYSTEMS

Drafts and Drips

Whenever a blower or fan operates, the air pressure is higher on the downstream (supply) side than on the upstream (return) side, because air is being removed from the return and pushed into the supply ducts. The air pressure inside the supply ducts is higher than the air pressure outside the supply ducts, and the air pressure inside the return is lower than the air pressure outside the return. Air moves from conditions of higher pressure to conditions of lower pressure, so if there are openings in the ducts, air leaks out of the supply system into the surrounding space, leading to loss of heating and cooling efficiency. Air can also leak into the return system from the surrounding space, creating the potential for spread of airborne contaminants.

If the blower is located in an uninhabited space such as a basement, a mechanical room above a loading dock, or a dusty attic, contaminants from these areas can enter the return system through openings in the ducts or around the filter enclosure, if it's leaky. And more often than not, the filtration is not adequate to prevent the particulates from reaching the supply ducts. Even the best particle filter will not stop gases (such as combustion products from idling diesel engines at a loading dock, which I discuss later in this chapter) from entering the supply ducts once the contaminants are in the return airflows. Any system that has a blower can also distribute odors, which are gases and vapors. In one office where the ceiling plenum was used as a return, there was an entire ceiling tile missing in the bathroom; thus most of the return airflow came from the men's room, creating some embarrassing moments.

If an outside wall communicates with (is open to) a return plenum, exterior air can leak into the wall cavity through construction gaps and around the frames of windows and doors. If this exterior air is humid and enters the cooler wall cavities in an air-conditioned building, moisture can condense on cooler building components (if they are at or below the dew point), including cold metal studs as well as pipes carrying cold water. Condensation can lead to microbial growth—one reason why larger buildings should be positively pressurized overall and the ceiling return plenum should be completely isolated from the cavities of the exterior wall (i.e., the drywall at exterior walls should extend up into the plenum to the underside of the floor above). Any time there is a leak from a cold-water pipe above a drywall or drop ceiling, mold can grow on both the top side of the ceiling (the side facing the floor structure above) and the bottom side of the ceiling (the side facing the room below).

When mold grows on the top side of the ceiling and the plenum is used as a return for the HVAC system, spores or musty odors can be disseminated. And sometimes service technicians will stand on a ladder and move a ceiling panel in a drop ceiling in order to work on phone or communication cables in the plenum; if the tiles are moldy, a large number of spores can become airborne this way.

Miscommunication

Sometimes wall partitions are shifted when new tenants move into an office or commercial space. When this happens, people don't necessarily pay attention to the relationships established between the supply and return ducts. In one building I investigated, a second smaller office had been carved out of a much larger space. Originally the large space had its own supply and return system, with the fan coil located in the ceiling plenum. Under the new arrangement, the two offices (one small, one larger) shared the system, so air for the smaller office still came from the larger office. Three women who didn't smoke worked in the smaller office, and a cigar smoker occupied the larger office. The women were constantly bothered by the smell of cigar smoke, because airflows carried this contaminant from the larger space into the smaller space.

Toasty or Frosty

In bigger buildings, the heating and cooling of spaces is usually divided into *zones:* one or more rooms heated or cooled by the same plenum-mounted fan coil or heat pump, controlled by a single thermostat. The location of a thermostat in a zone can affect thermal comfort. If hot or cool supply air is blowing directly onto the thermostat, it will reach its set point too soon, leaving the rest of the spaces in the zone either too hot or too cool. If an occupant in one of the rooms installs a copier or a second computer or printer, the operation of the new equipment can warm that room, and the occupant might then lower the thermostat. People in other rooms in the zone may then feel cool. In many buildings, the thermostat is covered by a locked box so that no one other than the maintenance personnel supposedly has access. Of course, the box must have openings to let air in so the thermostat can measure the temperature of that air. Many employees learn to make their own adjustments to the thermostat by fashioning widgets that can be inserted into those holes.

There are other reasons why a zone may seem too hot or too cool. Thermostats can malfunction or require recalibrating because the set points are either greater than or less than the room temperature actually achieved by that setting. Soiling and corrosion can impede the movement of mechanically operated louvers and dampers, and an overloaded filter or clogged coil can restrict airflow. Too much air coming out of a supply can make people who work near or in the path of the air feel too hot or too cool, depending on the season. Finally, thermostats may have to be moved when partition walls are moved, supply diffusers are relocated, or office equipment is purchased.

Bigger Is Not Always Better

Builders and air-conditioning designers or installers are often worried that an AC system will not have the capacity to cool a building on the hottest days. To avoid complaints, they install an AC system that has more cooling capacity than is most of the time needed. As a result, the air is cooled very quickly, and the spaces within the building rapidly reach the set point. Not enough moisture is removed from the air, and the relative humidity is undesirably high.

If the blower speed is lowered, the air will move more slowly over the cooling coils. The air will still be cooled to a lower temperature, but more airborne moisture will be removed, ultimately resulting in a lower relative humidity at the set point temperature in the cooled space. In addition, since there is less movement of cold air, the compressor doesn't turn on and off as frequently and has a longer run time, saving wear and tear on the equipment. But there is a limit as to how much the airflow can be reduced, because airflow warms the coil. If a coil stays too cold, the condensed water may freeze, and if enough ice builds up, the airflow through the coil will be blocked completely.

The Moldy Mansion

In 2000 the Governor's Mansion in South Carolina was renovated at a cost of approximately $5.6 million. In January 2003 the new governor moved in. In August he and his family returned from vacation to find mold growing on the clothing in their closets. Surfaces and clothing were cleaned, and steps were taken to reduce the relative humidity, but in June 2004 the governor and his family moved out after air testing revealed the presence of *Stachybotrys* mold. The First Lady declared that she had had a headache ever since moving into the house, and that her children had developed allergies and coughs.[1] Staff members who worked in the mansion also complained of chronic coughs, aches, and rashes.

Richard Bennett, the mold remediation specialist leading the cleanup efforts, said that the air-conditioning system had been left on while the building was being renovated, and sawdust and other construction debris contaminated the ducts and other components of the air-handling system. In addition, the AC system that was installed was too large for the space, and thus the system shut off before the air had been properly dehumidified, leading to conditions of high relative humidity conducive to microbial growth.

Bennett quoted an initial estimate of $400,000 for remediation efforts, which he thought might keep the governor and his family out of the mansion for three months.[2] Ultimately, the state spent more than $1.5 million on remediating the mansion and two other buildings in the complex. Most of the money was spent on improvements to the mechanical system.

VENTILATION

Modern buildings are fairly airtight, yet fresh air *must* be supplied to the interior and stale air exhausted to the exterior, either by the heating or cooling system itself, or by a separate ventilation system.

ASHRAE's Standard 62 recommends that fresh air be supplied at a rate of 20 cubic feet per minute per person in offices and 15 cfm/person in schools. Another way to express ventilation is in terms of the maximum difference in concentrations of carbon dioxide in indoor air versus outdoor air. The suggested maximum difference between CO_2 concentrations in office buildings and the CO_2 concentrations outdoors is about 500 ppm, corresponding to a delivery rate of fresh air of 20 cfm/person. Architects use these ASHRAE guidelines to design ventilation systems for buildings.

Smaller, single-story office or commercial buildings may have a passive ventilation system consisting of a vertical duct that extends from the ceiling plenum through the roof and is hooked over like an upside-down J at the top. The hot-air mechanical system in the building reduces the air pressure in the ceiling plenum (the return side of the system), and outside air is then drawn into the plenum from the ventilation duct, increasing the air pressure in the plenum and in the building. To balance the air pressure within the building envelope, the bathroom exhaust system is conveniently used to vent air out of the building. (A problem with this arrangement is that warm, moist air can enter a cold return plenum, leading to condensation.)

I once investigated a one-story retail building with this kind of ventilation system. I stood on a ladder, slid away one of the tiles in the drop ceiling, and peered into the plenum with my flashlight. The first thing I saw, directly in front of me, was the dried-up remains of a submarine sandwich. Who in the world, I wondered, could have eaten lunch in such a place? When I looked more closely, I could see that the bread appeared to have been pecked at. Then I noticed feathers scattered around the sandwich. I looked up at the bottom of the roof deck above and saw that the open end of the fresh-air duct was directly above the sandwich. I realized that a pigeon or sea gull must have settled down inside the open end of the vent at the roof to enjoy a sumptuous meal and then accidentally dropped the food down the duct. Usually a metal mesh covers the exterior open end of a ventilation duct like this, to keep birds from getting in. In this case the mesh was missing, and I guess there was one frustrated bird as a result.

A similar form of ventilation used in midsize buildings consists of a screened opening on the return side of a rooftop unit. Because the air pressure is greater on the outside of the building than in the return duct, exterior air is drawn through the opening into the return (with the flow controlled by a damper or louvers) and then distributed by the blower into the supply ducts and diffusers. Again, stale air is drawn out through the bathroom exhaust system. In this type of arrangement, the incoming fresh air is conditioned.

In larger buildings with plenum-mounted heat pumps or fan coils, fresh air is drawn in through a separate ventilation system, often located at the roof. The air is then distributed to each floor through branch ducts from a central, vertical duct. (This fresh air should be heated in the winter and dehumidified in the summer.) There is often a separate building exhaust system.

In this type of fresh-air distribution system, the branch duct may terminate in the ceiling plenum close to the center of the building, far from a remote fan coil or heat pump at the building's perimeter. The return airflow through the ceiling plenum is slow, so the fan coils or heat pumps near the end of a fresh-air duct receive the greatest amount of air. An office served by a fan coil or heat pump at the perimeter of the building, far from the central ventilation duct, receives very little fresh air. It is therefore a much better idea to provide each separate fan coil or heat pump unit with its own fresh air duct within about 10 feet of the return intake.

Ventilation is essential for providing and maintaining fresh air indoors, but it also serves another purpose: to positively pressurize the building interior. This pressurization prevents infiltration of unconditioned air and moisture from the outside environment. To keep the air pressure indoors slightly higher than the air pressure outdoors, more fresh air must be supplied than stale air exhausted.

PROBLEMS WITH VENTILATION

It's Suffocating

One kind of HVAC system, called *constant air volume,* supplies a constant flow of heated or cooled air and varies the air temperature according to the thermostat's demand. One advantage of this type of system is that fresh air can be continuously supplied. Another type of system, called *variable air volume,* supplies warm or cool air only when called for by the thermostat. If the thermostat is satisfied, there is no airflow and thus no supply of fresh air; this has led to air quality problems in buildings with variable air volume systems.

Sometimes HVAC equipment, including the fresh-air intake, is installed on a roof (a rooftop unit). Since most mechanical systems burn either oil or gas for energy, combustion products can be drawn into the building *(entrained)* if the fresh-air intakes are too close to the chimney or another combustion vent. Ventilation intakes located near kitchen and bathroom vents, as well as plumbing stacks, can draw in sewer gases and other odors. In college buildings or offices containing laboratory hoods that exhaust to the roof, intakes sometimes entrain dangerous chemicals.

When tar and gravel roofs are replaced or membrane roofs installed, asphalt fumes or the vapors from evaporating hydrocarbon solvents (see chapter 5) used for gluing the membrane or its seams can be drawn into the building. Water can pond on roofs with poor drainage, and mold, bacteria, and insects can flourish in the stagnant puddles. Odors and dried dust from this growth can enter the ventilation system through the roof intakes. In several buildings I have inspected, pigeons were nesting in the fresh-air intakes and rooftop heating and cooling units, and allergenic bioaerosol (feathers, fecal material, and mite allergens) spread through the ventilation systems. A number of serious respiratory illnesses can occur after exposure to dust containing high levels of bird droppings.

To ventilate a large building, a lot of air has to be taken in somewhere. Unfortunately, ventilation grilles are not very pretty and the airflows can be noisy, so architects are loath to put the intakes where they can be seen or heard. As a result, many ventilation grilles are located at the rear of a building near the loading docks, where they can draw in combustion products, including soot, from idling delivery trucks, most of which are diesel fueled.

Diesel engines produce more soot than gasoline engines do, and the soot can contain unburned fuel. Soot particulates are very small (from 0.01 to 0.12 micron) so they are respirable (see chapter 6). A press release from University of California Los Angeles noted that the number of ultrafine particulates downwind from a busy highway, on which about 25 percent of the traffic consisted of diesel-powered vehicles, was twenty-five to thirty times higher than the number of ultrafine particles upwind. At a distance of 330 feet from the roadway, the concentrations of particulates fell by 30 percent.[3]

One day while I was driving on a highway in light traffic on a clear day, I opened my windows so that the outdoor air could mix with the air in the car. As I drove, I measured the aerosolized particulates with a laser particle counter. The concentration of particles above 0.5 micron was about 500,000 per cubic foot of air (17.7/cm^3). Every time a truck or bus with a diesel engine drove by, the particle counts more than doubled to over a million per cubic foot. Coincidentally, for the first time in my life I noticed that I could detect a slight fuel odor after each diesel vehicle passed, and the instrument reading increased. I suspect that some unburned fuel remained on the soot, which is why I could smell diesel fuel in the exhaust. Diesel combustion products can affect those who are sensitized.

Stuck Open or Closed

In larger buildings, the amount of fresh air is controlled with sophisticated equipment. Sensors monitor temperature, pressure, and humidity differences, and louvers and dampers linked to pneumatic controls open and close to regulate the airflows. Sometimes dirt and rust accumulate, or the louvers and dampers are not properly maintained, and then they can become stuck in either an open or a closed position. If stuck shut, the introduction of fresh air into the building will be limited. If stuck open, more fresh air can be drawn in than is needed, leading to higher energy use because this air must be heated or cooled.

Ventilation is costly. In the summer, air that is hot and humid must be dehumidified. In the winter, air that is cold and dry must be heated and possibly humidified. During the energy crisis of the 1970s, one of the first cost-saving measures taken by many maintenance departments was to shut down the fresh-air intakes. As we saw in chapter 1, this occurred on the University of Massachusetts Boston campus and was in part responsible for the air quality crisis that developed there in 1994.

One very cold December I traveled to Washington, D.C., to give a presentation on indoor air quality. I stayed near the Capitol at a comfortable hotel constructed in a horseshoe shape. The "arms" of the horseshoe consisted of sixteen floors of rooms. Eight floors of meeting rooms, the restaurant, the lobby,

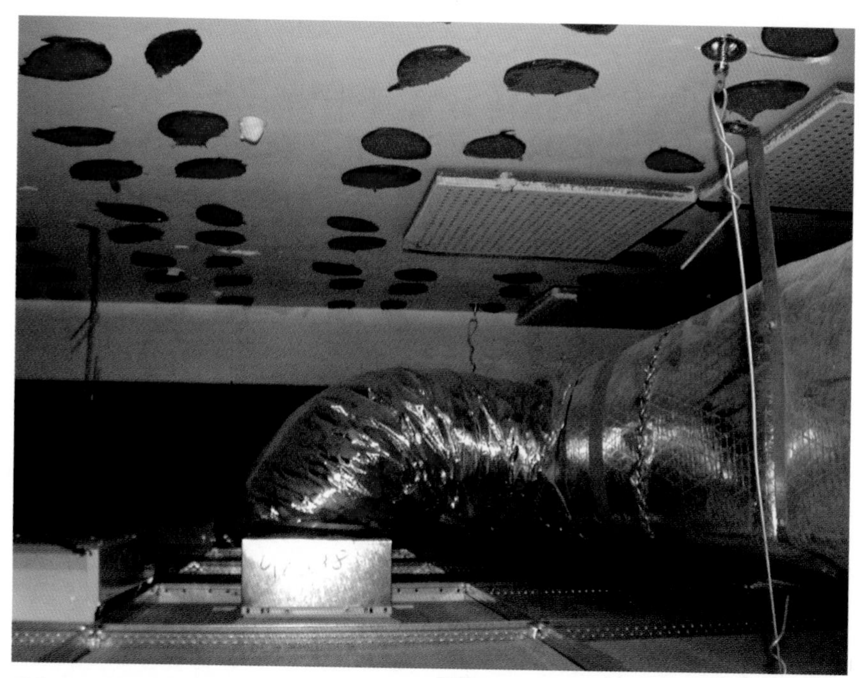

FIGURE 3.1. Inside a ceiling plenum in an older building. At the bottom of the photograph is a suspended ceiling. The wires at the right and left support the ceiling grid that holds the ceiling tiles. At the top of the photograph is the older, original plaster ceiling with oval flattened dollops of adhesive that once held acoustical tiles, two of which are still visible. At the center of the photograph is a supply duct. Immediately to the left is the top of a fluorescent light fixture (a metal box). This ceiling plenum tells a story: the original ceiling could have become damaged, so acoustical tiles were glued on. Those tiles probably became loose, and a suspended ceiling was installed. The space between the original ceiling and the suspended ceiling then served as a return for the mechanical system. *May Indoor Air Investigations LLC*

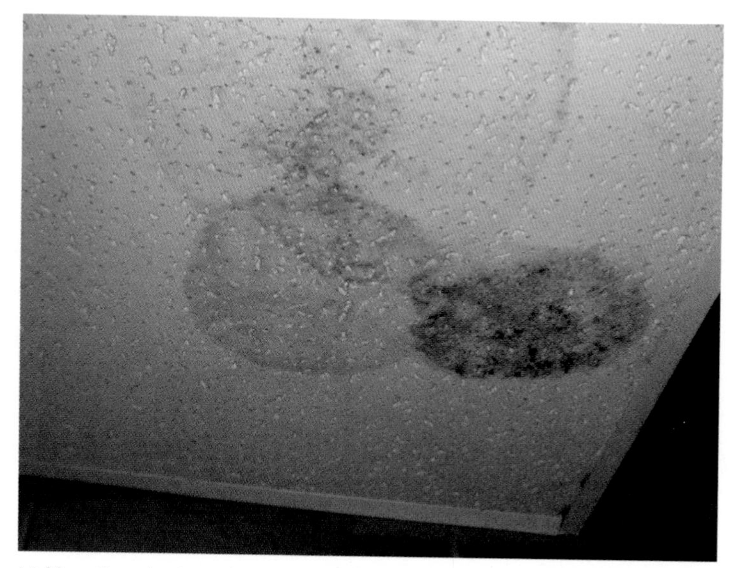

Moldy ceiling tile. Stained and moldy ceiling tiles like these are often ignored, but they can be a source of allergens. *May Indoor Air Investigations LLC*

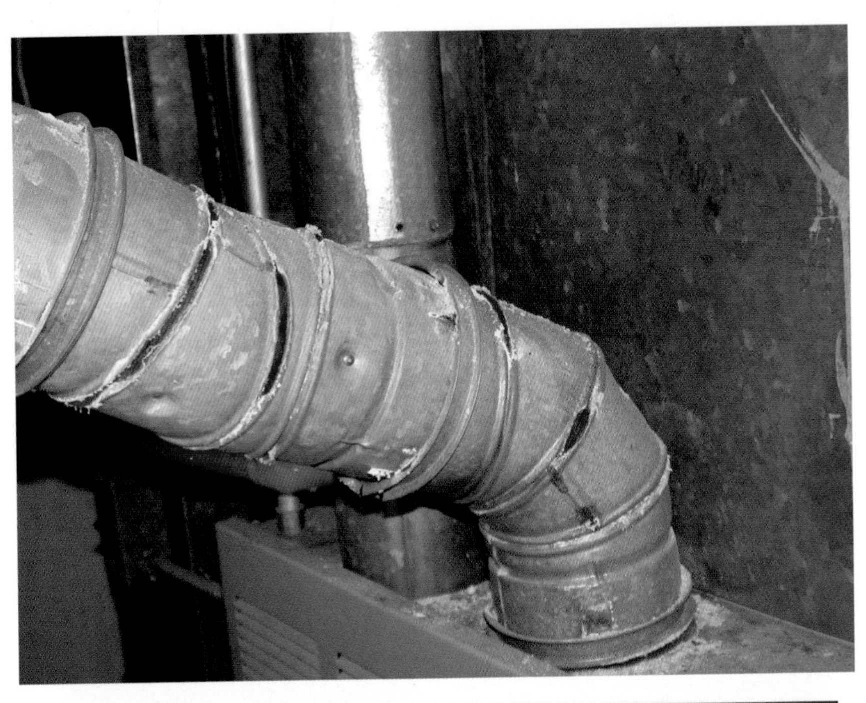

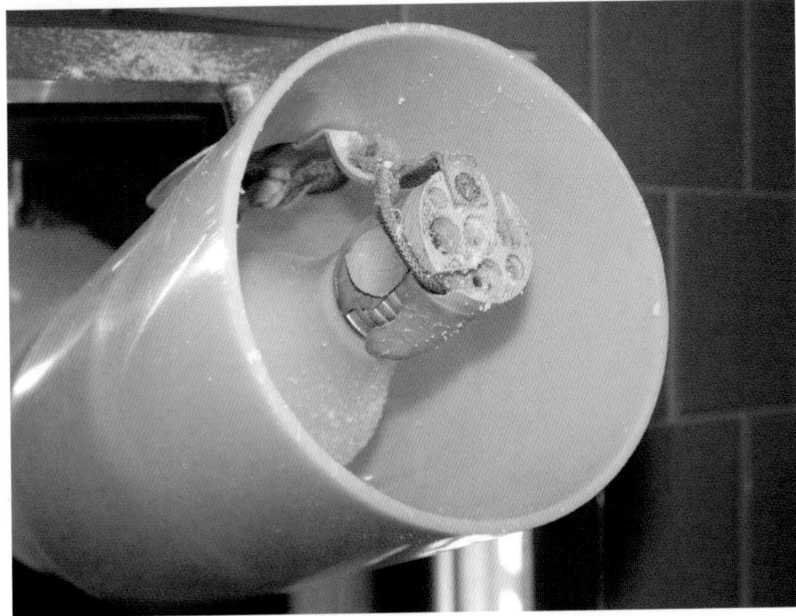

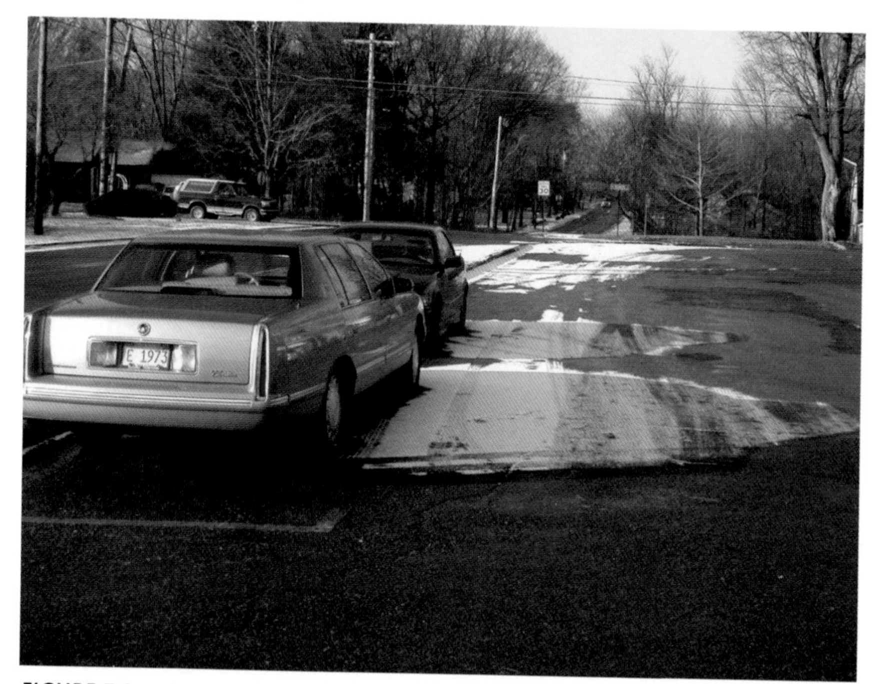

FIGURE 7.2. Cold car shadows. In the early morning, light snow fell on the asphalt in this parking lot. The rising sun cast long shadows. Radiant heat from the sun melted the snow, except where the cars' shadows fell on the ground, blocking the sunlight. *May Indoor Air Investigations LLC*

Facing page:

FIGURE 5.3. Corroded vent pipe. This pipe carries toxic combustion gases from a furnace into a chimney. The pipe is made of galvanized iron (iron coated with zinc metal). Metals corrode and form oxides when they combine chemically with the oxygen in air. There are two types of corrosion visible in the joints of this pipe. The white fluffy material is zinc oxide; the darker material is iron oxide (rust). Eventually, holes will develop in the pipe and combustion gases will leak out. *May Indoor Air Investigations LLC*

FIGURE 5.4. A putrid light fixture. This fixture caused a foul, dead-fish odor in a bathroom. You are looking at the fixture from the back; the light bulb is partially visible at the left. The plastic base is burned and broken. *May Indoor Air Investigations LLC*

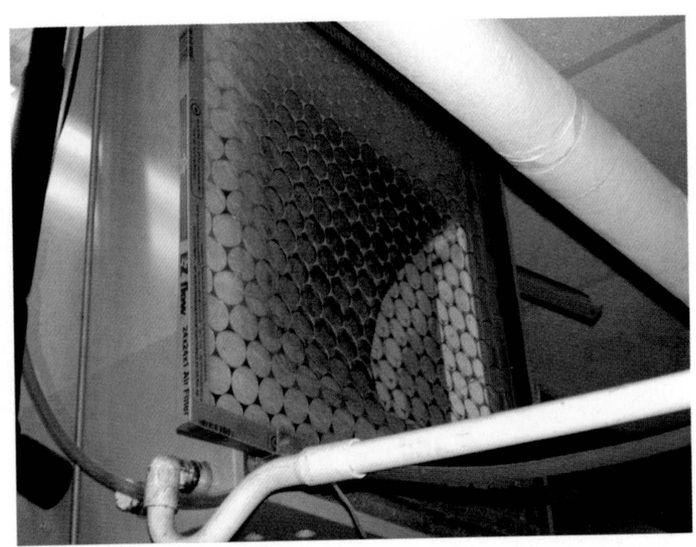

FIGURE 7.4. Clogged, damaged air-conditioning filter. The filter on this ceiling-mounted AC unit had not been changed for a very long time. The filter was so clogged and soiled that air couldn't pass through it. Thus the airflow forced the right side of filter backward, out of its frame (at the light, U-shaped area) and into the unit, leaving a gap in the filter. *May Indoor Air Investigations LLC*

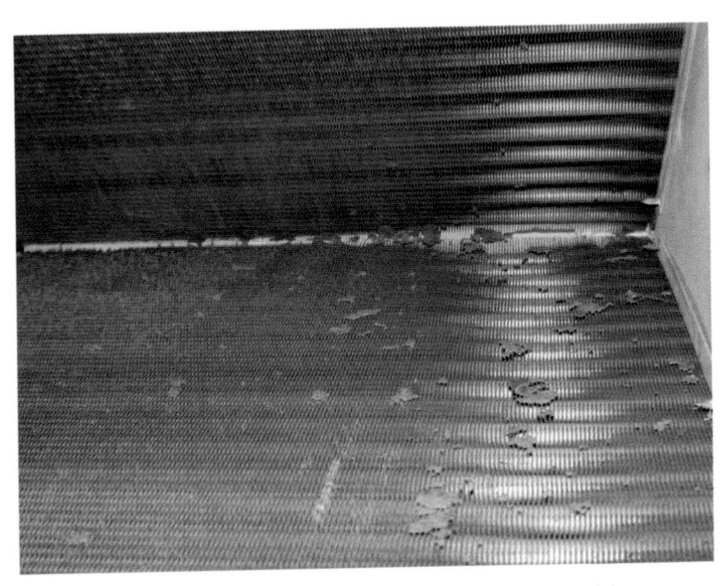

FIGURE 7.5. Clumps of dust on an air-conditioning coil. Because of the gap in the filter (see figure 7.4), unfiltered air flowed over the AC coil. Dust accumulated on the coil, and mold grew in the damp dust. *May Indoor Air Investigations LLC*

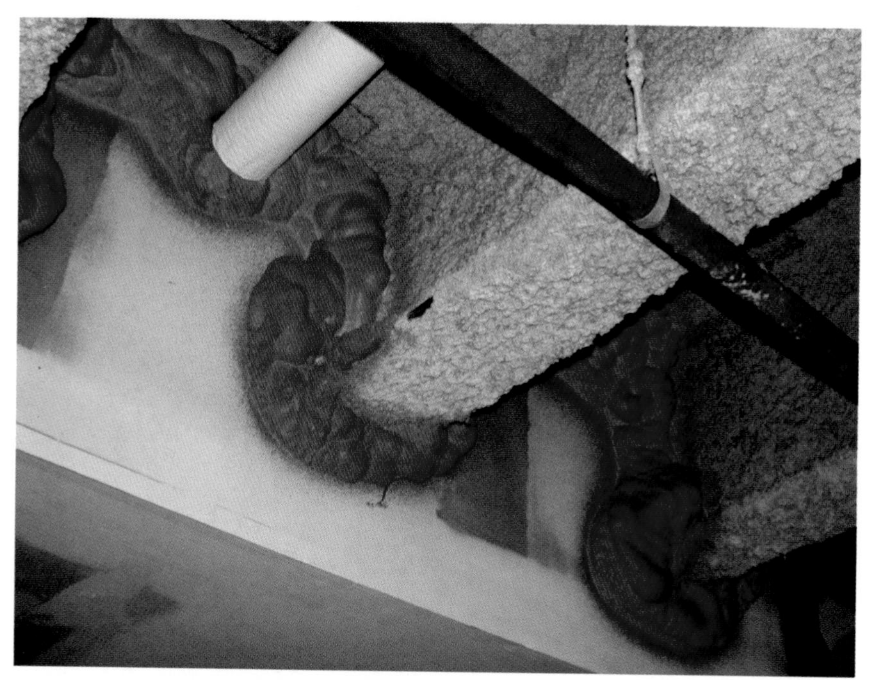

FIGURE 9.2. Various types of insulation. Three different types of insulation appear in this photograph. The steel beam in the middle is coated with sprayed-on fibrous insulation, which is gray and looks fuzzy. The pipe in the upper left-hand corner is wrapped in fiberglass insulation, coated with white paper. The lumpy material that snakes around the end of the pipe and beam is a sprayed-on foam insulation, applied to seal air gaps. On the bottom of the steel beam is a small dark spot where some of the insulation has fallen off. When chunks of insulation hit the floor, they can crumble from the impact as well as from foot traffic and then release irritating aerosol. *Jeffrey C. May*

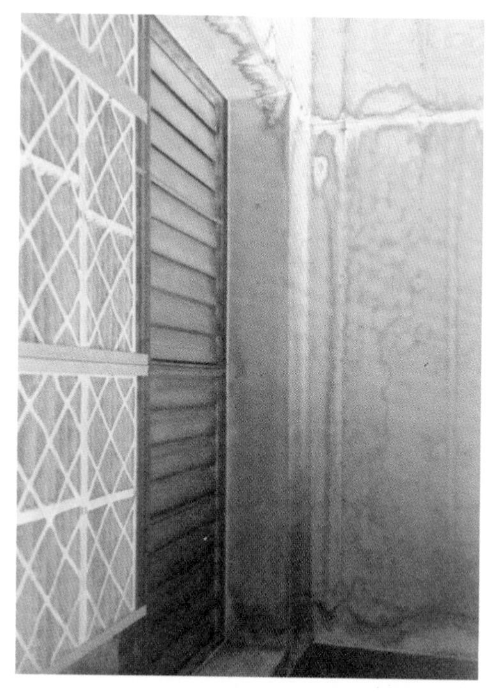

FIGURE 10.1. Moldy air-intake plenum. This air-intake plenum, part of a hospital's ventilation system, is located in a rooftop mechnical "penthouse." To the right (not visible in the photograph) is a louvered opening through which sunlight and fresh air are streaming in. Visible at the left is a bank of filters placed in front of preheat coils that help keep the coils clean. The motorized bypass dampers (metal louvers in the wall, adjacent to the filters) open when there is no need to preheat the air. The penthouse roof leaked, and snow and rain were sucked in through the open louvers. Water stains and mold growth are visible on the drywall in the right half of the photograph. One hopes that the downstream prefilters and filters in the air handler (not visible in the photograph) remove aerosolized mold spores and hyphae before the air enters the hospital. *Wagdy Anis AIA, SBRA Consulting*

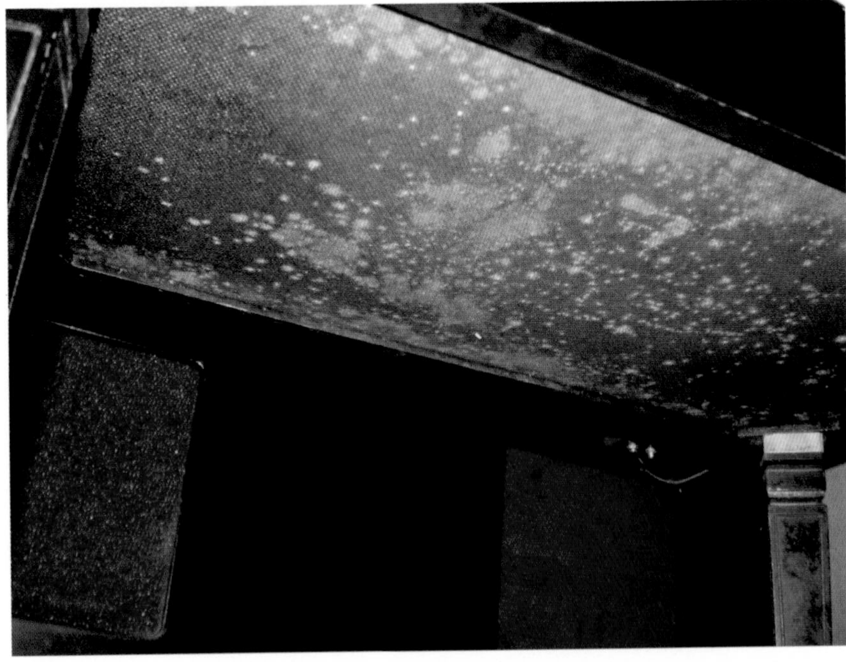

FIGURE 12.1. Excess moisture in a pool. This is the outside of a building on a cold, dry winter day. The building housed a large indoor pool. The air pressure inside the building was greater than the air pressure outside, so warm, moist air was moving from the pool area into the wall cavity behind the brick. Water condensed on the back of the brick, dripped down the wall, and exited at the crack between the concrete and the brick. Stains of efflorescence are visible on the concrete. *May Indoor Air Investigations LLC*

Facing page:
FIGURE 10.3. A decorated wall. This photograph was taken in the hallway leading from the basement playroom of a day care center. The staining on the floor is due to leakage of ground water through the foundation wall, a small part of which is visible at the left edge of the photograph. The water moved along the floor and was soaked up into the drywall, eventually leading to extensive mold growth (the spatter patterns on the wall). *May Indoor Air Investigations LLC*
FIGURE 11.2. A moldy oldie. Mildew grew on the underside of this used piano bench while it was stored in a damp basement. The mildew was readily visible, if anyone had thought to look. The bench was then sold to a pianist, who experienced symptoms whenever he sat on the bench to play his piano. *May Indoor Air Investigations LLC*

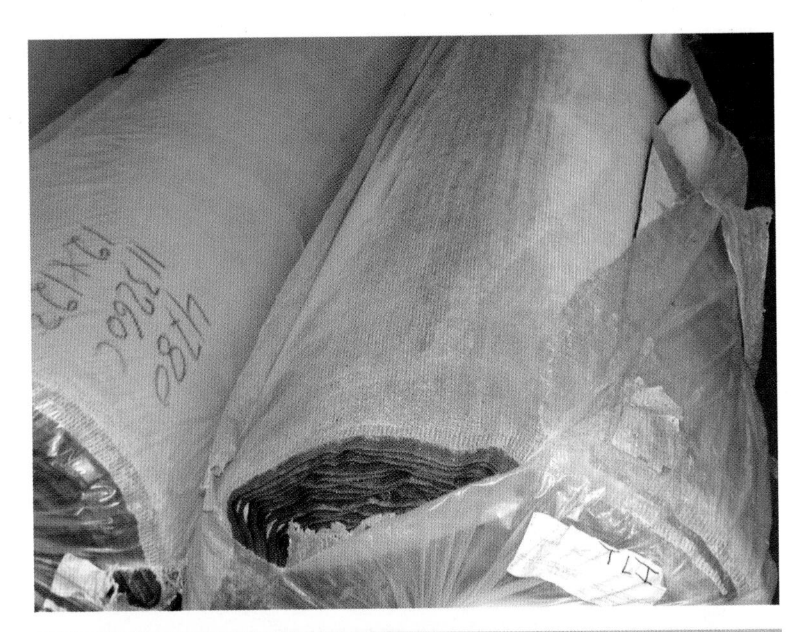

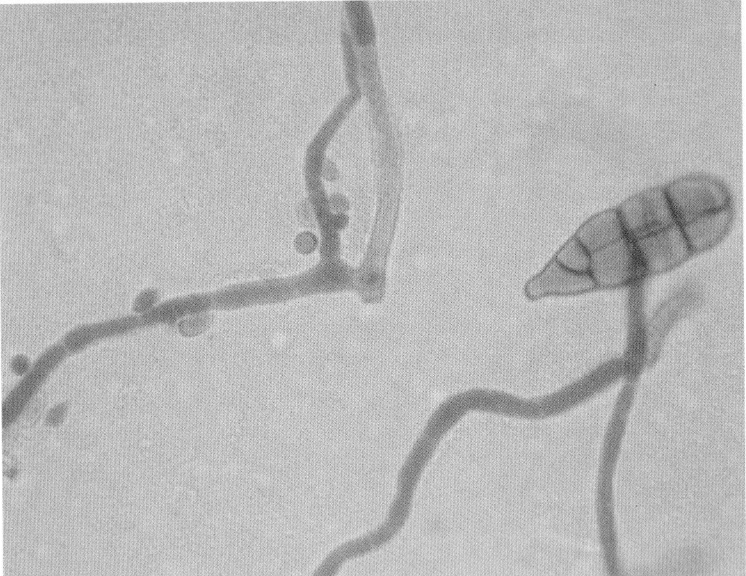

FIGURE 12.2. Doomed from the start. *Top panel:* Two rolls of new carpet, awaiting installation, sit on the floor in a hotel lobby. The plastic wrap on the roll at the right is torn, and there are water stains on the carpet backing, suggesting that the carpet had been sitting in a puddle of water. *Bottom panel:* This photomicrograph (a photograph taken through a microscope, in this case magnified about 500 times) depicts mold hyphae and two different types of mold spores that were found in the dust adhering to the carpet: a large *Alternaria* spore at the right, and several smaller oval and round *Cladosporium* spores at the left. This carpet was contaminated with mold before it was even installed. *Jeffrey C. May*

and the health club sat in the middle of the horseshoe. My room was on the fifteenth floor and my window faced inward, so I could see the roof of the lower structure. Several rooftop units were within view. One of them looked wounded because it was bandaged in multiple strips of duct tape. Cardboard had been taped onto the fresh-air intake to minimize the entrance of cool exterior air into the ventilation system—no doubt to save heating costs.

The Martin County Courthouse

The Martin County Courthouse complex in Florida opened in January 1989. Within months employees were complaining that the indoor air seemed muggy. Some people were even experiencing sick-building symptoms, including eye and throat irritation, headaches, fatigue, and allergy. In December 1992 the chorus of complaints became so loud that the complex was abandoned.

Species of *Aspergillus* and *Penicillium* molds were found growing on drywall behind vinyl wallpaper. The mold was able to grow because exterior humid air had leaked into wall cavities, where the air pressure was lower than the air pressure outdoors. Moisture then condensed on the cooler backsides of the interior walls, moved by capillary action through the drywall, and became trapped behind the vinyl wallpaper. Consultants also found *Stachybotrys* mold on the backs of ceiling tiles that had been soaked by condensation from poorly insulated pipes carrying chilled water.[4] Rainwater penetrating through exterior walls was also fostering mold growth.[5]

Problems with the ventilation system were also partly to blame for the conditions that led to microbial growth. Ron Bailey, an indoor air quality professional, believed that humid outdoor air was being introduced into the building envelope without being dehumidified, leading to conditions of high relative humidity. Other problems he mentioned included uneven air supplies to various parts of the building, poor placement of thermostats, and inadequate ventilation.[6]

After four years of extensive repairs, the complex was reopened. The renovation cost was over $26 million, more than twice the original cost of the complex.

MAINTAINING AN HVAC SYSTEM

All the air we breathe in a modern, "tight" building is supplied by the HVAC system, so whatever circulates inside the air-conveyance system has the potential to enter our lungs. It is therefore essential that these systems be filtered, maintained, and cleaned to the highest standards. While you are probably not involved in this line of work, just knowing what needs to be done can help you safeguard your health.

Changing the Filters

In buildings in which offices or other spaces have their own unit ventilators or ceiling fan coil units, occupants can keep written records of filter changes. Filters have to be changed regularly, once or twice a year or more often, depending on the type of filter used and how dusty the environment is. (Pleated media filters should be used.)

In larger office buildings, the ceiling plenum on a single level may contain twenty or thirty fan coils or heat pumps requiring filter changes. On any given occasion the HVAC technician may not know where all these units are located. Someone in the building needs to know the location of each unit, and the locations should be marked, either at the ceiling or on a floor-plan diagram that is readily accessible when needed. Knowing where the units are located can also help you determine the source of a particular odor.

Unfortunately, such monitoring is not possible in buildings with centralized systems. In many larger buildings there may be whole rooms full of filter banks consisting of pleated media filters, bag filters, or even electronic filters. Unlike most filter materials, which become more efficient as they become clogged (though they restrict more airflow), electronic filters are very efficient when clean but ineffective when soiled, so electronic filters should be kept dust free. (Some electronic filters produce ozone, which can trigger asthma symptoms; see chapter 3.)

Keeping the System Clean

The airflow at most ceiling diffusers (supplies in the ceiling) creates a soiling pattern, often consisting of soot, skin scales, and other particles from the air. In systems with air conditioning, this dust may also contain microbial growth, because the temperature of the metal grille may be below the dew point of the room air (when the blower turns off, moisture from the room air will condense on the cooler surfaces and wet the dust). Condensation like this should be prevented, though prevention may require the use of supplemental dehumidification in the room. Diffusers that are moldy can be cleaned with a dilute bleach or detergent solution (when the airflow is turned off). People doing this kind of work should wear a NIOSH N95 mask, gloves, and eye protection.

There should be no visible dust on a cooling coil (though unfortunately, most of the coils I have seen have been coated with a mat of dust), and the coil should be checked for soiling every time a filter is changed. A technician should also never see water dripping or leaking from any mechanical equipment, but particularly from a fan coil or heat pump in a ceiling plenum, because then there is the potential for microbial growth in the soaked lining material within the unit and on the damp ceiling surfaces under the unit. Such overflowing is often caused by a condensate pan drain clogged by microbial sludge. And if the lining material is soaked, cleaning the clogged line may not be adequate. Lining material containing microbial growth usually has to be replaced.

Microbial growth in duct dust is not likely unless there is water leaking onto soiled fiberglass or other duct-lining material, or unless there is excessively humid air (well over 75 percent relative humidity) passing through the ducts. If there are air quality complaints in a building with an air-conveyance system, however, the ducts should be investigated as a possible source of contamination. Many ducts can only be inspected by making a hole in the duct and inserting a borescope (a periscope with a light) or other device into the hole. Most professional duct-cleaning companies also have fiberoptic or robotic equipment that can move through the ductwork and transmit images of the conditions back to a video monitor.

With proper filtration and maintenance, ducts that were clean to begin with should remain clean. In forced hot-air systems in smaller residential buildings, however, ducts may need to be cleaned every ten years or so, because returns can accumulate biodegradable dust. And in any type of building, air-conditioning coils may need more frequent, even annual cleaning, although MERV 8 filtration should minimize the need for coil cleaning.

Ducts that are soiled or contaminated should be cleaned only by professionals. Metal ducts are smooth inside and thus can be cleaned with brushes and vacuum devices. Ducts that have coarse or fibrous lining materials are difficult to clean, but these lining materials can be sealed with a thick polymeric (plastic) coating. The uneven, spiral-shaped interiors of flexible ducts are also difficult to clean. Flexible ducts are inexpensive and easy to install, however, so it is usually cheaper to replace contaminated flexible ducts, if they are readily accessible, than to try to clean them.

Disturbing moldy, fibrous interior lining material or cleaning moldy ducts can aerosolize large numbers of allergens. Great caution should be exercised, therefore, when filters are changed or any soiled components are cleaned, particularly if individuals with allergies or mold sensitivities are working nearby. The air-conveyance system should also be shut off when such work is in progress.

A recent study conducted in Canada concluded that ultraviolet germicidal irradiation (UVGI), or the use of ultraviolet germicidal lights, in HVAC systems can reduce microbial contamination.[7] The use of such lights has been shown in many previous studies to reduce airborne contamination, and the results of the Canadian study are being used by manufacturers of UVGI equipment to promote sales. Still, I believe that the Canadian study was flawed, for several reasons. First, the devices ("coupons") used to collect spores lacked sticky surfaces. Second, the coupons were exposed directly to the UVGI, whereas microbes on an actual HVAC surface would have received only incident UV light at a variety of angles, the intensity of which would be attenuated by the dust accumulations on surfaces within the mechanical system. Third, the data and results for different seasons were not separated. The heating season is longer than the cooling season in Montreal, and in the heating season there is no condensation of moisture within the HVAC system to foster microbial growth. And last, even though workers within the buildings included in this study reported a reduction of symptoms indoors during the "UVGI-on periods," no statistically significant differences were reported in the indoor air concentrations of microbes at work stations; thus the authors were left with no explanation for the reported reduction in symptoms associated with UVGI.

Though UVGI may serve as an adjunct in disinfecting exposed air and reducing growth on irradiated surfaces, the impact of UVGI alone on overall air quality should not be overstated. To prevent microbial growth due to moisture or high relative humidity in HVAC systems, *the most important components of hygiene will always be proper design to begin with, then adequate filtration and regular maintenance.*

In a sense, the quality of indoor air depends on an equilibrium between opposing forces: the rate of generation of contaminants within or the introduction of contaminants into the building envelope, and the rate of removal of these contaminants through ventilation and filtration. As long as the latter exceeds the former, the building will be healthy for most of its occupants. The design and proper maintenance of the mechanical system are therefore of the greatest concern.

SOME PRACTICAL STEPS

- Know the locations of thermostats, filters, and ventilation intakes.
- Ask that moldy ceiling tiles be replaced and soiled diffusers be cleaned.
- Find out the schedule for filter changes and for coil and duct cleaning, to ensure that these occur on a regular basis.
- Dust from any components of a mechanical system should be handled with caution, because the dust may contain microbial growth that can become airborne and cause problems for those who have allergies or asthma.
- When ceiling tiles have to be moved to access the plenum, they should be handled carefully to avoid aerosolizing irritants or moldy dust. If several soiled ceiling tiles have to be moved, as many tiles as possible should be HEPA-vacuumed before being disturbed.
- If there is inadequate airflow or too much airflow at a clean ceiling diffuser with manually operated louvers, adjust the louvers.
- If the temperature of your workspace seems stratified, use a digital thermometer to corroborate your theory. Operating a small fan may work to mix the air.
- If you are concerned about indoor air quality problems, try to find someone who understands how the mechanical system operates

and who can communicate your concerns to HVAC contractors or the building management.

- Building management personnel should be aware of any projects outside the building (application of pesticides, construction or demolition, reroofing) that might generate airborne contaminants that could enter the ventilation system. Filters may have to be changed more frequently, or intakes of the HVAC system that could take in these contaminants may have to be temporarily sealed.

PART

II

Daily Life

Many of the air quality problems in office buildings, schools, hospitals, city halls, retail spaces, and hotels and motels stem from similar sources, including gases and particulates, excessive or inadequate relative humidity, contaminated heating, ventilation, and air-conditioning equipment, and inadequate ventilation, all of which I discussed in detail in part I. Part II focuses on indoor air quality problems that are common in specific types of buildings and describes some of the dramatic stories of those who have suffered because of poor IAQ.

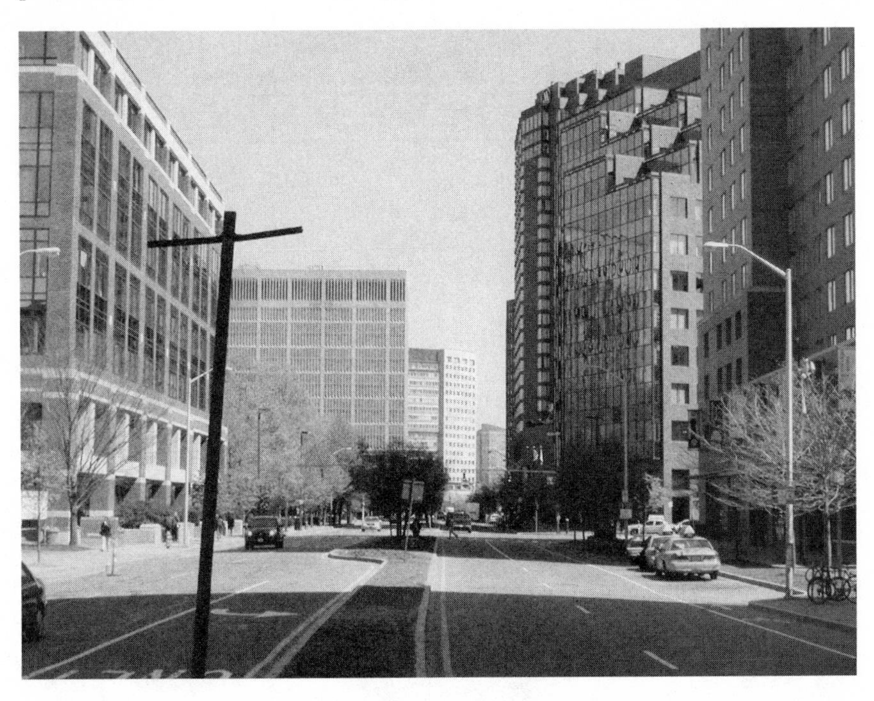

CHAPTER

8

Schools

Our Children, Our Future

When I was in high school, most students and faculty dreaded the day when chemistry classes added acid to sodium sulfide to produce hydrogen sulfide gas, which smells like rotten eggs. There are a number of sources of air quality problems in schools. Some sources, like science labs, are obvious; other sources are not so obvious.

A MALIGNANT MIX

Welding, automotive and machine shops, and even kitchens can be intermittent sources of volatile organic compounds (VOCs) and combustion gases. Administrative offices contain copiers and printers that may exhaust irritating chemicals; in many schools these machines are placed in unventilated closets. Irritating VOCs from fragrances and cleaning products, and even solvents (such as xylene) from permanent and erasable marker pens, can be a problem for students and teachers who are chemically sensitive.[1] And as in all buildings, off-gassing from paint, adhesives, or building materials can cause short-term or even long-term air quality problems.*

Wherever there are people, especially teenagers (if you consider them people!), there is food. And where there is food, there are cockroaches and other pests. Cockroach allergens are a significant cause of asthma symptoms; from 40 to 60 percent of people with asthma who live in urban areas are sensitized.[2]

* The Collaborative for High Performance Schools, or CHPS, has several manuals that provide guidance on the best practices for construction and renovation in school buildings (www.chps.net).

While cockroach body parts are allergenic (cause allergies), their fecal material is the primary source of the allergens. The fecal pellets can be large (up to one-eighth of an inch) and friable (easily broken up), and they are not readily aerosolized unless crushed and disturbed. Still, in a study of schools in Baltimore, 69 percent of the buildings contained measurable levels of roach allergens in dust.[3] Similar results have been observed in schools elsewhere, suggesting that exposure to roach allergens from dust in schools can be very significant, even though the allergen is rarely detected in air samples (see chapter 14).

Pest infestations lead to pest allergens and the need for pest control. Pesticides are often applied in school cafeteria and kitchen areas, and even outdoors on playing fields. I recall hearing about members of a football team who became ill after playing on a grass field that had just been treated with pesticide.

A study led by scientists from NIOSH and the EPA tracked illnesses associated with exposure to pesticides used in school buildings, on school property, or on nearby farmland. The incidence rates between 1998 and 2002 were found to have increased and "were 7.4 cases per million children and 27.3 cases per million school employee full-time equivalents."[4] More than 2,500 children were sickened: 3 cases of illness were severe, 275 were moderate, and 2,315 were of low severity. About one-third of the illnesses were associated with the use of insecticides. The authors recommended that practices be adopted to reduce the drift of pesticides, that pesticide "buffer zones" be established around school buildings, and that schools adopt integrated pest management (IPM) programs.

The ideal approach to pest problems is a technique called *integrated pest management (IPM)*. This approach uses monitoring and record-keeping to determine the type and extent of a problem, and then site-specific (rather than broadcast) application of effective, but to occupants the safest pesticides (those least toxic) in the smallest amounts and only when needed. Short-lasting rather than long-lasting pesticides, as well as nonvolatile rather than volatile pesticides (or solid dust), are preferable. Other commonsense practices of IPM include using weather stripping, caulk, and screens to keep pests out; keeping food, garbage, and trash in closed containers; and repairing leaks quickly. See the Resource Guide for the EPA's guide to pest management in school buildings.

Dust mites can also be present in schools, in carpeting, upholstered furniture, and stuffed animals. Dust mite allergens can thus be a problem, particularly for kindergartners who sit on carpets, lie on pillows, and play with stuffed animals. In 2002 a study of sixty elementary schools in Houston, Texas, revealed high levels of dust mites in 20 percent of the rooms.[5]

School buildings also seem particularly prone to mold growth due to water from leaks. Most modern schools are low and spread-out with flat roofs, and roof leaks are common. Many school buildings have classrooms below grade, and if the foundation has cracks or if there is a high water table or poor grading and drainage, water can penetrate. And the air in a classroom may contain allergens from pest infestations and fungal growth, if the classroom is located over a damp, contaminated crawl space.

CARPETING

Many schools are carpeted throughout, even in or near entryways where people track in moisture from rain and snow, again leading to microbial growth in the dust. In addition, carpeting is often laid on the concrete slab in below-grade spaces, or on the concrete floor above the crawl space. Many schools are closed in the summer and not air-conditioned or dehumidified, so unless there is a vapor-impermeable layer on top of the concrete, moisture can diffuse through to moisten the carpet dust. And if the relative humidity of the air near the concrete is 75 percent or higher (see chapter 4), fungi can sprout in the carpet dust. I investigated one school building that was built on a slab, and the carpeting on the concrete was so badly contaminated with mold that hoards of mold-eating mites had moved in. It was a music building, and some students and teachers who spent time there experienced hoarseness and breathing difficulties. Needless to say, chorus rehearsals didn't go very well!

It is common practice in schools to wash carpets during summer vacation, when the buildings are not in use and are thus closed up. Because of the lack of ventilation and the presence of hot, humid summer conditions, carpeting can remain damp long enough for microbial growth to occur in the dust. I know of one elementary school in Massachusetts in which all the carpeting had been washed during a two-week period in the summer, when the outdoor relative humidity was over 80 percent. After the carpets were washed, the windows and doors were closed, and the classrooms became musty as fungi sprouted. When the superintendent of schools was informed of what had happened, he had all the carpeting replaced.

Unfortunately, most school budgets are inadequate, and maintenance repairs are often postponed. Moldy ceiling tiles remain in place for years, and carpeting and carpet pads that have been soaked by flooding are all too often dried out and reinstalled rather than replaced. Allergens from microbial growth on dampened carpet dust remain in the carpet after it has been dried, and the allergens can continue to be aerosolized for years by foot traffic.

In an investigation I did of a school building, one of the teachers was about to retire because of respiratory problems she experienced in her classroom. I was walking down the hallway with the principal, discussing some of the problems in the building. The hallway had VCT (vinyl composite tile) flooring, but ahead of us beyond a pair of swinging doors was a carpeted section

Some experts continue to deny that carpeting can be a source of bioaerosol. According to Alan Hedge, a professor of design and environmental analysis at Cornell University, "Concerns that carpeting in schools is contributing to an increase in respiratory problems, allergies and asthma in schools are unfounded."[1] Some data seem to support that view. For example, in one study, airborne particulate matter was measured in both a carpeted gym room and an uncarpeted gym room.[2] The results suggested that some cleaning practices, such as sweeping with push brooms (without using sweeping compound) and using high-speed burnishing devices on VCT flooring, rather than types of floor covering themselves, are responsible for elevated levels of aerosolized particulate matter. Yet in another study, in which particulate mass concentrations were measured both outdoors and indoors (in a limited number of carpeted and uncarpeted classrooms), the data suggested that "carpeted floor coverings may present an increased exposure risk to children from particulate matter harbored on the flooring material as compared to hard-surfaced flooring."[3] Despite the conflicting conclusions of these two studies, common sense tells us that hard-surfaced floors can never contain as much dust, and thus allergens, as carpeted ones (see chapter 3). And like many studies, these two looked only at the amount of particulate matter (dust) and not what the particulate matter consisted of, so there is no way to know whether the dust was allergenic or even toxic.

1. S. Lang, "CU Expert: Carpets in Schools Benefit Air Quality," *Cornell Chronicle*, 29 March 2001.

2. W. Turner et al., "Realtime Measurement of (PM-10) Dust Levels in a Carpeted and Non-Carpeted School Gym Room," *Proceedings of Indoor Air 2002, the 9th International Conference on Indoor Air Quality and Climate*, Monterey, Calif., 30 June–5 July 2002.

3. R. Shaughnessy et al., "Preliminary Study of Flooring in School in the U.S.: Airborne Particulate Exposures in Carpeted vs. Uncarpeted Classrooms," *Proceedings of Indoor Air 2002*.

of hallway—the hallway that led to the retiring teacher's classroom. As soon as we passed through these doors and started walking on the carpeting, I began to cough. The principal turned to me with a serious look and asked, "If you were a teacher, you wouldn't be able to work here, would you?" And he was right. Both the teacher and I were sensitized to allergens from microbial growth (mold and bacteria) in the carpet dust. As students and teachers walked on that carpet, the allergens became airborne.

Should school buildings be carpeted? People who support the use of carpeting claim, and rightly so, that carpets add sound-proofing, soften the interior, and provide a welcoming and warm ambiance. On the other hand, carpets in school buildings are usually vacuumed with inefficiently filtered vacuum cleaners that aerosolize allergens and any contaminants that may be in the carpet dust (see chapter 3). In view of all the risks, I believe that the use of carpeting in schools should be very limited, despite the advantages of this floor covering.

UNIVENTS

Many classrooms have unit ventilators or *univents* (mentioned in chapter 7). A univent is a metal box, usually placed against an outside wall, with a room air intake at the bottom (with a filter) and a grille at the top, which supplies conditioned air. An access panel is located at the front of the box; if you were to remove this panel, you would find a heat exchanger and one or more blowers inside.

Classroom debris can fall through the grille at the top of a univent. Sometimes teachers put plants or even bread mold experiments on top of the grille. Then leaves and crumbs may land on the top of the heat exchanger below the grille and stay there until some pest or mold spore dines on the biodegradable material.

The dust on the fiberglass insulation on the access panels in univents often becomes infested with microbial growth and can be a major source of airborne allergens. Soiled fiberglass insulation should be replaced with either solid-surfaced foam insulation or fiberglass insulation that has an aluminum foil surface. Such surfaces can be cleaned, and they prevent the insulation from becoming saturated with moisture.

The hot-water piping for the univents is often routed through a crawl space.

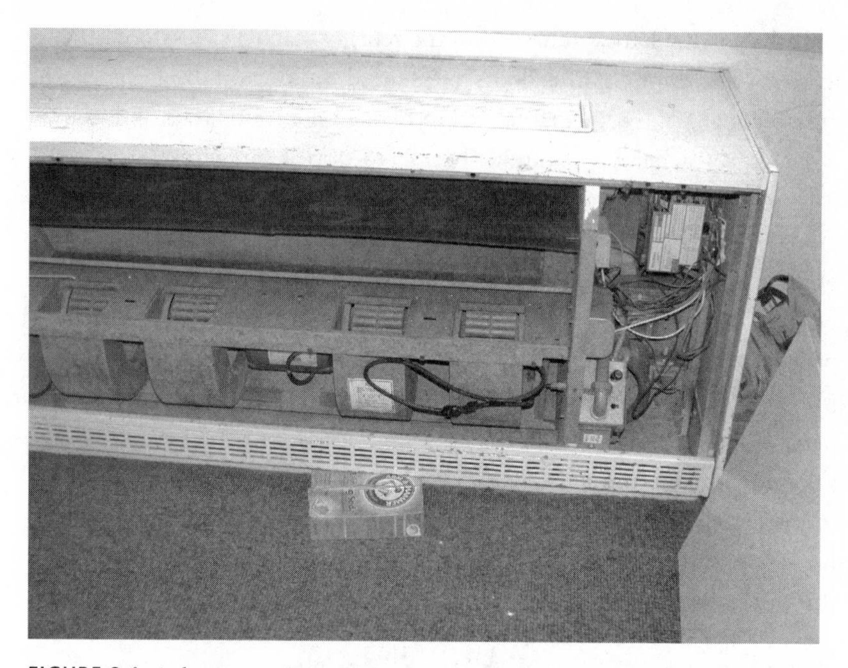

FIGURE 8.1. A classroom univent. This univent was at the exterior wall of an elementary school classroom. The teacher had been complaining about allergy problems, so the custodian had already cleaned the blowers (visible in the photograph just above the grille at the bottom) and the coil (just above the blowers). The univent access panel is at the right. Unfortunately, the fiberglass insulation on the inside of the panel had never been cleaned and was covered with mold. *May Indoor Air Investigations LLC*

The holes in the floor through which the piping passes between the crawl space and the univent are usually larger than the diameter of the piping, and these holes create pathways for airflows that may contain contaminants (including mold spores) present in the crawl space.

In some classrooms the piping carrying hot water to the univent does not pass through the crawl space but rather is installed behind shelving along the bottom of the exterior wall. There is about a 3-inch space beneath and behind the shelving. Some sections of the pipes, called *fin tubes,* have fins (rows of very thin parallel metal plates) that function as heat emitters. Grilles on the top and along the bottom of the shelving allow airflow. Heated air rises up out of the back of the shelving by convection, and cooler air is drawn in at the bottom. Unfortunately, the metal grille at the bottom usually cannot be removed, and thus there is no access to clean the fins or remove the dust that in many cases has accumulated for decades. In most schools I have investigated, this dust is severely contaminated with mold growth.

To provide ventilation, a univent draws in outside air through a louver at the exterior side of the unit. The amount of fresh air being introduced is often controlled by dampers. Unfortunately, it is common for maintenance personnel to close the fresh air dampers to prevent water in the piping from freezing, as sometimes occurs in cold weather if the boiler does not have the capacity to keep the water hot enough or if the heat is turned down at night. As a result, univents rarely deliver enough fresh air—and lack of fresh air is a common problem in schools.

MCKINLEY ELEMENTARY

The story of the air quality crisis at the McKinley Elementary School in Fairfield, Connecticut, illustrates how air quality problems in schools can lead to personal tragedy.

In the fall of 1991 Joellen Lawson, a veteran teacher and specialist in attention deficit disorder (ADD), was transferred to the McKinley Elementary School to work as a part-time special-education teacher.[6] She had just earned her second master's degree in health education and was looking forward to being a member of her new school community.

In her first year at McKinley, Joellen taught in a second-floor classroom. In her second year she worked mostly in room 118, a windowless space located at grade with wall-to-wall carpet laid on the concrete slab. After a while she began to feel ill. By noon on many days she had a headache and burning eyes and felt tired. She also began coughing. She had never had any of these health problems in the six school buildings she had previously worked in. Having suffered from asthma and allergy as a child, though, she thought something in room 118 was responsible for her symptoms, and she asked to be moved.

In 1993 Joellen was assigned to a small room located in the school's library/media center. The room had a window, and she began to feel better until the 1994–95 school year, when she became a full-time teacher and thus spent more time in the building. The following year her chronic cough became so severe that she herniated a disc in her back. She also experienced tingling and muscle spasms and developed a tremor, particularly noticeable in her hands.

In 1997 she was at last assigned her own regular classroom, room 116—another space at grade. The room had been vacated by a teacher who had taught there for years and who never removed her materials from the storage closet when she was transferred to another school. Joellen didn't use the closet, not only because it was full but because to her it smelled musty. And her teaching assistant said that she sometimes felt as if she might pass out when she opened the closet door. After she began working in the classroom, the assistant experienced sinus and nasal congestion and discharge from her eyes and nose, and she developed asthma for the first time in her life.[7]

In May 1998 Joellen finally got around to cleaning out the closet, working for four days before school, during her breaks, and after school hours. She worked alone because she didn't want her teaching assistant to be exposed to the closet's dusty contents. She filled twenty plastic garbage bags with moldy papers and other teaching materials, some of which dated back to the 1960s. On the second day of her cleaning project, Joellen felt dizzy and sick to her stomach. On Sunday, June 1, she woke up and her bedroom seemed to be spinning. "From that day onward, my life was never the same," she said.

The following day she still felt dizzy. She vomited and had tremors. She went to the emergency room, where the staff suspected a case of food poisoning. Like all dedicated teachers, Joellen was conscientious, so she returned to work several days later to complete the school year even though she was still fighting vertigo. She hoped summer vacation would bring a return to good health, but her symptoms continued. She experienced night sweats, low-grade fevers, and migraine headaches. She had trouble focusing her vision and found loud noises painful. Sometimes there was even mild bleeding from her ears.

Joellen had always been physically active. She had practiced yoga regularly and done aerobic exercise several times a week, but now her health was clearly in decline. She began an odyssey that summer, traveling from one physician to another, hoping to find the cause of her vestibular dysfunction (dizziness, vertigo). The possibilities mentioned to her included multiple sclerosis, a brain tumor, lupus, and Lyme disease. She saw fourteen doctors but still didn't know the cause of her suffering.

She tried returning to work the following fall for the 1998–99 school year, but her symptoms were so severe that on two occasions her parents, who lived nearby, had to come pick her up and take her away from the building. "Once

I asked my father to call my classroom assistant and tell her what happened, so she wouldn't worry when I disappeared," Joellen said. She began to suffer from memory loss and word retrieval problems. She would sometimes forget the names of students she had been working with for two or three years. She was embarrassed and alarmed by her cognitive dysfunction and kept hoping she would get better, but she didn't. She was granted a medical leave for the 1999–2000 and 2000–2001 school years, absences that ultimately turned into a disability retirement. On her last day at McKinley she was so weak and shaky that friends had to help her to her mother's car. Unlike many people who retire, Joellen didn't feel as if she had reached the celebrated end of a wonderful professional life; rather, she felt forced into an early leave-taking from a career she loved and to which she had been committed for twenty-three years.

While Joellen was struggling with her symptoms, Dr. John Santilli, an allergist who had been practicing medicine in the Fairfield area for almost three decades and who had yet to hear about or to meet Joellen Lawson, had been treating students and teachers from the McKinley school. Every September the number of cases of bronchitis and sinus infections would increase, and Dr. Santilli's office staff hypothesized that contagious students infected others in the first few weeks of school. Events that unfolded over the next few years, however, led Dr. Santilli to consider mold exposure as a cause of many of these symptoms.[8]

The McKinley building had been suffering from delayed maintenance. According to Charlotte Leslie, a McKinley parent and president of the McKinley PTA at the time, "The Board of Education and Central Administration were in charge of not only our children's education, but also the buildings that they learned in. When they would go before the Boards of Selectmen and Finance and the Representative Town Meetings and the budgets would be cut, it seemed that the maintenance of the buildings would suffer. Our building, part built in 1928, in 1952, and in 1973, suffered more than most." The building also had a history of roof leaks. "It had been raining inside the building for years," Charlotte Leslie added.[9]

In the summer of 2000, two years after Joellen Lawson stopped working in the building, a new roof was installed. In part because the gutters in the older section of the building weren't functioning properly, water still cascaded down the exterior of some parts of the building and entered wall cavities whenever it rained heavily. In the fall after school started, musty odors in a few of the rooms led to the removal of some carpeting while school was in session. A thirty-eight-year-old custodian who assisted in this work developed asthma and a severe cough (he is now on disability leave).[10] During this period a second teacher at McKinley, a thirty-one-year-old woman with a history of allergies, asthma, and sinusitis, was taken by ambulance twice to the emergency room for treatment.[11]

After a student developed asthma within weeks of starting school, parents demanded air quality testing, and on September 28, 2000, a consultant from the Connecticut Department of Labor's Division of Occupational Safety and Health (CONN-OSHA) met with school officials, conducted a walk-through inspection of the building, and undertook sampling for indoor air fungal levels. The consultant found that a "musty odor was apparent throughout the Media Center" and that there were "water-damaged ceiling tiles in office areas, damp wall coverings, and cracks in the wall structure near the rear exit." Yet the results from the first round of testing revealed "that the indoor air fungal levels did not exceed the outdoor air fungal level in any of the areas sampled," and thus the results were inconclusive. The consultant returned to the building on October 2 to retest. At that time she found that the "total number of viable particles found in the indoor sample collected from the Faculty Room between Rooms 221 and 222 was three times greater than the total number of viable particles found in the outdoor . . . air sample"—a finding that suggested a mold problem.[12]

CONN-OSHA only tested for fungal spores that were viable or culturable (alive and capable of growing). But in this case, as in so many others, the number of dead spores in both indoor and outdoor air may far outnumber the number of airborne living spores present. And all spores, whether living or dead, contain allergens that can cause symptoms in those who are sensitized. Testing only for culturable spores therefore does not paint a complete picture of the number of spores and of the amount of allergens (or microbial toxins) to which those who are sensitized may be exposed.[13] In this case, even though the number of viable particles was greater indoors than outdoors, the results still underestimated the true total counts of all the spores present, dead as well as living.

By the middle of October the "cafeteria, library, two classrooms and a music room [were] closed due to high fungal levels caused by excessive moisture," and "two children [were] hospitalized . . . after suffering allergic reactions, while dozens more have said they felt ill."[14] A watchful school nurse kept a log of the students and staff who had health complaints or symptoms that might have been caused by environmental exposures in the building. She stated that "approximately 40 percent of the students, teachers, and staff reported the following symptoms: fatigue, dizziness, post-nasal drip, sinus headache and pressure, nasal blockage, skin rashes, earache, eye itching and burning, sore throat, wheezing, sneezing, chest tightness, and green or yellow nasal mucus."[15] Symptoms seemed to "cluster around a few areas of the building including Rm. 105, the Media Center, Cafeteria, Rm. 117, and the upper floor of the 1928 wing."[16] And students and teachers from the school continued to file through Dr. Santilli's office.

Dr. Santilli's office had been consistently sampling the outdoor air for mold spore counts since 1978, but during this period he became increasingly convinced of the connection between his patients' symptoms and the school's *indoor* air quality.* He urged many McKinley students to stay away from the building: "I won't let them go back to school," he said.[17] The absentee rate in the student body climbed to almost 25 percent. Parents were asking if the school was safe for their children. "We don't have an answer to that," replied the superintendent of schools.[18]

According to Charlotte Leslie, "On Wednesday, October 18, approximately 130 children out of a population of 348 did not report to school."[19] The school was closed the next day, and a contingency plan that had been developed was put into action. McKinley students were brought by bus to the school grounds, as usual, but from there they reboarded separate buses and were redistributed among six other schools. "We adjusted to having the children stand outside in tents in all kinds of weather while they regrouped to be sent on to their host schools—for many children that meant two bus rides each way per day," Charlotte Leslie said. It was a disruptive and difficult time for everyone.

In November a private environmental consulting company conducted additional sampling throughout the school. Dr. Santilli remarked that "once we

* Dr. Santilli is now involved in several studies of "sick" schools. One of the questionnaires he is using is designed to uncover a connection between allergy symptoms from exposure to mold and cognitive impairment.

started getting the testing results back it became obvious that McKinley was not a problem but a huge problem."[20] Needless to say, people were concerned.

The consultants found that the total spore count (which includes both living and dead spores) was 53,000 fungal spores per cubic meter of air (counts/m^3) in room 107 and 6,500 counts/m^3 in the gym, as compared with 1,900 counts/m^3 outdoors.[21] In other words, the indoor counts ranged between three and more than twenty-five times the outdoor counts. Some indoor air quality investigators consider indoor spore levels over 1,000 counts/m^3 to be reason for concern.[22] (I discuss air quality testing and test reports in chapter 14.)

The consultants also found that much of the carpeting in the building was contaminated by microbial growth (yeast and fungi). The original McKinley school had been built in wetlands, and when the old building was torn down and the ground excavated for the new foundation, the hole filled with water like a lake.[23] In the part of the building constructed in 1928, where room 118 was located (in which Joellen worked much of the time in her second year in the building), excess moisture was coming through the floor slab, creating conditions of high relative humidity in the carpet. In addition, custodial personnel reported that the carpeting took more than twenty-four hours to dry after being washed. The carpet in room 118 contained over 20,000,000 colony-forming units of mold per gram of dust (cfu/gram), including 560,000 cfu/gram of *Aspergillus glaucus,* 6,000,000 cfu/gram of *Cladosporium* species, and 13,000,000 cfu/gram of *Wallemia* species.[24] (*Wallemia* mold is sometimes found in agricultural settings. One species, *W. sebi,* produces a mycotoxin, walleminol. *W. sebi* has been associated with allergy, asthma, and the hypersensitivity disease known as farmer's lung.)[25]

The results of the sampling in room 118 illustrate another problem with culturable sampling. In the CONN-OSHA report of sampling in room 118 undertaken on October 2, no *Wallemia* colonies were reported, yet the consultants' November 15 testing of dust from the carpet in the room found 13,000,000 colony-forming units of *Wallemia* mold per gram of carpet dust. It is impossible for this many spores to be present in the dust and not be present in the air, so why didn't the culturable sampler pick this up? It is not uncommon for *Wallemia* spores to go undetected, because species in this genus of fungi require drier conditions than those found in the petri dish cultures used.[26] So even if there were many viable spores present on the surface of the medium, they would grow so slowly that other colonies could grow over and conceal them.

The consultants' report stated,

> Fungus and bacteria are normally found in the outdoor and indoor environment. Reported amplified indoor sources in the range of 1.0×10^5 [100,000] cfu/gram to 9.9×10^5 [990,000] cfu/gram of bulk material sampled from *indoor* environments are hypothesized to potentially affect the health of people who are known asthmatics, suffer from certain allergies, or are immunocompromised, should repeated exposures to the source occur. Amplified indoor sources at or above 1.0×10^6 [1,000,000] cfu/gram of fungus have been known to be capable of affecting the health of non-immunocompromised individuals, should repeated exposure occur. Certain specific types of fungus may affect the health of occupants at levels lower than those cited above.[27]

In six rooms, including room 118, the concentration of microbial growth in the carpeting was above 1,000,000 cfu/gram. And in about 70 percent of the classrooms tested on all floors of the McKinley school, the concentration of fungi and yeast in the carpeting was greater than 100,000 cfu/gram. Rooms like these are like giant petri dishes full of microbial growth flourishing in the nutrient, in this case the carpet dust.

In the media center (where Joellen had moved years earlier after feeling ill in room 118), books were covered with active mildew growth, mostly *Aspergillus* species along with some *Penicillium* and *Cladosporium* species. The carpet in this area had already been removed, because teachers and students had complained of musty odors and allergy symptoms. The consultants' report suggested that the high humidity that had developed over the summer in the media center was responsible for the fungal proliferation. (During the summer the rooftop air-conditioning unit for the media center was not operated, and therefore there was no dehumidification.)

Water that was leaking around windows, entering wall cavities, and wetting the finished sides of walls was causing microbial growth within the wall cavities. This wouldn't necessarily have caused an air quality problem if the by-products of this growth had remained within the wall cavities, but because the air pressure within the classrooms was generally less than the air pressure outdoors, air flowed from the exterior into the wall cavities, and then into the interior of the building.

By design, fresh air was to be blown into the McKinley classrooms through the unit ventilators. In the 1928 section of the school, though, all the fresh-air vents in the unit ventilators had been closed off to improve heating efficiency and thus save money on fuel. Part of the ventilation system consisted of rooftop exhaust fans that removed air through ducts from every classroom. As that air was removed, replacement air had to come from somewhere, so it infiltrated from the wall cavities where mold growth was located.

There was yet another problem caused by the reduced ventilation: there wasn't enough fresh air in the classrooms tested. As the consultants' report stated, "At current ventilation recommendations Classroom 109 could handle a population of 6, Classroom 202 a population of 2, Classroom 218 a population of 12, and Classroom 117 a population of 7."[28] Obviously, many more children than that occupied these rooms during the school day, so elevated levels of carbon dioxide and other contaminants would have been present.

In the CONN-OSHA report, the carbon dioxide concentration in room 109 was 434 parts per million in the morning and 620 ppm in the afternoon. During both measuring periods, windows were open and there was only one person present (the investigator had no control over the conditions in the rooms). The carbon dioxide concentration in room 218 was 410 ppm in the morning and 770 ppm in the afternoon. That room was empty when the morning measurement was taken but contained nineteen people when the afternoon measurement was taken, and in both instances, windows were open.

According to the CONN-OSHA report, only two in-use classrooms were tested for carbon dioxide when the windows were closed and people were present: rooms 216 and 220. There were eighteen people in room 216 and 1,040 ppm of CO_2. There were also eighteen people in room 220 and 1,180 ppm of CO_2.[29] In other words, most of the CONN-OSHA testing for CO_2 was undertaken when the windows were open or occupancy low, so the results do not reflect potential concentrations of carbon dioxide in full classrooms in the winter when windows would be closed. The consultants' report, on the other hand, clearly indicates that in many classrooms the ventilation was inadequate for typical winter use. When the rooms were at full occupancy, they must have seemed stuffy. As you remember from chapter 5, elevated levels of carbon dioxide can make people feel drowsy. For schools, the American Society of Heating, Refrigerating, and Air-Conditioning Engineers recommends a minimum of 15 cubic feet of fresh air per minute per person, and a difference of no more than about 650 parts per million of CO_2 between the indoor and outdoor air.

Where to Go from Here?

As is often the case with indoor air quality crises, there were multiple sources of contaminants in the McKinley school and many problems to address. The consultants recommended that the carpeting be removed and replaced with a solid flooring such as tile, and "under no circumstance should carpet be installed in Room 121, 118, 117, or 116 (on the ground floor of the 1928 wing). The concrete floor slab has been found to have high moisture emission rates."[30] Other consultants recommended improving the ventilation, eliminating leaks around windows, replacing some of the drywall near the floor in classrooms at grade, and running the air conditioning in the media center during the summer to dehumidify the space. The land outside the building would have to be regraded to keep surface water away from the slab and exterior walls. Cracks in the foundation would have to be sealed to prevent water penetration. There was also leakage at the parapet wall (the upward extension of an exterior wall, usually at the perimeter of the roof) as well as elevated mold and moisture in the crawl space under the wing built in 1952.

Throughout that year school board members wondered what made more sense: to spend millions of dollars remediating the school or to tear it down and build a new one. Initially the school board asked the town for $2.5 million to clean up the mold as well as to remove asbestos floor tiles under the carpeting, with an additional $3.5 million for work required to bring the building up to code.[31] The school department hoped that two wings would be ready for school's opening day in the fall of 2001 and planned to import twelve portable classrooms to provide space while the rest of the building was being cleaned and repaired.

The $2.5 million request was approved that spring, but some people remained unsure of the correct action to take. Though she had supported the appropriation, "Board of Finance member E. Penny Hug said she still was apprehensive about approving funds for a school that might be torn down in the

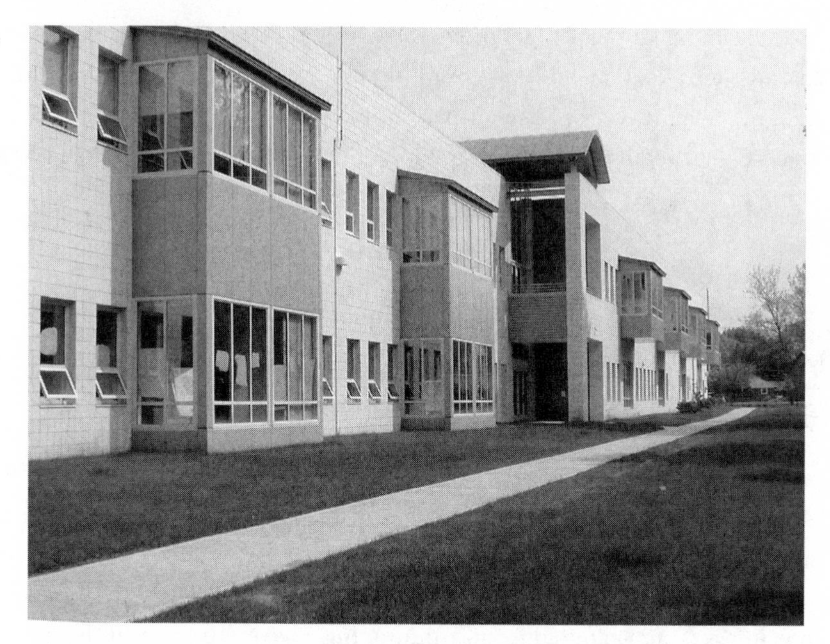

FIGURE 8.2. The new McKinley school. This is the back of the new school building. *Jeffrey C. May*

near future."[32] Partly because the extent of the cost of remediation is difficult to determine in advance, the decision was finally made to demolish rather than remediate the McKinley school and to build a new facility at a projected cost of $21 million.

McKinley parents had hoped that the school's community would be reunited in one space rather than continue to be divided up among six schools, and the school community was finally reunited in another building while the new McKinley school was under construction. For some people, however, the experience had taken a psychological as well as medical toll. Representative Town Meeting member Charlene Sabia Lebo said that many children were now afraid to go to school.[33]

The community now has a new school, but a number of people have illnesses from which they will continue to suffer for years to come. Joellen Lawson has problems with her sight and hearing and can't drive a car because of her vertigo. She has chronic fatigue and must rest every three or four hours during the day. She has almost no tolerance for VOCs in the environment, in-

Public Act 03-220, enacted in Connecticut in 2003, requires environmental assessments for proposed school-building sites, the operation of HVAC systems in accordance with existing standards, and inspection and evaluation programs for new construction or additions. The act also encourages the establishment of committees to increase awareness among staff and students about indoor air quality issues, among others.[1]

1. Connecticut General Assembly, Public Act 03-220 for Substitute House Bill 6426, www.cga.ct.gov/.

cluding fragrances and many cleaning compounds. One of her greatest losses is that she can no longer practice the profession she loves. And an illness like Joellen's doesn't belong just to her. As she has had to adjust her life, so has her husband. Their income has declined, they lead more isolated lives, he has had to take over many of the chores they used to share, and on the days when she feels particularly ill he is her caregiver.

Joellen is still an educator and a fighter, though, and her influence has spread far beyond that of many healthy people. Along with other victims of sick schools, she started a grass-roots organization called the Canary Committee.* According to the organization's mission statement, "Far too often the discovery and remediation of indoor environmental pollution does not occur until after the health of school occupants has been harmed. . . . Overall, the mission of the Canary Committee is to promote practices, policies and resources that will protect children and school personnel from harmful substances found in schools."[34] The committee was instrumental in getting air quality legislation passed nearly unanimously in the state of Connecticut after several prior efforts to get the legislation through the State Senate and House of Representatives failed. I hope that other state legislatures will take this step as well.

AN INDEPENDENT SCHOOL

A friend of mine asked me to investigate the library of an independent school in the greater Boston area. He had just been hired as the librarian, and after a

* She also founded the Connecticut Foundation for Environmentally Safe Schools (see the Resource Guide).

few months at his new job he began to feel disoriented during the day and to have headaches. Thinking that something in the indoor air was bothering him, he began keeping a window partway open, but he still felt ill when in the room and better when he was away from the library.

Under the library was the school's art room, where students worked with oil paint and other art supplies. Vapors from the paints and thinners were moving with airflows up into the library above (partly via a connecting stairway). Air flowing out the open window depressurized the library, and then even more air flowed up from the art room below. I suspect that my friend the librarian had become sensitized to the solvents.

THE ISLAND SCHOOL

Several kindergarten teachers had been experiencing headaches and complaining of odd odors in an elementary school on an island. Another indoor air quality professional had visited the site and made a number of recommendations, which had been followed. Carpets had been HEPA-vacuumed and unit ventilators had been cleaned. One teacher in particular was still feeling ill in her classroom, however, so I was asked to undertake more extensive air and dust sampling.

The vice principal, the director of maintenance, and a member of the town's Health Department met me when I arrived. When we walked into the entranceway next to the cafeteria, I was struck by a strong chlorine-like odor that permeated that part of the building. The director of maintenance told me that the kitchen area had just been washed down with diluted bleach.

The welcoming committee took me on a tour of the building, which was carpeted throughout except in the cafeteria and the gym. Like many schools, this building was constructed over a crawl space, with a newer wing for the middle school and two older wings for the younger students. The newer classrooms had a centralized ventilation system, and the older rooms had unit ventilators. Every classroom except the computer lab had a door to the exterior as well as wide windows that looked out onto fields and trees beyond. The building was one of the most pleasant, best-ventilated, and cleanest schools I have visited.

As we walked around, I could see students working in groups in the classrooms and in the library, and teachers greeted us as we moved down hallways and peeked in doors. Art projects seemed to be an important part of the curriculum, because every classroom in the lower grades had easels and shelves of paint, and art work hung on classroom and hallway walls. There was a sense of happy and productive activity throughout the building.

By the end of our tour, the school day was drawing to a close. Teachers were greeting parents who were beginning to arrive to pick up their children. Even though doors to the exterior were opening and closing, I could still smell that chlorine-like odor—strongest in the kindergarten and first- and second-grade classrooms. In one room several easels were propped up in a corner where students had just been working with finger paints. Large sheets of paint-covered paper were drying on a rack, and jars of paint were still open. In this room, the odor was overwhelming.

Holding the jar of paint a foot or so from my nose, I moved my hand over the opening at the top to push airflow in my direction. I took one whiff and my eyes watered; here was the source of the chlorine-like odor. Even though the paint was labeled nontoxic because it was water-based rather than oil-based, it contained a chemical preservative that was off-gassing irritating fumes to which students and teachers were exposed on a daily basis.

My sampling uncovered a few other problems, including a univent full of moldy dust. I also recommended that the cleaning staff avoid using chlorine bleach and ammonia in the same space at the same time (see chapter 3), and that the teachers stop using fragranced cleaning sheets to wipe down surfaces. The major culprit in the school's air quality problems, however, was the paint. Luckily, it was clear right from the start that people wanted to do all they could to take care of any air quality problems. In this school community, at least, sufferers had many advocates on their side.

AND MORE . . .

Ever since I decided to write this book, I have been collecting stories about air quality problems in school buildings. Here are a few examples.

The West Carrollton High School and Middle School in Ohio

One teacher claimed that there were leaks in her classroom and that the mold growth that ensued left her with reduced respiratory capacity, sinus infections, a cough, and memory problems. She felt better when she was away from the building. An article published in January 2002 stated that "more than half of the school's 73 teachers have complained of eye, nose and throat irritation, headaches or fatigue." And as typical with air quality problems, particularly when children are involved, the situation quickly became a crisis and accusations were flying. "In December more than 300 of the 1,140 students left classes in protest, demanding that the school administration improve conditions at the high school."[35]

A public forum was held in the school auditorium, and over three hundred concerned parents attended. A consultant reported that 62,000 cfu/gram of dust was present in the library carpet and 385,000 cfu/gram of dust in the computer room carpet. Ironically, dust from the duct supplying air to the auditorium where the meeting was held contained as much as 115,000 cfu/gram.[36] The most common genus of fungi present in the duct was *Penicillium*.

Jefferson Forest High School in Virginia

In the fall of 2000 the ceiling tiles in teacher Linda Higgins's classroom fell, and the water on the carpeted floor stood more than 2 inches deep. Trash cans were positioned throughout the room to catch rainwater. "I joked and told people I lived in the rain forest," Higgins said.[37] During that year she became so hoarse that she could no longer sing in her choir. She also lost her sense of smell and experienced headaches and fatigue. Other teachers and students reported frequent bronchitis and pneumonia.

Eventually, *Stachybotrys* mold was found in five rooms. The mold growth was fueled, people believed, by water entering through roof leaks. The school building, constructed in 1972, had a history of leaks and flooding, and the roof had been replaced three times. The school was closed early for summer vacation, and in the cleanup work that followed, all the contaminated ceiling tiles and carpeting were removed.

Battery Creek High School in South Carolina

After the ducts in the school were cleaned and sealed, Christine Callahan, who had been teaching in the building for seventeen years, suffered from "tremors, skin sensitivity, coughing, dizziness and an inability to walk properly." She sued the company that had done the cleaning, claiming that they "did not properly prepare ducts in the school before cleaning or sufficiently ventilate classrooms, used chemicals that cause health problems and did not warn Callahan and other school staff of possible injury from the chemicals."[38]

A spokesman for the school district said, "We've done everything we have been told was appropriate" and claimed that the work had been done according to EPA guidelines. A number of other teachers also experienced symptoms, however, and as a local attorney said, "It doesn't take a rocket scientist to figure out that if 14 people get sick on the same day with the same symptoms . . . something is wrong with the air."[39]

Charlotte Leslie, president of the McKinley school's PTA, said that she was "shocked to find how widespread the mold, air quality, radon and asbestos problems [in schools] are, not just in Connecticut, but nationwide. We owe

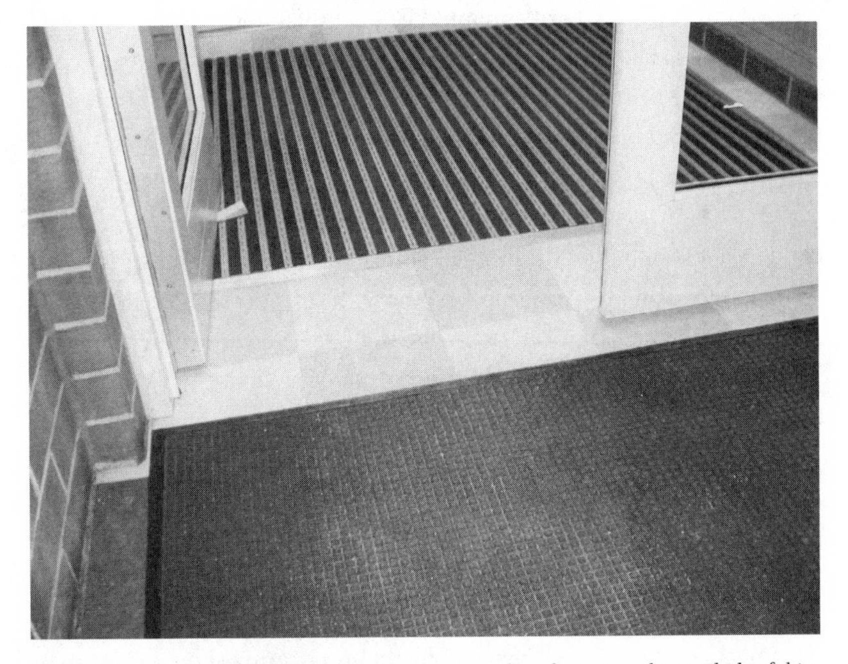

FIGURE 8.3. Elementary school entry. As students and teachers enter the vestibule of this school building (upper half of the photograph), they step across a metal walk-off grate. Then they pass into the hallway and cross a walk-off mat (bottom half of the photograph). The grate captures some of the dirt, and the mat absorbs the water from people's shoes. The pan under the grate can be cleaned and the mat can be vacuumed or periodically replaced. *Jeffrey C. May*

it to our children and their teachers and staff to be educated on this issue and to advocate on their behalf."[40] If exposures to bioaerosols could be eliminated, the concentrations of VOCs reduced, and adequate fresh air introduced, school buildings would be much healthier places for our children and their teachers.

SOME PRACTICAL STEPS

- The gaps around the piping running between crawl spaces and univents should be sealed.
- If your classroom is above a crawl space, monitor the relative humidity in the crawl space with a hygrometer (see chapter 4). If the RH is above 75 percent, mold can grow.
- Do not block univents or convector grilles with books, papers, or plants.
- All fins, coils, and grilles should be kept dust free.
- Fiberglass insulation on univent access panels is often covered with moldy dust. To minimize the spread of contaminants, this insulation should be cleaned (outside or in an isolated, unoccupied space inside) or replaced with foil-faced insulation or with foam insulation that has a cleanable, nonporous surface.
- Surfaces should not be cleaned with sour-smelling or musty sponges or mops (see chapter 3) or with strongly scented products.
- Carpeting must not be cleaned by wet methods unless the carpeting will be thoroughly dry within twenty-four to forty-eight hours.
- Children should not enter a school building directly onto permanently installed carpeting. A replaceable mat can be placed on top of or used instead of carpeting at entranceways.
- If dry carpeting in a space seems to be the source of an indoor air quality problem and removal is not an immediate option, the floor can be temporarily covered with 4- by 8-foot sheets of a stiff material that can be joined at the seams. This covering should be nonslip and splinter free and should not off-gas. The carpet can also be temporarily covered with adhesive-backed polyethylene, sold to painting and other contractors and available in rolls of different widths.

- If you are concerned about a particular carpet, get a vacuum dust sample and send it off to a lab for microbial analysis (see the Resource Guide and part III).
- Have plumbing and roof leaks repaired and moldy ceiling tiles replaced as quickly as possible (see chapter 7).
- It is not a good idea to keep a pet in the classroom if any of the students are allergic to that animal.
- Refer to the EPA's "Tools for Schools" for an overall indoor air quality plan for schools (see the Resource Guide).

CHAPTER

9

Nine to Five

Where We Work

Tinted glass clads the exterior of many office buildings. On a sunny day the glass reflects the sky and the walls of adjacent buildings; in twilight the glass allows us to peer inside the building. We have the visual impression that these massive structures are part of the sky—light and airy. Little could be further from the truth. Such buildings are sealed from the world, and the occupants within may suffer from a lack of fresh air—the air that is just on the other side of their inoperable windows.

VENTILATION FRUSTRATION

David Bearg, a Professional Engineer and Certified Industrial Hygienist, joined me to investigate the offices of a company that occupied two floors in a seventeen-floor building less than ten years old. The chief executive officer (CEO) was experiencing allergy problems in his expansive office. Other employees complained of minor symptoms of sick-building syndrome (SBS; see chapter 1), particularly in the conference room at the perimeter of the building.

This building had about fifteen heat pumps per floor, mounted in the ceiling plenum. Because it was difficult to tell where each heat pump was located, not all had been properly maintained: the coils and some of the filters were soiled, and some units had no filters at all.

There was a mechanical room on the roof with a boiler and a preheater for the fresh air supplied by a blower to every floor. The fresh air was divided into four equal flows and directed through vertical ducts at each corner of the rec-

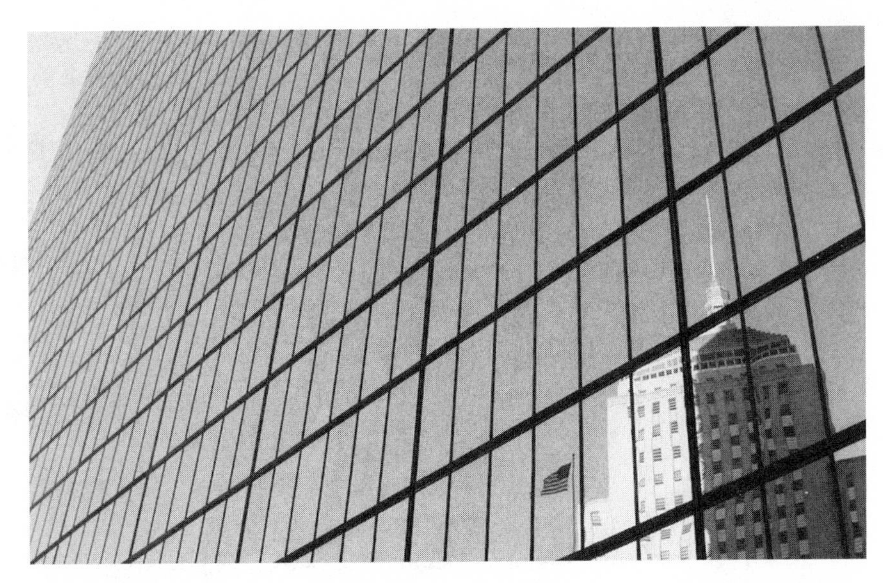

FIGURE 9.1. Reflections. The glass facade of Hancock Tower in Boston reflects a neighboring building. *Jeffrey C. May*

tangular building. A branch of the duct system (called a *T*) supplied fresh air to the plenum on each floor.

I set up a ladder on the fourth floor, removed a ceiling tile, and looked into the plenum toward an exterior wall where the CEO's office was located. As I expected, I could see that the drywall at the exterior perimeter wall extended all the way up to the steel decking above the plenum. But I could also see that the partition walls for the CEO's office also extended all the way up to the steel decking. His ceiling plenum was therefore completely isolated (disconnected) from the rest of the plenum space, except for some small gaps around cables and the supply ducts that passed through the upper part of those partition walls.

The heat pump that supplied heated and cooled air to the CEO's office was not located in the plenum above that room. As the heat pump operated to supply conditioned air to his office, it was removing air from the plenum above the rest of the offices on that floor but not air from his isolated plenum. As a result, there was little difference in air pressure between his ceiling plenum and his office; thus airflows from the office up into the plenum were minimal. Since little air was being removed, not much entered, and the room seemed stuffy. The same situation existed in the conference room where meetings were held, and where many people were breathing in oxygen (O_2) and exhaling carbon dioxide (CO_2). It is no surprise that people felt lethargic during long meetings (and not because the discussions were dull!).

We also found elevated levels of CO_2 throughout both floors of the office building occupied by this company. On workdays in this building, the concentration was low in the morning before people arrived (around 550 parts per million) but still greater than the concentration outside (360 ppm), indicating that the building hadn't been adequately ventilated overnight. As the workday wore on, the CO_2 concentrations indoors rose. Around 4:00 P.M., as people started leaving for the day, these concentrations peaked at about 1,200 ppm. This is far from being an unsafe level of carbon dioxide; still, air containing such levels of CO_2 can seem stuffy. (ASHRAE recommends that carbon dioxide concentrations in offices should not exceed the outdoor concentration by more than about 500 ppm.)

The carbon dioxide levels in this building fell to the outside concentration only at the end of the weekend, when the building had been unoccupied for two days. Bearg's data suggested that fresh air was being supplied to the offices at a rate of about 13 cubic feet per minute per person—not bad compared with many other buildings, but still less than ASHRAE's suggested 20 cfm (see chapter 7).

We recommended that fresh air be carried by ducts from the corner supplies to within a few feet of each of the heat pumps, and that openings be created in the partition walls in the ceiling plenum above the CEO's office and the conference room, to allow communication (airflow) throughout the ceiling plenum on that level. We also suggested that some of the heat pumps be operated in the fan-on position rather than the fan-auto position. In the *fan-auto* position, fresh air is distributed only when heating or cooling is called for by the thermostat; otherwise, the heat pump blower is off. In the *fan-on* position, the blower runs continuously, not only providing hot or cool air as needed but also constantly providing some outdoor air.

Fan On versus Fan Auto

It is common in many office buildings for fresh air to be supplied through the ductwork only when the blower is operating to supply heated or cooled air, though in more sophisticated HVAC systems, fresh air is supplied continuously (see chapter 7). In one building I investigated, in which occupants were complaining that the air seemed stuffy, I was amazed by the difference it made to run the fan all the time.

The offices in question were on the same level as the mechanical room, which in turn was open to the ceiling plenum. An open-ended duct in the mechanical room wall, located at the level of the plenum, supplied a strong flow of fresh air from the roof. The return for the system was located at the base of the fan coil. The fan switch was in the auto-fan position rather than fan-on position, and the building suffered from inadequate ventilation during the fall and spring, when heated or cooled air was not needed and thus fresh air not distributed.

I visited the site in the spring and found the air stale. I was standing in a room with four other people and suggested that they allow me to flip the fan switch on the thermostat from the auto-fan to the fan-on position. I went to the mechanical closet to see if the blower was operating. By the time I returned to the room where the four employees were waiting for me, everyone was smiling in relief to be breathing the fresh air. (Continuously operating the blower may require supplemental dehumidification during the cooling season, because as condensed moisture on the cooling coils is reevaporated into the airflow, the relative humidity rises. This can lead to mildew problems.)

Air in the Bathroom: Good and Bad

Another interesting problem turned up outside a men's room in one of the corners of the building David Bearg and I investigated. Fresh air was dumped into the ceiling plenum near the bathroom. Ordinarily this air would have been distributed to a number of rooms, but in this case the bathroom was receiving most of the fresh air.

The bathroom exhaust pulled air out of the bathroom, lowering the pressure in that room. Air then flowed from the hallway through gaps around the door, lowering the pressure in the hallway. Normally the air pressure in a ceiling plenum is lower than the air pressure in the rooms below, because air is being drawn into the heat pump returns. In this case, though, there was so much fresh air being supplied to that corner of the plenum that the air pressure was greater in the plenum than in the hallway, particularly since air was flowing from the hallway into the bathroom (because of the bathroom exhaust). Some of the fresh air was therefore being short-circuited (moving through the more direct route) into the hallway and from there into the bathroom, rather than being distributed to other rooms. The fresh air was then being exhausted to the outside. The air quality in the hallway outside the men's room was probably the best on the floor!

Air flowing *from* a bathroom into an adjoining space because of pressure differences caused an unpleasant problem in a 150-year-old six-story brick building that had been converted from an abandoned factory into high-end office space. In view of the historical significance of the building, the original windows were all replaced with new operable sash windows with insulated glass, rather than with "decorative windows" that do not open. The developers assumed that people would open windows for fresh air, so no provisions were made in the mechanical system for bringing fresh air into the building. The windows were left open in the summer, but in the winter they remained closed.

I was asked to investigate because some employees on the fourth floor were complaining about a nauseating odor that appeared briefly at the start of each workday. Some people seemed even to be suffering from SBS symptoms. A number of them had formed an "air team" that distributed questionnaires to all the workers in the office to see what symptoms they were having and with what frequency. Headaches and fatigue were very common, as well as eye and throat irritation toward the end of the day. In addition, most mentioned that they had colds and bronchitis more frequently. One employee had no complaints, but she worked mostly off-site. Everyone else who filled out the questionnaire agreed that within hours of leaving the building, they felt better.

Most of the workers' symptoms were typical for buildings with inadequate ventilation. After the investigation, people started to open windows. The nauseating odor on the fourth floor, however, was present for another reason. The bathrooms in the building were equipped with heat supplies and exhaust fans, except the bathroom on the fourth floor, which had a supply but no exhaust fan. In consequence, the air pressure in the fourth-floor bathroom was higher than the air pressure in the adjacent workspace. Whenever the bathroom was used (and the use was heaviest first thing in the morning), odors moved with airflows through the louvers in the door from the higher air pressure (bathroom) to the lower air pressure (adjacent workspace).

To solve a number of problems in the building, I recommended that a ventilation system that could warm air in winter and dehumidify it in the summer be installed to introduce fresh air, that media filters be installed on the existing rooftop units, and that the fourth-floor bathroom be connected to the exhaust system.

A similar problem occurred in another office when several employees were eating lunch in a meeting room, and three of them suddenly began to feel nauseated. One of the three also experienced a tingling sensation. The fan coil and the large return grille for that part of the building were located in the ceiling plenum directly outside the bathroom door. The return lowered the air pressure outside the bathroom door. Once again, the air pressure in the bathroom was greater than the pressure outside the room, and air flowed from the bathroom into the adjacent space and then into the ceiling plenum return. From there, it went into the lunch room through the supply ducts.

There was an air freshener spray in the bathroom, and someone must have used it a little more liberally than usual during the lunch hour. Bathroom odors and volatile organic compounds (VOCs) from the air freshener were rapidly distributed by the mechanical system into the lunch room, causing the people's symptoms.

THE COSTLY CROWN JEWEL

The $170 million Ruggles Center project is an example of the effect an indoor air quality crisis can have on an entire community. The center—intended to be the crown jewel in the redevelopment of Roxbury, Massachusetts—was to consist of a hotel, a parking garage, and three office buildings, one of which would be occupied by the Massachusetts Registry of Motor Vehicles (RMV). In May 1991 a ceremony was held in front of the newly built Ruggles subway station to celebrate the start of the project. Governor William Weld, who had signed the bill moving the RMV to the Ruggles Center, delivered a speech. "This is an area that desperately needs investment," he said. "The . . . project will bring . . . 2,000 construction and 3,000 nonconstruction jobs . . . [to] a long underdeveloped area of the city."[1] Potential lenders questioned whether the center would attract tenants, however, so the developers had some difficulty financing the project. Finally, the Bank of Boston rose to the occasion and provided $26 million for the first phase.

Construction started in June 1991, and in April 1994 the first building was completed: the nine-story 157,000-square-foot facility that would house a single tenant, the state-of-the-art Registry of Motor Vehicles. In a portent of what was to come, on the RMV's first day of occupancy most of the over six hundred employees lost the use of their computers and telephones because a contractor who was installing computer lines accidentally disabled a phone cable. But the communication problems and frustrations experienced on opening day paled in comparison with the events that followed.

In the first week of June a number of Registry employees, most of whom worked on the fourth floor, began to complain of nausea, skin irritation, and itchiness. A consultant, the first of a parade of about fifty to be brought into the building, noted that inadequate ventilation at a printer on the fourth floor might be causing the SBS symptoms. At about the same time, employees noticed moisture dripping from ceiling tiles and a sweat-sock odor in some parts of the building. By mid-July eighteen more employees had fallen ill, and the union was calling for evacuation of the barely four-month-old building. Registrar Gerald A. Gnazzo said that the problems had not begun until May, when the heat pumps were first used for cooling. An RMV spokesman, Aubrey Haznar, commented, "The building is safe. You just have this permeating smell which causes people to get sick to their stomach."[2]

In mid-July 1994 the Registry hired a full-time nurse and physician to take care of the mounting numbers of people falling ill inside the building. Within weeks the nurse, Ann Zaia, had become ill herself. "My chest felt tight and I had severe shortness of breath," she said. "It felt just like an elephant was sitting on my chest."[3] They moved her into a trailer in the parking lot, where she continued to see sick employees (up to 120 people a day). She herself felt better a week after she vacated the building.

Employees continued to work in the building while the union complained that Registry officials were being indifferent to unbearable conditions. By the end of June over two hundred people had lost work time to go home sick or to go to the hospital. The *Boston Globe* reported that "Registry employees became accustomed to ambulances pulling up to the entrance to cart away ill colleagues."[4]

At the time, the majority of Roxbury's residents were African-American, and when the events at the Ruggles Center first began to unfold, some peo-

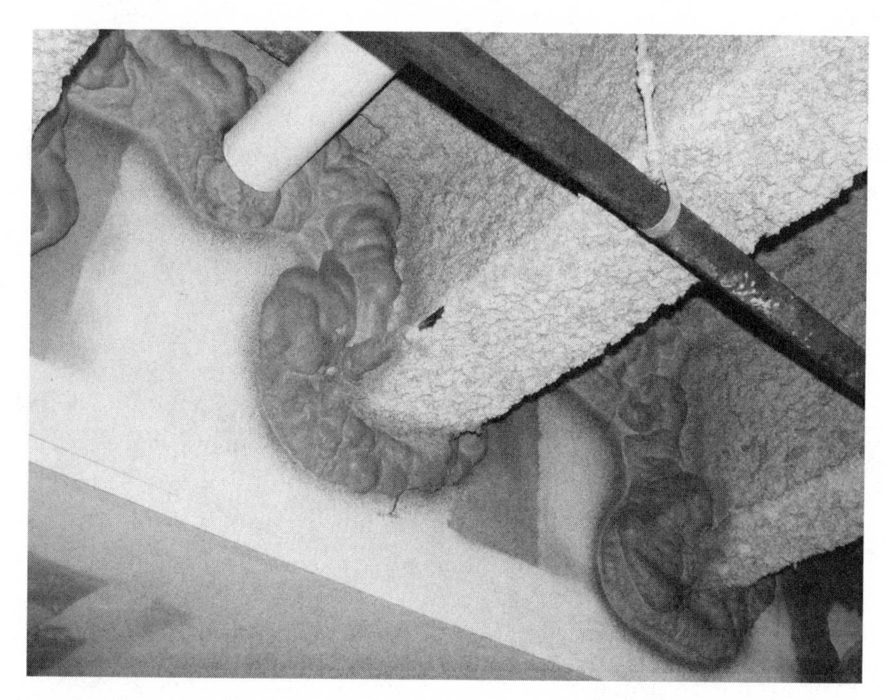

FIGURE 9.2. Various types of insulation. Three different types of insulation appear in this photograph. The steel beam in the middle is coated with sprayed-on fibrous insulation, which is gray and looks fuzzy. The pipe in the upper left-hand corner is wrapped in fiberglass insulation, coated with white paper. The lumpy material that snakes around the end of the pipe and beam is a sprayed-on foam insulation, applied to seal air gaps. On the bottom of the steel beam is a small dark spot where some of the insulation has fallen off. When chunks of insulation hit the floor, they can crumble from the impact as well as from foot traffic and then release irritating aerosol. *Jeffrey C. May*

ple suspected that racism was fueling the complaints—that some of the workers were "feigning illness because they resented relocating to a minority neighborhood."[5] But as the months went by and more and more employees complained of symptoms, many became fearful about working in the building, including those who were not ill.

Between 1994 and 1995 over $14 million was spent to determine and eliminate the causes of the air quality problems in the Ruggles Center. Because skin irritation was a common symptom, suspicion was initially focused on the mineral wool fireproofing that had been sprayed onto the steel structure in the ceiling plenum. The building owner claimed that cable installers hired by the Registry had loosened the insulation. Others accused the developers of trying to cut costs by omitting a key step in the application of the fireproofing: spraying the insulation with a sealant that would have prevented the release of fibers. Whatever the cause, fibers from the fireproofing were found on the backside of the drop ceiling tiles as well as in the dust on desk surfaces in office spaces below.

What else was wrong with the building? Some consultants thought that the ventilation system was at fault. A rooftop unit took in fresh air and blew it down a vertical duct in the core of the building. The duct was open to the ceiling plenum of each floor. This fresh air flowing into each plenum may have disturbed the insulation. In addition, whenever fresh air is dumped at one location (such as the center of a ceiling plenum), there is no way to be certain that it will be distributed to all of the heat pumps, some of which may be remote from the fresh air supply. In such cases there may be areas with inadequate fresh air. There may be no odors present, but the air will seem stale. (The original building plans had specified that ducts be installed to provide fresh air to the individual heat pumps, but those ducts were eliminated to save money.)[6] And at the Ruggles Center that spring and early summer, the fresh air from the rooftop unit was not dehumidified or cooled, yet the plenum was cooled by the building's air conditioning. Moisture from the warm spring air may have condensed in the cold plenum, fueling microbial growth.

There were other sources of moisture for mold and bacterial growth. Some of the heat pump units suspended in the ceiling plenum had been incorrectly pitched, so the condensate pans didn't drain as intended. Water therefore overflowed and dripped out of these units and onto the ceiling tiles. Once the angles of these heat pumps were adjusted, the dripping ceased. Although very little microbial growth was observed on the coils within the heat pumps, I believe that the most likely source of the sweat-sock odor noted by some of the workers was the growth of bacteria and yeast in moist dust on the coils. The ceiling tiles, which emitted the characteristic sickening smell of butyric acid due to bacterial growth, represented another source of odor.

In July 1995, little more than a year after the building had opened, a NIOSH representative said that the Registry of Motor Vehicles was "one of the worst buildings we have ever encountered."[7] In July 1996, representatives of the workers' union sued to have the building closed. The Department of Health ultimately issued an order to vacate the building, and fifteen months after moving into the Ruggles Center, the RMV moved most of its employees back to its cramped old quarters in downtown Boston. Once workers were out of the building, most of their symptoms disappeared, though some who were diagnosed with occupational asthma may remain permanently afflicted by this illness. The state terminated its lease during the summer of 1996. The building owners could not pay their mortgage, and the bank foreclosed that fall. Soon afterward the entire parcel went up for auction and was purchased by Northeastern University for $17 million.

After foreclosure and before Northeastern purchased the building, the heat pumps were cleaned, the crumbling insulation and suspended ceiling tiles were removed, and the carpets were replaced. Rather than fresh air being randomly dumped into the ceiling plenum, the air was piped directly to the returns of the heat pumps through ducts that connected to the vertical supply shaft. The fresh air then mixed with the rest of the supply air from each heat pump and was more evenly apportioned to every diffuser. These steps not only improved the distribution of fresh air but also prevented the disturbance of the insulation.

The building is now occupied, and as far as I know there have been no indoor air quality problems.[8] But the planned hotel and other two office towers
were never built. The failure of the development project was a financial blo
to the Roxbury community and put an end to some of the dreams for t
neighborhood's redevelopment. As Michael Grunwald wrote in the *Bos*
Globe, "There was nothing wrong with Roxbury; the problems were inside
building, where defectively maintained fireproofing was making workers
every day."[9]

As so often happens in such cases, the indoor air quality crisis at R
provoked social, political, and psychological turmoil. The developers
representatives, contractors, subcontractors, and employees becam
up in a blame game and mired in negotiations over who was finan
sponsible for the debacle. And the ongoing litigation prevented th
semination of the lessons learned: if IAQ investigators, scientists,
chitects, HVAC designers, and building managers are to prev
problems from occurring in other buildings, they need to under
thing that went wrong at the Ruggles Center.

TAXING WORK IN THE REVENUE OFFICES

In an attempt to better understand the relationship between respiratory illness and mold growth indoors, NIOSH studied a number of buildings where there was a high rate of building-related illness (BRI). The Connecticut Department of Revenue Services in Hartford fit the criteria.

A number of workers in the building were reporting symptoms such as coughing, burning eyes, and respiratory discomfort. Kim Harris was one of them. When she first moved into her new workspace, Kim experienced headaches and felt dizzy. Soon she was coughing and wheezing. Diagnosed with asthma, she became unable to work and had to depend on workmen's compensation. Her income dropped so drastically that she was forced to move her family of four into a one-bedroom apartment.[10] Soon after moving into her seventeenth-floor office, another employee, Arlyce Walker, began to experience a sore throat as well as a burning sensation in her mouth when she ate certain foods. Some days she even lost her voice. She was diagnosed with *sarcoidosis,* an inflammatory lung disease. Dr. Eileen Storey, director of the Center for Indoor Environments and Health at the University of Connecticut Health Center, commented that sarcoidosis "traditionally . . . has not been thought of as an environmental disease, but in the last 10 years, there is increasing evidence that it is allergic."[11] Dr. Storey's clinic ended up treating approximately a hundred people who worked in the building.

The building had a history of problems with rainwater penetration, resulting in damp walls and carpeting. The concentrations of mold and bacteria in preliminary air and dust samples taken in the building raised some concern.

As we have seen, in some sick office buildings, the impact on workers' health can be significant. In one such office building with water-intrusion and mold problems, NIOSH researchers, as well as other scientists, found that both the rate of adult-onset asthma and the rate of relief from sick-building symptoms away from work were more than three times higher than in the general population. A survey of 247 people revealed that respiratory symptoms accounted for one-third of the sick days taken.[1]

1. J. Cox-Ganser et al., "Respiratory Morbidity in Office Workers in a Water-Damaged Building," *Environmental Health Perspectives* 113 (April 2005): 485–90.

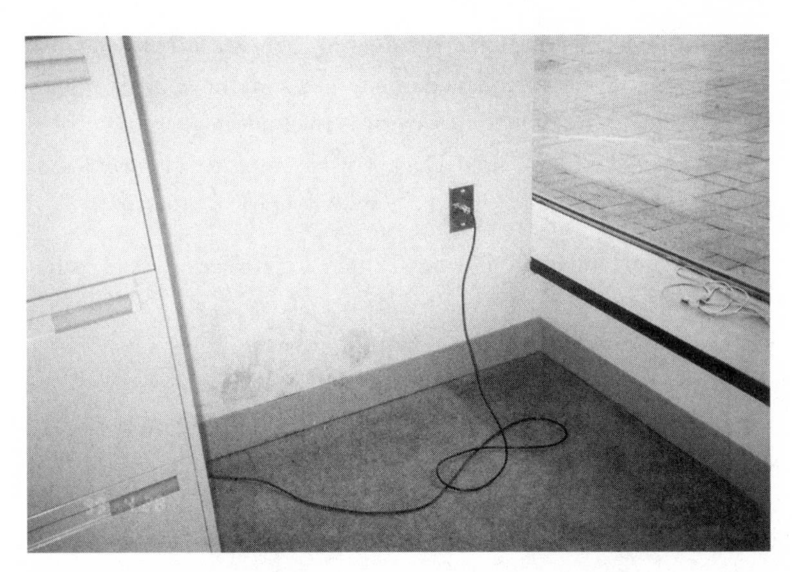

FIGURE 9.3. Office asthma files. This photograph isn't very dramatic, but this small corner in a large office space exacerbated the asthma symptoms of two employees who worked at nearby desks. In the upper right-hand corner is a large glass panel looking out over an outdoor patio. Water leaked in at the bottom of the panel and soaked into the carpet and drywall, leading to mildew growth (not visible in the carpet but visible as splotches on the lower portion of the wall). Foot traffic disturbed mildew growing in the carpet dust, and spores were aerosolized. Two filing cabinets were concealing the wall mildew, which was discovered only when the cabinets were moved.
May Indoor Air Investigations LLC

On the other hand, T. R. Anson, the state public works commissioner in charge of maintaining state buildings, acknowledged the building's moisture problems but did not believe that microbial growth was necessarily the cause of the BRIs. "We know the air inside that building is better than the air outside the facility," he said.[12]

Again: disagreements, denials, and turmoil while building occupants continued to suffer.

CARPETING CATASTROPHE

Built in 1970, with additions constructed in the 1980s, the Waterside Mall complex in Washington, D.C., was home to the United States Environmental Protection Agency, an organization that almost quadrupled in size during its first twenty-five years of occupancy. A major renovation was undertaken in

1987, during which nearly 30,000 square yards of new carpeting was installed. About sixty employees complained of chronic symptoms, including a handful who ultimately could no longer work in the building because of chemical sensitivity. The EPA commissioned an extensive employee survey. Here are excerpts from some of the histories the employees provided:

> *History #5:* On January 20th, 1988, I entered my office at 7 A.M. and noticed a strong acrid smell from the carpet that had been installed with adhesive the previous afternoon. Within fifteen minutes, my eyes, face, ear canals, and lungs were burning. My voice became hoarse and disappeared and I had great difficulty breathing. I was disoriented and dizzy. My eyes and nose were running. . . . I left the building and stayed away for a number of days until I felt somewhat better. My doctor said that I had a severe allergic-type reaction to the carpet fumes.
>
> *History #7:* In May 1988 I went to a person's office in the basement of the East Tower to give research assistance. The office had been carpeted in January. Within minutes, hives started to break out on my fingers and arm.
>
> *History #8:* When my work area was recarpeted in early 1988 I experienced severe headache, body weakness and pain, and eye and throat irritation. My symptoms are specific to Waterside Mall.
>
> *History #9:* At 4:30 P.M. on Friday, April 22nd, 1988, EPA removed the old rugs from my office 932B in the East Tower and replaced them with new ones. . . . I returned to work at 6 A.M. on the following Monday. I had sustained a very severe headache by 3:30 and went home. The headache ameliorated over the evening. I went to work at 6 A.M. on Tuesday and by noon the headache had returned, my throat had swelled, I had difficulty breathing and was dizzy and light-headed. I had shortness of breath, my voice became hoarse, and my eyes were red and irritated.
>
> *History #14:* My branch's office is on the third floor of the Mall at Waterside. The office was remodeled and new carpets were installed during Winter 1987–1988. We moved back to our office in January 1988. There was a noticeable odor in the office. We tried to vent the office by leaving the corridor doors open and running fans for a couple of weeks.

The odor lasted for over six months. Around the corner fifty yards from our office, a sensitive person who is not in our branch had to leave her office because of the emissions coming from our remodeled space. Throughout the first half of 1988, five out of the seven people in my branch complained of headaches and throat and eye irritations. . . . I have not reported my health problems to EPA's Health Unit because I am uneasy about my anonymity being preserved.[13]

The building had had air quality problems in the past, most likely associated with the inadequate supply of fresh air combined with typical VOC emissions from office equipment, maintenance chemicals, and the like. (The design ventilation rate was for about 5 cubic feet of air per minute per person, rather than today's ASHRAE guideline of 20 cfm/person, and the building was heavily populated.)

Still, some people argued that the symptoms were psychogenic. In response to the complaints, the Carpet and Rug Institute funded a literature review of 350 technical articles about chemicals in carpet emissions. Alan Hedge, professor of design and environmental analysis at Cornell University, and Rodney R. Dietert, director of the Institute for Comparative and Environmental Toxicology, undertook this review and produced a 156-page report. Hedge commented that anxiety could be fueling people's ailments: "Many people who report symptoms may unknowingly be responding to odors they believe are related to toxicity; once one feels threatened by a strong odor, the increased anxiety may result in hyperventilation, nausea and dizziness. Concerns about toxic exposures may also lead to headache, weakness, vomiting and burning in the throat and eyes, all symptoms associated with SBS and IAQ. Such cases of mass psychogenic illness are well documented in the medical literature."[14]

A lot of money was at stake. In 2003 the carpet industry installed almost 2 billion square yards of carpeting.[15] Carpet mills generate about $12 billion of wholesale volume a year, and carpet retail businesses probably generate more than twice that amount. It is understandable, therefore, that the carpet industry was concerned about allegations that carpeting was causing health problems at the Waterside Mall and invested resources in proving otherwise.

Millions of people live and work symptom free in spaces with wall-to-wall carpeting. Nevertheless, many people claimed that chemicals off-gassing from carpeting were the source of the air quality problems in the Waterside Mall. The chemical 4-phenylcyclohexene (4-PC) is often the major VOC emitted from carpeting, as I discussed in chapter 3. After installation of new carpeting, air concentrations of 4-PC in buildings typically range from 0.3 to 2.6 parts per billion or 2 to 17 micrograms per cubic meter. During an industrial hygiene survey of the Waterside Mall EPA headquarters in areas where new carpeting had been installed, concentrations of 0.9 ppb (6 mcg/m^3) were found in the offices and 1.5 ppb (9.7 mcg/m^3) in the mall area. And it was estimated that at the time of installation, the concentrations might have been five to ten times higher. (The reported odor threshold for 4-PC is 0.3 ppb, or 2 mcg/m^3, so people would have been able to smell the chemical at the con-

One measure of the toxicity of a chemical is its LD_{50}, the lethal dose at which 50 percent of exposed research animals would die. One of the most famous experiments to measure the effect of carpet emissions on animals was done by Rosalind Anderson of the former Anderson Laboratories in Dedham, Massachusetts. Utilizing ASTM Method E981 (a method for testing the toxicity of chemicals on mice), she exposed mice to an airstream that contained fumes from a sample of heated carpet that was considered "toxic."[1] Approximately a quarter of the mice died, while others exhibited neurotoxic effects.[2]

Dr. Yves Alarie, who devised ASTM Method E981, obtained similar results, but other laboratories were unable to reproduce them (in one case, probably because air from the carpet was bubbled through water and thus "filtered" before entering the mouse chamber), so Anderson's work was discredited. Some people even claimed that the mice had died because they choked in their restraints.

To determine the LD_{50} of 4-PC, another scientist exposed rats for six hours to 60 ppm (400 mg/m^3) of the chemical, levels more than a thousand times greater than the mathematically estimated levels of airborne 4-PC in the newly carpeted areas of the Waterside Mall.[3] The LD_{50} could not be determined from this test (a 50 percent mortality rate among the rats was not reached), and so concerns about toxicity at the mall were discounted.

1. J. Waytiuk, "Piling It On: Are Your Carpets Harboring Health Hazards?" *Green Living Eco-Home* 8 (March–April 1997), www.emagazine.com.

2. R. Anderson, "Toxic Emissions from Carpets," in *Proceedings of Indoor Air 1993, the 6th International Conference on Indoor Air Quality and Climate,* Helsinki, Finland, 4–8 July 1993, 1:651–56.

3. K. Haneke, *4-Phenylcyclohexene, Review of Toxicological Literature* (Research Triangle Park, N.C.: Prepared by Integrated Laboratory Systems for the National Institute of Environmental Health Sciences, July 2002), iv.

In my opinion, the major issue with new carpeting is not toxicity but rather a hypersensitivity to a chemical or chemicals. For comparison, consider the allergic hypersensitivity to peanuts. Millions of people eat peanuts without any problem, but a few out of every thousand people can eat a single peanut and die. We don't consider peanuts to be toxic, however, and they are not. Nonetheless, in schools where peanut-allergic children are present, peanuts and foods made with peanuts are often banned.

centrations measured.)[16] Still, none of the chemical emissions were toxic per se, nor were the concentrations at the mall at a toxic level.

It seems clear, nonetheless, that many of the most serious symptoms experienced by EPA employees began with the installation of the carpeting. Ultimately, after the EPA replaced all of the styrene-butadiene-backed ("latex"-backed) carpeting with urethane-backed material, most of the complaints disappeared. (Each time I have encountered situations in which people began to suffer symptoms soon after carpeting was installed, in every case they felt better after the offending carpeting was removed.)

The carpet industry has taken concerns about toxicity very seriously and has instituted a "green label" testing program. To meet the criteria for a green label, carpets are tested by an independent laboratory and must have low emission rates for 4-PC, styrene, and formaldehyde.[17] (Unfortunately, few individual carpets are actually tested, and off-gassing can vary from batch to batch.) Most carpeting today has significantly lower VOC emissions than carpets installed in the 1980s, but some people still complain that "new-carpet smell" makes them experience sick-building symptoms.

SOME PRACTICAL STEPS

- Carpeting should be chosen very carefully. It is best to avoid styrene-butadiene ("latex") backing as well as adhesives with high emission rates of VOCs.
- Use the foil test (described at the end of chapter 3 under "Some Practical Steps") if you suspect that a surface in your office might be off-gassing.

- If bathroom or sewer gas odors are a problem, check to see that there is water in the waste-line traps, that toilet seals are tight (no toilet should be loose; see chapter 3), that every bathroom has an exhaust, and that air is flowing from the surrounding space into the bathroom rather than vice versa.
- If you are sensitive to mold, avoid working in a carpeted below-grade space. If working elsewhere is not an option for you, be sure that the space is consistently heated (to at least 64°F in the colder months) and dehumidified (no more than 50 to 60 percent relative humidity in the warmer months).
- There should be no visible mold in the workspace.

CHAPTER

10

Infirm Infirmaries and Coughing Courthouses

Since the terrorist attacks of September 11, 2001, Americans have a renewed respect not only for those who serve our country in the armed forces but also for those who serve the public on the home front. Firefighters battle flames, police officers subdue armed suspects, and doctors and nurses work around the clock to treat the sick and injured. Those who dedicate their lives to helping others face danger and crises every day. They should not also have to deal with poor indoor air quality, a more insidious and often unrecognized threat.

HOSPITALS

All medical facilities should be vigilant about the quality of indoor air, but hospitals face a special challenge. Most office buildings and schools are used only during business hours, and most of the people within are healthy. Hospitals, however, are heavily used around the clock, and they treat people who are ill and thus potentially more susceptible to indoor contaminants. And sometimes, unfortunately, the doctors and nurses who are supplying the cures become victims of poor hospital air quality.

Disinfectants and Sterilizing Agents

Because of the need to minimize the presence of pathogenic organisms in medical care facilities, disinfectants and sterilizing agents are an invariable part of the environment. Glutaraldehyde, a disinfectant also used in developing X-ray film, is an irritating liquid very likely to cause allergic sensitization.

Ethylene oxide (C_2H_4O), a sterilizing agent used in many hospitals, is a carcinogenic gas that may be associated with increased risk of spontaneous abortion (miscarriage).[1] Disinfectants and sterilizing agents are lethal to cells, because they combine chemically and irreversibly with essential components of either cell metabolism (such as enzymes) or cell replication (such as DNA)—bad for bacteria, but not so great for us, either. Even the residues of sterilizing gases found in the treated gowns of operating room staff can cause symptoms and skin rashes. When sterilizing agents and disinfectants are used, excess gas must be vented directly to the roof or to an area where the gas cannot be inhaled or entrained (carried back into the building on airflows).

The air pressure in operating rooms and other treatment areas is usually higher than the air pressure in adjacent rooms, to prevent the infiltration of air that might contain pathogenic microorganisms like bacteria and viruses. This pressure differential, however, may cause the spread of operating room

Over the course of approximately three years in a Veterans' Hospital in Denver, six chemotherapy patients, whose immune systems were suppressed, acquired fungal infections caused by *Aspergillus* mold.[1] The source of the illness was identified when the same species of *Aspergillus* mold found in the patients' lungs was also found growing in a crawl space under the hospital. As a result of the stack effect (see chapter 4), air from the crawl space was entering the elevator shaft. Hospital officials hypothesized that air exiting the elevator shaft and flowing into the hospital wards was carrying spores from the mold found in the crawl space soil. In other cases of nosocomial (hospital-induced) aspergillosis in bone-marrow transplant units, the source of the *Aspergillus* spores was traced to hospital showers. Unlike people whose immune systems are compromised by chemotherapy or disease, people with healthy immune systems can breathe in *Aspergillus* spores every day and never become infected.

1. A. Imse, "VA Cites Cleanliness Problem at Hospital, Officials Say Fungal Infections May Be Linked to Dirt Floor," *Rocky Mountain News*, 30 December 2004.

Over 200 of the 541 members of a hospital cleaning department in Denmark had occupational skin disease at some point in their employment. Allergic contact dermatitis was often due to contact with sterilizing agents such as glutaraldehyde and formaldehyde. Causes of irritant dermatitis included contact with detergents and bleach.[1]

1. K. Hansen, "Occupational Dermatoses in Hospital Cleaning Women," *Contact Dermatitis* 9 (September 1983): 343–51.

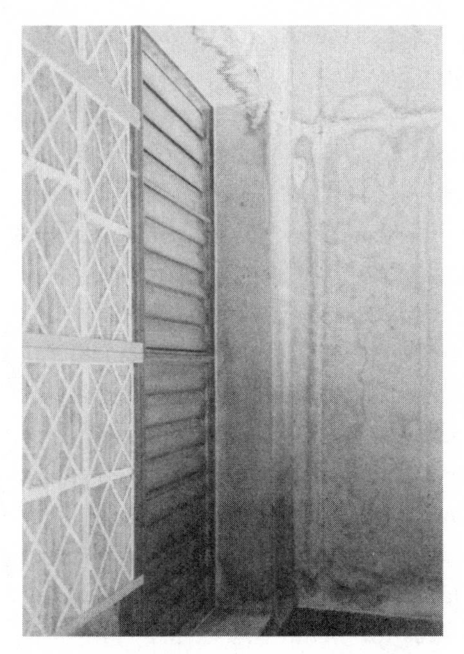

FIGURE 10.1. Moldy air-intake plenum. This air-intake plenum, part of a hospital's ventilation system, is located in a rooftop mechanical "penthouse." To the right (not visible in the photograph) is a louvered opening through which sunlight and fresh air are streaming in. Visible at the left is a bank of filters placed in front of preheat coils that help keep the coils clean. The motorized bypass dampers (metal louvers in the wall, adjacent to the filters) open when there is no need to preheat the air. The penthouse roof leaked, and snow and rain were sucked in through the open louvers. Water stains and mold growth are visible on the drywall in the right half of the photograph. One hopes that the downstream prefilters and filters in the air handler (not visible in the photograph) remove aerosolized mold spores and hyphae before the air enters the hospital.
Wagdy Anis AIA, SBRA Consulting

gases (including sterilizing agents and vapors from disinfectants) from treatment areas into adjacent rooms.

Medical facilities are cleaned more frequently than any other type of building. Because cleaning agents can produce VOCs from the fragrances or solvents they contain, only unscented or low-VOC-emitting products should be used (see chapter 3). Renovation work, which generates dust and an offgassing of solvents from adhesives and paints, often takes place while hospital spaces are occupied—when, after all, are they not? (See the Resource Guide for a reference on renovating hospitals.) Bioaerosol can also be present if there are conditions conducive to microbial growth in carpeting or HVAC equipment. And ventilation is of the utmost importance in medical facilities. The exhaust vents and intake vents should be far enough away from each other to avoid re-entrainment.

Latex Allergy

Latex gloves are made from rubber that is derived from rubber tree sap, which contains protein allergens that adhere to the latex in the finished gloves. When someone is wearing latex gloves, skin on the hand is in constant contact with the allergens. In addition, latex gloves are dusted on the inside with cornstarch ("donning powder"), making it easier to slide the sticky gloves on. The latex allergens from the glove surface coat the microscopic cornstarch granules, which can then act as surrogate allergens. When people snap the gloves while putting them on or taking them off, the starch particles can become aerosolized. If inhaled, these airborne particles can even cause anaphylactic shock in already sensitized individuals.

Allergy to latex used to be rare, but since the 1990s the fear of acquiring HIV/AIDS has become widespread, and all medical professionals, including dentists and emergency medical technicians, have begun wearing latex gloves. The rate of latex allergy has climbed as a result of this greatly increased exposure to latex allergens. It is now estimated that 7 percent or more of all nurses have developed allergy to latex from contact with protective gloves; some nurses have even had to leave the profession because of it. Fortunately, many hospitals have eliminated the use of latex gloves and switched to nonlatex or powder-free gloves. Nonetheless, since many other items used in medical procedures may contain latex, hospitals can still be dangerous places for people who have latex allergies, and most medical facilities have special carts loaded with supplies that are all latex free.

Brigham and Women's Hospital

Boston's Brigham and Women's Hospital, one of the world's best-known medical facilities, has about eighty-five hundred full-time employees, spread out in several interconnected buildings on a large campus occupying a city block. For several years in the early 1990s, employees who worked on floor L1, a below-grade level that contained operating rooms and sterilizing and X-ray labs, complained of health symptoms including eye irritation and upper respiratory problems.[2] Then, in the spring of 1993, fourteen employees in the coronary care unit (CCU) on the twelfth floor of the hospital began to suffer from rashes, sneezing, and hives.[3] At least seven of the fourteen were ultimately diagnosed with latex allergy but were able to return to work after nonlatex gloves started being used.

In July, five of Brigham and Women's thirty-two operating rooms were shut down when nurses and doctors experienced headache and fatigue. Suspicions focused on the ventilation system and the chemicals present in the operating room. Margaret Hanson, a clinical vice president, said, "We've pulled the ventilation system apart, and keep finding little things in the operating room environment that [we think] might cause sensitivity, but everything keeps coming up negative."[4]

The hospital hired a company called Environmental Health and Engineering to investigate. Jack McCarthy, an indoor environmental consultant and president of EH&E, commented that most hospital operating rooms are "like small chemical laboratories."[5] In November the operating room ceilings were cleaned of all lint and dust. The hospital also planned to improve the operating room ventilation. Prior to the ventilation improvements done to the L1 rooms, an exhaust hood for the sterilizing agent glutaraldehyde vented into the ceiling plenum.[6] Still, the glutaraldehyde concentration on L1 was in the range of 0.7 to 6.6 parts per billion[7]—mostly below the reported odor threshold of 40 ppb.[8] An ethylene oxide sterilizer was also leaking into occupied space on L1, though none of the testing ever detected the gas in the air. (Because chemicals may be present in air on an intermittent basis, a test indicating that a chemical is not present at a particular time does not necessarily mean that the chemical is never present.)

At first the hospital reported low numbers of sufferers. Margaret Hanson had noted that "fewer than a hundred" out of approximately three hundred nurses and several hundred anesthesiologists and surgeons who worked in thirty-two operating rooms had reported symptoms.[9] Increasing numbers of nurses fell ill, though, and by the summer of 1994 eighty nurses, eighteen of whom worked on the twelfth floor, were on disability leave. Kathleen Delaney, a cardiac nurse, was one of the eighty. Her symptoms included headaches and respiratory problems. The *Boston Globe* reported, "Delaney said she has remained so ill since departing the Brigham that she rarely leaves home. 'Why didn't anyone tell me?' she said. . . . 'If someone had told me, maybe I wouldn't be as sick as I am.'"[10]

By February 1994, three hundred of the hospital's eighteen hundred nurses were reporting symptoms, and more than fifty hospital employees were suing the HVAC contractors, "charging they developed severe health problems because of poor air quality."[11] Nurses, like teachers, are dedicated care providers, and many were upset that their symptoms prevented them from doing their jobs. The *Boston Globe* reported, "Marie Mannion, of Derry, N.H., one of the nurses disabled by the hazards . . . [which have] forced her from her job as a bone marrow specialist, said she has been devastated. 'I loved my job, I can't make it through [the television show] ER without crying, I miss it so much.'"[12]

Diane (last name withheld at request), a nurse for over twenty-five years who worked at the hospital, was among those suffering symptoms. She had a history of allergies as a child, and her sensitivities to VOCs (see chapter 5), including fragrances, solvents, and the vapors from a particular electroencephalogram paste, were exacerbated by her exposures at Brigham and Women's. (She noted that other co-workers were also bothered by the paste fumes.)[13] She finally had to leave the profession.

The hospital's air quality problems ended the twenty-year career of another nurse from the CCU on the twelfth floor, Kathy Sperrazza, who had a "set of health problems ranging from asthma and pounding headaches to numbness in one leg and confusion."[14] She blamed her illness on latex gloves and on the many chemicals present in a hospital environment.

Like Joellen Lawson (see chapter 8), Kathy was a fighter. Despite her illness, she represented the nurses as chairwoman of the Massachusetts Nurses Association (MNA) bargaining committee. In addition to expressing air quality concerns, the MNA requested a number of improvements for the nurses, such as more job security, pay raises, and better health insurance coverage. For months Sperrazza "stood in the lobby of the Brigham, handing out thousands of leaflets and buttons."[15] By the end of the summer of 1996, when negotiations with the hospital stalled, the MNA leadership took a step extraordinary for a hospital union: they called for a strike. About fourteen hundred (80 percent) of the nurses voted, and twelve hundred agreed to strike, forcing a marathon, last-ditch effort to negotiate. If an agreement was not reached, the nurses were ready to walk off their jobs.

As the *Boston Globe* reported, "Sperrazza led a group of 16 union representatives into a closed door meeting with 10 hospital officials. The meeting began at 9:30 a.m. Thursday and ended 4 a.m. Friday."[16] An accord was reached, part of which included a buyout program for the seventy-five to one hundred nurses who had been disabled by the air quality problems at the hospital. Sperrazza estimated that the cost of the buyout might be as high as $5 million, though the figure ultimately proved to be lower.[17] One of the nurses who accepted the buyout was Sperrazza herself, who at the age of forty-four left the

In April 1995, before the cleaning, dust samples taken from above suspended-ceiling surfaces at the twelfth floor of Brigham and Women's Hospital contained between 122 and 364 micrograms of latex allergen per gram of dust and as high a concentration as 119 micrograms of latex allergen per gram of dust on the lower ceiling surfaces. "The outside reviewers noted this to be a 'troubling finding' and recommended cleaning." The cleaning was successful, and samples taken in June 1996 had no detectable levels of latex allergen.[1]

1. M. Kawamoto et al., *Health Hazard Evaluation Report HETA 96-0012-2652, Brigham and Women's Hospital, Boston, Massachusetts* (Washington, D.C.: NIOSH, September 1997), 19.

profession she loved. She went on to get two master's degrees, one in occupational health and the other in labor relations, and she is now a member of the MNA Congress on Health and Safety.

The problems that arose at Brigham and Women's Hospital were due to the presence of chemicals and latex allergens, compounded by the lack of adequate ventilation. The hospital spent a great deal of money to improve the quality of its indoor air. The twelfth floor was closed and cleaned twice, and plans were made to clean the whole facility, top to bottom, within a year, at a projected cost of more than $500,000 per floor. Hospital officials pledged about $8 million for the work to be done.[18] Part of the purpose of the costly floor-to-floor cleaning was to eliminate settled dust that contained cornstarch granules coated with latex allergens. Fresh air is now delivered to every area of the hospital. The use of toxic sterilizing agents such as glutaraldehyde has been reduced, and where such agents are used, efficient local exhaust ventilation has been installed. The hospital's occupational health and safety programs, as well as its environmental services, have been expanded.

Brigham and Women's Hospital has become a model for responsible management of indoor air quality. The steps the hospital took have influenced procedures followed at hospitals all over the country.

The Dizzy Dentist

I once received a call from an orthodontist who began to feel dizzy and nauseated one afternoon while he was working on a patient. A colleague in the same office often had headaches. The treatment area consisted of a large open room where as many as six orthodontists worked simultaneously. To one side of the treatment area was the waiting room, and to the other side was a small lab where plastic orthodontic appliances (such as bite plates and mouth guards) were fabricated.

Typically the office was relatively quiet until around 3:30 in the afternoon, when as many as twenty teenagers would show up after school to have their braces adjusted. They were often accompanied by their parents. From 3:30 until the end of the day, the space was crowded with as many as thirty people.

The building was a fairly new, rather airtight wood-frame structure. A furnace with an air-conditioning coil was located in the attic. There was no mechanical ventilation system, nor were there any pathways for adequate amounts of fresh air to enter the space when the windows were closed. There was also no exhaust in the lab, so when the mixtures of chemicals were heated and cured to form plastic shapes for oral appliances, chemical fumes entered the workspace.

The office had another problem: an elevated level of carbon dioxide (CO_2) due to the lack of ventilation. When I measured the CO_2 level, at a time of day when there were only about a dozen people in the office, I found a concentration of 1,500 ppm, which is above the ASHRAE Standard 62 guideline of about 1,000 ppm. I suspect that the concentration was much higher in the afternoons, when more people were in the space.

I concluded that the orthodontists suffered symptoms of sick-building syndrome because the air was stuffy and full of vapors. I recommended that an exhaust system be installed for the lab, to vent the chemical fumes outside instead of keeping them inside. I also suggested that the orthodontists bring some fresh outdoor air in through the duct system to replace the air being exhausted and to lower the CO_2 concentration.

MUNICIPAL BUILDINGS

News about indoor air quality crises can spread slowly or quickly, depending on whether the buildings involved are public or private, well trafficked or secluded. Municipal buildings are public and in a way belong to us all, so information about IAQ problems in buildings such as courthouses is likely to be disseminated quickly.

Fumes in the Courthouse

The lengthy IAQ crisis at the Suffolk County Courthouse, a high-rise building in Boston's Pemberton Square, began in October 1993 with a $9.9 million contract to waterproof the exterior of the occupied building. The *Boston Globe* followed the story for over five years.

1994—June: "A defense attorney nearly fainted at the opening of a trial and a court stenographer was out of work for two weeks with pneumonia-like symptoms." People suspected that fumes from the waterproofing material were entering the building envelope and making people ill.

July: A person was hospitalized "for treatment of a diabetic condition that his doctor blamed on inhalation of the fumes. . . . [He] vomited for 22 hours and was unable to eat as required to keep his diabetes under control. He was rushed to Milton Hospital . . . where he was unconscious for a day and then awoke to see a priest standing over him, giving the last rites."

August: The cost of the crisis was mounting: $200,000 "to move two offices out of the courthouse and to pay for an independent occupational hygienist," $101,934 for "moving the . . . criminal clerk's office," $45,000 "to relocate the . . . probation office."

1995—February: Janice Boyle, a twenty-seven-year-old probation officer who was pregnant, left the building because she was worried about the fumes. "I've been healthy for 27 years and then all of a sudden I'm in this building for three months and come down with headaches, urinary tract infections, and liver problems," she said. In the words of Gary Wilson, an assistant trial magistrate in the building, "There's only so much of this you can take." The reporter noted that "as [Wilson] worked in a foul-smelling courtroom on the seventh floor last Friday, one of his eyes twitched."

July: Lawsuits were filed against the general contractor who was responsible for the waterproofing and against the architect who had planned the renovation of the building exterior. "In the lawsuit, the employees said they have suffered numerous health problems, including enlarged livers, asthma attacks, vomiting, nausea, diarrhea, chest pains, bronchitis, headaches, toxemia, pneumonia, skin rashes, migraines, disorientation, memory loss, insomnia, dizziness and chemical sensitivity."

November: "Five people who sat on the Suffolk County grand jury in the past several months have complained they suffered illnesses in the courthouse, the first indication that noxious fumes have affected people other than employees."

1999—January: "Seven companies have agreed to pay $3 million to 29 courthouse employees who contended they suffered various illnesses when chemical weatherproofing was applied to the exterior of the Suffolk County Courthouse in 1993 and 1995."[19]

What was wrong with the weatherproofing? The material used was Duramem 500, a paste with the consistency and odor of roof tar. The material contains the solvent xylene (see chapter 3) as well as residues (less than 2 percent) of two chemicals called *isocyanates:* methylene bisphenyl isocyanate (MDI) and toluene diisocyanate (TDI). Both are irritating and toxic. OSHA notes that

> MDI vapor is a potent respiratory sensitizer. It also is a strong irritant of the eyes, mucous membranes, and skin and can cause pulmonary edema. Exposure of humans to high concentrations causes cough, dyspnea, increased secretions, and chest pains. MDI and other diisocyanates cause pulmonary sensitization in susceptible individuals; should this occur, further exposure should be avoided, since extremely low levels of exposure may trigger an asthmatic episode; cross-sensitization to unrelated materials probably does not occur.[20]

Duramem 500 paste can be applied over exterior masonry to create a waterproof membrane; in this case, it was applied under a new building veneer. Unfortunately the paste is a moisture-cured urethane, which means that it must react chemically with water vapor from the air to achieve its final, elastic condition (to cure). In other words, water vapor from the air must diffuse into the paste. At 77°F and 50 percent relative humidity, Duramem 500 should take forty-eight hours to cure. At temperatures lower than 77°F and RH under 50 percent, the material takes longer to cure; it should not be applied when the temperature is below 40°F. While the urethane is curing (combining with water vapor), the xylene solvent in the Duramem 500 must evaporate.

The specification data sheet for Duramem 500 that formerly appeared on the manufacturer's website (it has since been removed) warned that the material should not be applied in too thick a layer. If painted on too thick (thicker than a tenth of an inch), "the result will be a retarded cure which in confined or poorly ventilated occupied areas can prolong the bituminous/solvent odor and emissions of vapor."[21] The contractors insisted that the weatherproofing had been properly applied, but consultants claimed that the material was too thick in some areas. "Joan Parker, a former industrial hygiene engineer with the state Division of Occupational Hygiene . . . , took a sample from the 16th-floor exterior wall that measured close to an inch [thick]"— ten times thicker than the maximum recommended.[22] And, as so often happens, the concentrations of contaminants within the building envelope, in this case the fumes from the weatherproofing material, were elevated as a result of the lack of ventilation at the time the Duramem was applied.

When the complaints began in November 1994, an industrial hygienist was called in to do some testing, and the concentration of isocyanates measured was 23 ppb. "The State's recommended short-term limit at the time was 5 ppb for industrial work environments," commented Joan Parker. "Exposure at levels close to 5 ppb could easily have elicited a severe respiratory reaction in already sensitized individuals." Despite the results of the November testing, more waterproofing was applied in June. More than twenty-four hours after the application, the isocyanate concentration remained as high as 19 ppb.[23]

The waterproofing material was finally removed, at an estimated cost of between $30 million and $40 million.

The Law of the Land

In 2002 a mold infestation forced the evacuation of a Chicago-area police station. Some theorized that mold growing in a bag of marijuana in the evidence room spread throughout the station and "chased the department away." Although the mold was most likely growing in the building for other reasons, such as elevated relative humidity, it is common to find *Aspergillus* spores in marijuana. The dried leaves of the drug can be as moldy as any other kind of dried leaf, including tobacco leaves—another reason not to smoke, especially if you have asthma or allergy to *Aspergillus* mold.[24]

In another police department building, located in Michigan, more than fifty people who worked on the seventh floor were moved out "after complaints about poor ventilation, leaky ceilings, mold, vermin and pigeon droppings." The building also had plumbing leaks and rodent infestations. Officer Ken Hayes commented, "We finally had our voices heard. . . . It's bad up there, and nobody's done anything about it for years." Sergeant Theresa Byrge, who worked in the property crime unit and who has asthma, said, "I've never been as sick this frequently in my life."[25]

In Connecticut, people who worked in a police department located in a below-grade space in a hundred-year-old building were becoming sick and missing days of work. Testing revealed mold growth in several lower-level office areas. Consultants undertook a more detailed evaluation and made a number of recommendations, including carpet replacement, improved dehumidification, and better control of rainwater on the exterior of the building envelope.

Dr. John Santilli, who had been treating people sickened by conditions at the McKinley school in Fairfield (see chapter 8), also treated several people who worked in this building. He noted that "80 percent of the 25 police department employees surveyed had 'significant' allergy problems and 60 percent of those surveyed experienced cognitive allergy problems." He added that the "normal rate for such allergy problems in the general population is 20 percent."[26]

I investigated a police station in which the chief of police experienced headaches and a general sense of fatigue. The building was small and had formerly served as a bank. The bank vault was now used as locked storage for weapons and evidence. Unfortunately, the climate in that geographical area was damp, and the slab-on-grade vault was not dehumidified. Everything in the vault was covered with *Aspergillus* mold. Whenever anyone went into the vault, spores entered the main office area. I suspect that the police chief was allergic to the mold.

Laws of the land may rule in the courts and police stations, but biology and the laws of physics and chemistry govern why mold grows and how contaminants spread within the building envelope.

OTHER PUBLIC BUILDINGS

The Renovated Library

A library building I once investigated consisted of a brick structure dating to the nineteenth century with a modern addition at the back. In 1990 all the

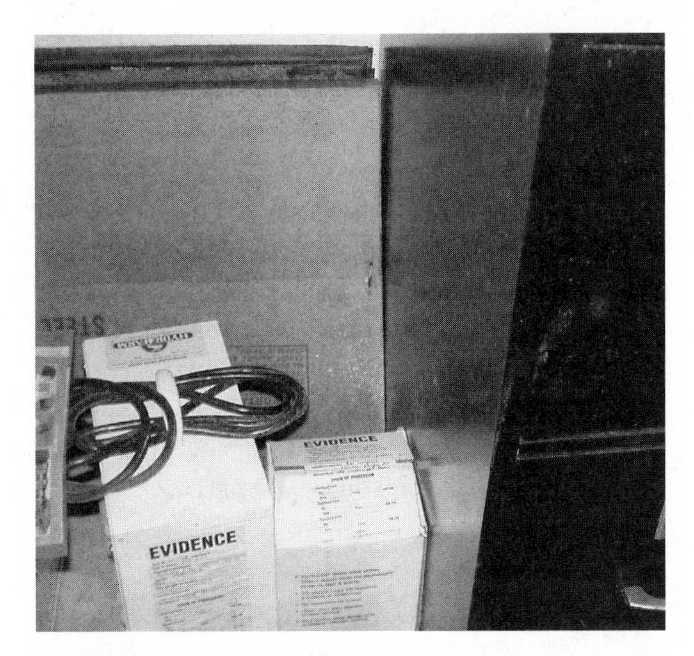

FIGURE 10.2. The *Aspergillus* case. These are some of the items in the evidence vault of the police station discussed in the text. White spots of *Aspergillus* mold are visible on the cardboard behind the evidence boxes, as well as on the filing cabinet and the looped electrical cord. *May Indoor Air Investigations LLC*

leaky old double-hung sash windows were replaced with airtight insulated-glass windows, and three large air-conditioning fan coil units were installed in the attic of the original building. After the renovation, the librarians started complaining that the air seemed stuffy; even when the library was nearly empty of patrons, the CO_2 concentration was 800 ppm. One librarian began to have asthma symptoms.

The library attic was full of loose insulation and over a hundred years' worth of dust that included insect and animal droppings. At the peak of the roof, visible from the outside, was a small square cupola with louvers on each of the four sides. A large duct in the attic terminated at the cupola. This duct had been in place for years and was originally installed as an exhaust for the library.

The air-conditioning installer had intended to supply each fan coil with fresh air from the exterior through that old duct, but there were several impediments to this plan. First, the old duct was longer than the newer ducts connecting the fan coils together. The longer the pathway for airflow, the greater the friction resisting that airflow. If only one fan coil was operating, return air was sucked through the shorter ducts connected to the fan coils that were not operating, rather than through the long fresh-air duct. Some of that air came from the attic and some from the library (air was being sucked back into the fan coil). Second, though the fresh-air duct would function when all three fan coils were operating at the same time, most of the air would still come from the attic, because there was a large opening at the top of the old duct that could not be seen from below. This hole allowed dusty attic air to enter the return system. In addition, the old, original exhaust fan was still in place inside the duct leading to the cupola, and the fan blades were blocking the flow of fresh air.

Below-Grade Is Often "Below Grade"

Air quality problems due to mold are frequently found in basement spaces that are used only intermittently and are therefore not kept consistently warm or dehumidified. Some church and synagogue basements are used only once a week for Sabbath school or are rented out for mornings-only day care programs, and toddlers as well as older children crawl and jump around on moldy carpets. Many library basements are converted into children's reading rooms, and books and even toys can be covered with mold. Such rooms are often (but not always) permeated by a musty odor.

I investigated a small library in Vermont in which the children's reading room was tucked into basement space. Next door was a musty unheated storage area containing books covered with mold. The walls of the children's space had been painted in colored stripes, and the blue, orange, and green bookshelves were low so that young readers could reach the books. The floor was carpeted, and beanbag chairs and large cushions were placed here and there so that children could settle in and browse through a good book. Unfortunately, the entire lower level was permeated with a strong odor of mold.

Finished below-grade spaces must be kept consistently warm in the winter (64°F or higher) and dehumidified in the summer (the relative humidity should not exceed 50 percent). Leaks that occur in basements used as habitable space should be quickly repaired. Wall-to-wall carpeting on concrete

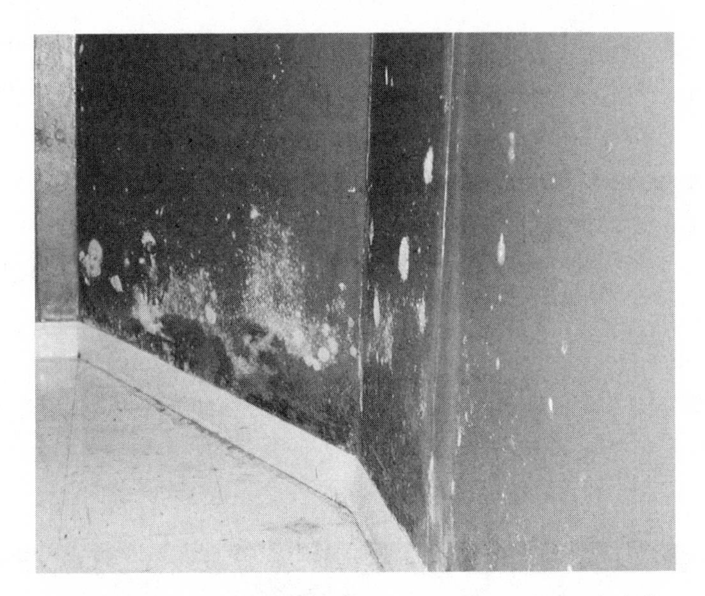

FIGURE 10.3. A decorated wall. This photograph was taken in the hallway leading from the basement playroom of a day care center. The staining on the floor is due to leakage of ground water through the foundation wall, a small part of which is visible at the left edge of the photograph. The water moved along the floor and was soaked up into the drywall, eventually leading to extensive mold growth (the spatter patterns on the wall). *May Indoor Air Investigations LLC*

should be avoided. And children should be allowed to spend time only in those finished below-grade spaces that are free of mold growth. Any moldy below-grade space should be professionally cleaned under containment conditions. (See the Resource Guide for guidelines on mold remediation.)

And More . . .

According to the World Health Organization, "about 30% of new and remodeled buildings worldwide might have poor indoor air quality."[27] It is therefore no surprise that my dismaying collection of stories about air quality problems in medical facilities, municipal buildings, and other public buildings continues to grow. It now includes the following:

In California: Nancy Mucciaccio had rarely been sick in her thirty years as a nurse. Then she experienced nerve damage in one arm and one leg.

"The source of her injuries, she said, is something most nurses aren't aware can harm them—common sterilizing and disinfecting chemicals used in hospitals."[28]

In Ohio: A city official who was a chemical engineer found mold in a building that housed a courthouse and the jail. A judge ordered the jail to be closed, saying that the facility was in a "deplorable and unsanitary condition."[29]

In Finland: A military hospital suffered severe water damage, and a major mold problem developed. Over ten employees reported health symptoms, including cough, asthma, and rhinitis.[30]

SOME PRACTICAL STEPS

- If you have a latex allergy, be sure everyone you work with knows about it. Just in case, keep a disposable NIOSH N95 mask with you, particularly when you enter medical facilities.
- Work areas in medical facilities in which toxic chemicals are used or plastics are cured or heated should be vented and exhausted to the exterior.
- Avoid exposures to elevated levels of disinfectants and sterilizing agents, particularly if you have allergies or respiratory problems.
- People with mold sensitivities should avoid spending time in a musty-smelling or moldy below-grade space. When such spaces can't be avoided, a respirator or a mask with a minimum rating of N95 should be worn.
- Musty smells can arise from mildew on small surfaces, such as the covers of a book, as well as from mildew covering larger surfaces, such as floors, walls, and ceilings. Use a bright flashlight held at an oblique angle (almost parallel to the surface) to inspect a smooth surface where you suspect mold may be growing.

CHAPTER

11

Retail Spaces

Shop Till You Drop

The retail world is served up to us in a multitude of enticing spaces, with about 15 million employees in the United States providing help for consumers.[1] As prospective buyers, we try on different coats to find the right size, squeeze melons to see which are ripe, and savor the offerings at a restaurant buffet. As retail employees, we answer customers' questions, stock shelves, and ring up sales. But buyers and sellers alike may be affected by asthma, allergy, or sick-building symptoms in a retail environment.

Some business establishments are particularly prone to microbial growth—if they are located below grade, for example, or if they sell goods that have been stored in moldy spaces. Specific kinds of stores may contain noxious fumes:

- —Automobile dealerships that are permeated by the strong, characteristic odor of rubber
- —Office areas of automobile body shops where paints and solvents are used
- —Shoe stores in which solvents from adhesives off-gas
- —Stores that sell furniture made of particle board, which off-gasses formaldehyde
- —Carpet stores in which carpet backing off-gasses 4-phenylcyclohexene, styrene, and other chemicals
- —Showrooms and office areas in manufacturing facilities, as well as dry-cleaning establishments, where volatile organic compounds may be present

—Hardware and building supply stores where paints are mixed and bags of fertilizer containing pesticides are stored

The chemical emissions and bioaerosol to which people may be exposed in retail spaces are typically within limits that are generally considered to be safe; nonetheless, some individuals, particularly employees, will have chronic exposures and thus may be at risk of developing hypersensitivities. Every possible step should therefore be taken to minimize exposures, including creating air pressure differentials by introducing more fresh air into certain areas of the building and by having adequate exhaust.

Let's start with a subject dear to everyone's heart: food.

RESTAURANTS

Ventilation Problems

Every now and then I am overcome by the urge to visit my favorite corner pizzeria. One time there was quite a commotion going on when I entered the store. There was a man standing behind the service counter covered with soot and talking with the owner. The owner told me that the man was a technician who had been working on the boiler located in the basement. Combustion gases from the boiler were being drawn up into the kitchen on the ground level. The heating technician had said that the pizzeria needed a new chimney—which sounded odd to me, because the chimney, visible at the exterior of the building, seemed to be in fine condition. I couldn't resist asking the owner if the basement door was normally kept open. Yes, he replied, because they kept many of the food supplies at the lower level.

Combustion gases are exhausted from a boiler into the chimney through a vent pipe (see chapter 7). The chimney draft must be sufficient to prevent *back-drafting* (when the combustion gases are drawn into the room where the boiler is located rather than into the chimney) but not so strong as to remove the heated gases too quickly. If the hot combustion gases are sucked out of the boiler too fast, then heat is drawn up into the chimney and wasted rather than transferred to the water in the boiler. Oil-fired boilers have a *barometric damper:* an opening in the vent pipe with a flap that can swing open, depending on pressure differences. When the chimney draft is too strong, the barometric damper opens and air in the mechanical closet or basement, or wherever the boiler is located, is drawn through the damper into the vent pipe and chimney. This reduces the flow of hot combustion gases through the boiler and out the vent pipe.

In this pizzeria, the exhaust hood above the stove and griddle reduced the air pressure in the kitchen area, and the kitchen's air pressure was lower than the air pressure in the basement. Air from the basement was flowing into the kitchen, acting as *replacement air* (also called *makeup air*) for the air that was being drawn out of the kitchen through the exhaust. In turn, as air flowed out of the basement, the basement air pressure became lower than the air pressure in the chimney. A back-draft occurred, and air containing combustion gases flowed out of the barometric damper into the basement from the chimney. These combustion gases were then carried with airflows up to the first floor. When the basement door was closed and the stove exhaust fan was running, very little replacement air came from the basement; rather, replacement air was supplied by infiltration around first-floor windows and doors, and by air flowing from the outside through the leaky enclosure for the "through-wall" air-conditioning unit located in one of the restaurant's walls.

I suggested that the owner of the pizzeria keep the basement door closed and install a source of combustion air in the basement instead of getting a new chimney; this approach solved his problem. In return, I got my next slice of pizza "on the house."

Depressurization leading to back-drafting is a common problem in restaurants because of the powerful kitchen exhausts installed over the griddles, designed to remove greasy smoke produced by cooking. Whenever a large exhaust fan is operating, makeup air must be supplied, either by a second fan blowing air down a shaft from the roof to the perimeter of the exhaust hood or by a vent open to the outside, located near the stove for a passive airflow supply.

When not tuned properly, an oil-fired boiler (such as the one in the pizzeria) produces quite a bit of soot but ordinarily only a small amount of carbon monoxide (CO). In contrast, a gas-fired boiler can produce large amounts of CO when it is malfunctioning. In another, much larger, restaurant I investigated, one with a separate, expansive dining area and at least a dozen people working in the kitchen, some employees were complaining of headaches. Again, the door from the kitchen to the basement was open, and the gas-fired boiler located in the basement was producing CO. The kitchen exhaust was pulling the CO along with other combustion products up into the kitchen from the lower level. The boiler needed to be cleaned and adjusted, combustion air had to be provided, the door to the basement had to be closed, and more makeup air was needed for the stove exhaust.

Smelly Flowers

I was once asked to investigate the source of an irritating odor problem that had been present intermittently for several years in a single-story retail block. The block housed several restaurants and stores, including a florist, a hairdresser, and a yarn shop.

Accusations were flying. The owner of the florist shop blamed the hairdressers, claiming that the chemicals used to remove nail polish were the culprit. Suspicion focused on the manicurist, who had been seen wearing a mask at work. (The hairdressers never noticed any odor, because the odor was masked by the perfumes and vapors from all the products associated with shampooing, dyeing, curling, and straightening.)

The florist created dried, lacquered floral arrangements in the basement workspace under her shop. Before I was called in, the employees of the yarn shop had complained that the fumes from the lacquer sprays were spreading throughout the building, so the florist had begun to do the spraying in the alley behind the building rather than in her basement. I suspected that she still did some spraying inside, though, because I saw over a hundred cans of paint spray in her basement, and it was hard to imagine her spraying floral arrangements in the exterior alley in rainy or cold weather. (If the yarn shop employees had kept an event log, including the weather conditions on days when they smelled the fumes, they might have been able to identify the source of the odors more easily.)

Each of the restaurants in the building had a powerful kitchen exhaust fan, all located close to the doors that opened from the kitchens into a common hallway running along the rear of the restaurants. Because the restaurants did not have adequate makeup air, employees kept doors to the hallway and the door leading from the hallway to the alley outside partially open for fresh air. Because of the kitchen exhaust fans, the air pressure in the hallway was lower than the air pressure outside, and when the florist sprayed her arrangements outdoors, exterior air flowing into the hallway carried in paint fumes.

I suggested that makeup air for the kitchen exhausts be provided to the hoods, and that the florist either move her spraying operation farther away from the building or install an adequate exhaust hood in her basement workshop so that she could resume spraying there. (When chemicals such as solvents are present, local exhausts or exhaust hoods should be used whenever possible to minimize the spread of vapors into the air. A localized exhaust for a vapor source is always more effective in removing the contaminant than attempts to dilute the contaminant once it has mixed with the air in a space.)

The people in the yarn shop had an additional problem: their heat pump was suspended in a ceiling plenum above drop-ceiling tiles. The return was not ducted, so air for the return came from the ceiling plenum, which was not airtight. As the heat pump supplied air from the plenum to the yarn shop, the air pressure in the plenum was reduced, and air infiltrated from the central hallway and from adjacent retail spaces into the plenum. The solvents from the florist's lacquer spray thus found their way from the hallway into the air supply for the yarn shop. I recommended that the yarn shop owner have a ducted return installed that would conduct air directly into the heat pump via a ceiling grille, so that the heat pump would circulate air from the yarn shop rather than from the hallway or adjacent retail spaces, and so that the ceiling plenum would not become depressurized. (Fresh air entered the yarn shop through infiltration.)

The manicurist in the hairdresser shop who wore the mask was a victim of still another problem. The hairdressing shop had a washer and a dryer in the finished below-grade space where the manicurist worked, and the dryer was vented to the inside rather than to the outside. Laundry lint coated with fabric softeners and detergent residues was entering the space. The manicurist had become sensitized to these chemicals, so she wore a mask to filter out the irritant dust.

A domino situation!

Other Unpleasant Odors

The characteristic cooking odor present in many restaurants stigmatizes these businesses as "greasy spoons." Many fast-food restaurants prevent the odors of grilling and deep frying from flowing into the dining room by exhausting air from the kitchen area. And kitchens can have odor problems of their own. Sinks in which grease may accumulate must have a reservoir that allows water to drain out but leaves the grease behind in the trap, so that the pipes won't become clogged. These grease reservoirs must be cleaned out periodically, because the grease can develop a rancid odor due to the action of bacteria. In one restaurant the grease trap was vented through a pipe that terminated at the dish-washing sink. Employees working at the sink were sometimes nauseated by the odor, because the low pressure in the kitchen caused by the stove exhaust fan pulled the foul-smelling gases out of the trap.

Earlier in this book I talked about how air pressure differences can carry odors from bathrooms into rooms nearby. A restroom odor in a restaurant can take a customer's appetite away, so the air pressure in the restaurant's bathroom should always be less than the air pressure in the dining area. In addition, to avoid leakage of sewer gas, damaged drain pipes and broken toilet seals should be repaired.

The odor of sewer gas almost put one restaurant out of business. The building was beautifully situated alongside a ferry slip on a picturesque river in a Southern tourist town. Customers entering the restaurant from the street could sit in booths in the long, narrow dining area, where smoking was not allowed, or walk through a connecting hallway to the bar in the back of the building, where they could smoke and sip mint juleps. Outside the bar was a large deck that overlooked the water, where customers could watch the riverboats dock and depart while they ate and drank. The kitchen and restrooms were off to the side of the dining room.

The stove exhaust system in the restaurant had two blowers: one to remove air and one to provide makeup air. But more air was supplied than removed, so the air pressure in the kitchen was greater than the air pressure outdoors. In addition, the air-conditioning system was unbalanced, so more air was being returned from the dining room to the rooftop unit than was being supplied to the dining room. In consequence, the air pressure was lower in the dining room than in the kitchen or the bar. Even though the stove had an exhaust system, air was flowing from the smoky cooking area toward the dining room. Air was also flowing from the bar into the dining area, carrying cigarette smoke with it.

Patrons sitting in the dining room might have been able to tolerate the smell of cooking food and even the cigarette smoke, but a sickening odor of sewer gas, drawn up into the dining room from the crawl space below, drove them away. The owner of the building had hired several experts to try to solve the problem, but it wasn't until he hired an experienced inspector, a member of the American Society of Home Inspectors (ASHI), that the source of the odor was identified. The inspector went into the crawl space and found an open waste pipe from which sewer gas was flowing into the crawl space and from there into the dining room through cracks in the floor and through openings around plumbing pipes.

The opening in the waste pipe was repaired, the exhaust blower was adjusted, and the air-conditioning distribution was changed so that the air pressure was higher in the dining room than in the kitchen, bar, and crawl space. At last the dining room air cleared. By then, though, word had gotten around town that the food was fair but the air was foul, and it took months to reverse that impression.

Cigarette Smoke

Many restaurants have a nonsmoking area located near the entrance doors and a smoking area located toward the back near the bar. While this separation is rarely completely effective, it does help minimize the amount of cigarette smoke in the nonsmoking area. Most bars have inadequate ventilation, though, and so they fill with cigarette smoke. Although most patrons don't spend long periods of time in a restaurant day after day, cooks and wait staff certainly do, and their exposure to secondhand smoke (ETS, or environmental tobacco smoke) can be substantial.

Some municipalities have banned cigarette smoking in public places, including restaurants and bars—a move I strongly support. Many people who own restaurants and bars are fearful that they will lose business if smoking is prohibited in their establishments, but sometimes smoking bans have actually increased traffic, because nonsmokers are more apt to eat and drink in smoke-free environments.

Smoking bans can cause political controversy. In Somerville, Massachusetts, Joseph A. Curtatone, a thirty-seven-year-old lawyer elected mayor in 2003 on a pro-business platform, made it clear in a *Boston Globe* article published several months before he took office that he did not support the smoking ban that was in effect in Somerville restaurants and bars: "Some of these businesses are down 40 percent. I just don't think it's fair. . . . And a large part of our tax base is made up of bars and restaurants." Curtatone's position on the smoking ban was already drawing criticism from members of Somerville's Board of Health. Two board members, the *Globe* reported, had said that "the incoming mayor endangered the health of bar and restaurant workers and undercut the board's authority when he made campaign promises to bar and restaurant owners that the smoking ban would be reversed."[2]

In January 2004 the *Somerville Journal* reported that Mayor Curtatone had replaced a Board of Health member whose term was expiring and who opposed a reconsideration of the smoking ban.[3] In February, Somerville Alderman Bill Roche "proposed an order that was passed by the Board of Aldermen asking the Board of Health to reconsider its decision not to hold a public hearing on the city's smoking ban which took effect last October."[4] In March, some restaurant owners were still citing loss of business, but complaints had died down. The struggle in the Somerville community was soon to be moot, however, because in July 2004 Massachusetts joined New York, Connecticut, Maine, Delaware, and California in instituting a statewide smoking ban.

Filtration systems designed to reduce the amount of smoke in restaurants and bars can be helpful but are not necessarily effective, particularly if they are not regularly maintained. In the end, the best way to protect nonsmoking patrons and employees is a No Smoking sign.

Cleanliness

Crumbs and liquids can be spilled by wait staff as well as patrons onto tables, chairs, and carpeting and even into return grilles. Flour particles can become airborne when cakes and breads are prepared and pie crusts dusted before being rolled. If carpets and other fleecy surfaces are not regularly and adequately cleaned (preferably HEPA-vacuumed) and mechanical systems are not adequately filtered, and if moisture is present from condensation or high relative humidity, mold and other microorganisms can flourish, including bacteria that can give a carpet a sour smell. It is therefore particularly important in restaurants, bars, and cafeterias to keep mechanical systems and surfaces clean.

Sometimes a sponge or cloth contaminated with microbial growth (usually bacteria) is used to wipe a counter or table. The surface may then reek—unpleasant, but not necessarily unhealthy. If the cloth drips water into food, how-

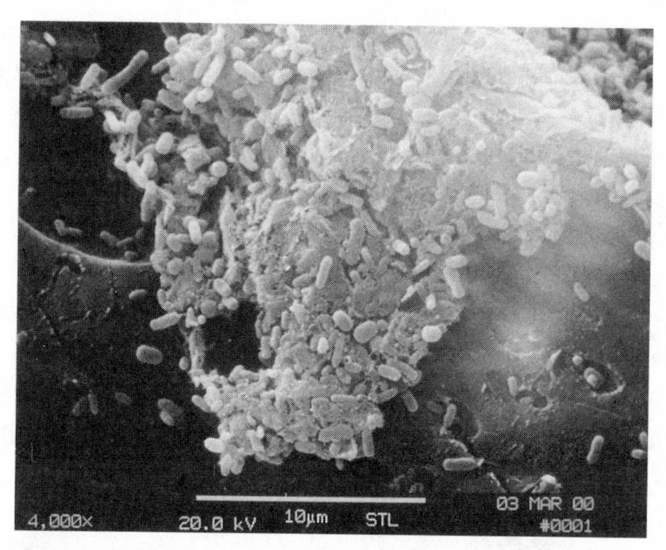

FIGURE 11.1. Bacteria on a sponge (SEM 4,000×). The smooth but slightly pocked sponge surface is visible at the lower right of the photograph. A skin scale was draped over the surface of the sponge but is now being digested by bacteria (the oval and cylindrical objects). The irregularly shaped gray bits in the middle of the photograph and the lighter area at the top right are all that remain (for now!) of the skin scale. *May Indoor Air Investigations LLC*

ever, or if your glass has been wiped with a sponge contaminated by bacterial growth, you can become ill. Foul odors coming from sponges or wiping cloths signal biological growth, and the sponge or cloth should be washed in a bleach solution or replaced.

Food and crumbs left on countertops and other surfaces can attract cockroaches and mice, which are associated with the spread of allergens and diseases. Rats too sometimes lurk in restaurant basements and other food storage areas. Rat excretions can impart a rank odor to the spaces the rodents occupy. This odor sometimes diffuses into foods such as cheese, tainting the flavor.

Disinviting Pest-Guests

Indoor pesticide use, including the use of wasp and bee sprays, should be as limited as possible. If pesticides are to be applied in a building where people work, research should be done to find out what treatments are options, how the pest control operator will apply the treatment, and what steps will be taken to prevent the spread of the chemicals to other areas of the building (see the first sidebar of chapter 8). Measures should be taken to protect furnishings, and the spaces to be treated should be vacated while the work is going on. Depending on the type of application, sufficient time should pass before the space is reoccupied.

All that being said, strategies other than pesticides (such as eliminating the pests' food and water sources) should be used whenever possible. If areas where food is prepared and served are kept clean, infestations from cockroaches and mice can be kept to a minimum if not entirely avoided. And unless there is a bee or wasp nest indoors—and then again that should be handled by professionals who explain their methods and do all they can to prevent the spread of sprays or powders used—a stray bee or wasp can be eliminated by opening a door or window rather than saturating the insect with a pesticide spray.

SUPERMARKETS

If not kept clean, supermarkets can also attract rodents and cockroaches, and supermarkets contain refrigeration equipment that can become contaminated if dust and food bits accumulate around compressors, where airflows and leaks can introduce moisture. In one grocery store a misting system was used to keep the fresh vegetables moist. The system became contaminated with *Legionella* bacteria, and several shoppers fell ill with Legionnaires' disease. Even if a misting system isn't contaminated, it sprays water onto food, and unless the shelves or racks are kept clean and the food fresh, microbes can flourish.

Food markets can be difficult places for people who are sensitized to fragrances and laundry chemicals. (People with chemical sensitivities usually avoid the aisles containing laundry products and scented candles.) Boxed laundry detergents and softeners can off-gas fragrances or leak irritating chemicals onto the shelves or floor, and the household aisle is usually stacked with perfumed candles and soaps. We can't avoid going into supermarkets, but if you are sensitive to fragrances, avoid certain aisles, and if a supermarket has a musty odor, shop elsewhere.

LAUNDROMATS

Liquid fabric softeners added to washing machines and fabric softener sheets used in dryers can bother those who are sensitized. Products used to wash clothes can also contain potentially irritating chemicals: *detergents,* which to a chemist are specific compounds that solubilize (dissolve) grease; *surfactants,* which facilitate the removal of soiling and are also used as fabric softeners; and proteolytic (digestive) *enzymes,* which aid in the removal of protein stains, such as those caused by egg and blood. Exposure to these chemicals is less likely to occur when liquid rather than powdered detergents are used, but still, liquids froth and bubble. Residues of any washing product (including enzymes) can remain on clothing after it is washed and dried, and this clothing can shed microscopic fibers that have chemicals adsorbed on the surface. And whenever a lint filter from a dryer is cleaned, some of the chemical-coated lint fibers become airborne.

Subtilisin is one of the most common enzymes added to laundry products. In the 1960s, when manufacturers first started incorporating these enzymes into their formulations for laundry products, they began to notice an increase in the asthma rate among their production workers. In some facilities the occurrence of allergic sensitization was as high as 50 percent as a result of exposure to subtilisin-containing dust, and a majority of those workers also suffered from occupational asthma.[5] Strict dust controls, as well as other changes in the manufacturing processes, were instituted to minimize worker exposures. (There are exposure limits for hundreds of synthetic chemicals, but at the present time subtilisin, derived from genetically modified bacteria, is the only *bioaerosol* for which there is an exposure guideline: 0.06 microgram per cubic meter.) Nonetheless, there have been cases of occupational asthma and even a case of hypersensitivity pneumonitis associated with the use of cleaning compounds containing subtilisin.[6]

When knowledge of occupational asthma among workers handling subtilisin-containing products became public, concerns were voiced about everyday exposures due to the use of laundry detergents containing subtilisin. In the early 1970s there was not a corresponding increase in the occurrence of consumer sensitization, according to one review.[7] However, the number of detergents that contain enzymes (mostly subtilisin, but other enzymes are also beginning to be used) has increased. Probably more than half the laundry loads in the country are washed with these products. I believe that significant numbers of individuals are sensitized to subtilisin, and that this hypersensitivity may be responsible for some of the allergic symptoms that people experience in laundromats, the laundry aisle in a grocery store, or even in the street, if they are downwind from a dryer exhaust.

Dryers can also cause air quality problems. In a tight building, dryer exhausts can remove enough air to depressurize a space. If there is a boiler present, back-drafting can occur. Dryers must have adequate makeup air to avoid back-drafting of other combustion equipment located nearby. In addition, dryers should always be vented to the exterior to avoid the emission indoors of excess moisture, laundry chemicals, lint, and even combustion products from a gas-fired dryer.

DRY CLEANING

In dry cleaning, a solvent called *tetrachloroethylene,* sometimes referred to as *perchloroethylene* or *PERC,* is used to dissolve grease stains. Most of the solvent is removed from the garment before it is hung on the rack. A residual amount of solvent remains in the item, however, and is responsible for the characteristic dry-cleaning odor. At one time PERC was used as a general anesthetic, because high concentrations can cause loss of consciousness. The chemical may also be carcinogenic, but according to the New York City Department of Health and Mental Hygiene, "the currently available information is not sufficient to determine the health effects from low levels of PERC exposure and whether PERC causes cancer in humans."[8]

Most dry cleaners do not do the cleaning on site. The concentration of tetrachloroethylene in such shops ranges from 10 to 20 milligrams per cubic meter of air,[9] less than 0.3 percent of the OSHA permissible exposure limit, or PEL (and still below the reported odor threshold of about 27 mg/m^3). When the dry cleaning is done on site, however, concentrations of this chemical on the premises are of course higher, and the air outside the shop, as well as the air in apartments located above such a facility, can still contain significant PERC concentrations.

Individuals who have chemical sensitivities may react even to residual amounts of chemicals, so dry-cleaning businesses should have adequate ventilation.

BEAUTY SHOPS

Dyes (such as para-phenylenediamine) and bleaches (such as ammonium persulfate) used in hairdressing salons are sensitizing agents that can cause asthma if particles coated with the chemicals are inhaled by people who are sensitized.[10] Most exposures to these chemicals are via skin contact, however, so it is essential for those who work in the beauty trade to protect their skin. (Ironically, exposure to hair itself can cause allergy in some people. In a study conducted in Finland, approximately 12 percent of those who cut hair were found to be allergic to the common yeast, a *dermatophyte,* that causes dandruff.)[11]

Some hairdressing shops schedule hair dyeing, curling, and straightening for certain days of the week, so that people who are just getting haircuts on other days will not be exposed. Other shops set aside a space, preferably exhausted and well ventilated, for such work. Such steps reduce potential exposures for customers and employees alike.

PHOTOGRAPHIC PROCESSING

The chemicals used in photography stores where film is developed and printed can cause allergy and asthma problems. Sodium sulfite reacts with water to produce sulfur dioxide, an irritating gas responsible for asthma symptoms (see chapter 5). Glutaraldehyde, also used in developing film (including X-ray films), is an irritant to mucous membranes and the lungs (see chapter 10). Hydroquinone and 4-(methylamino)phenol sulfate, as well as other chemicals used in developer, can cause skin allergies.[12]

GARDENING SUPPLIES

Building supply outlets and hardware stores sell fertilizer containing pesticides, a combination that saves a step in the application of both. According to the manufacturer's advertisement for one such product, a 25-pound bag of the fertilizer contains about 1 percent or 0.25 pound of the pesticide atrazine. Because exposure to pesticides can cause chemical sensitivities, fertilizers that contain pesticide should be packaged in containers that prevent the release of dust and vapor, and the containers should be stored outside under cover or inside only in well-ventilated areas.

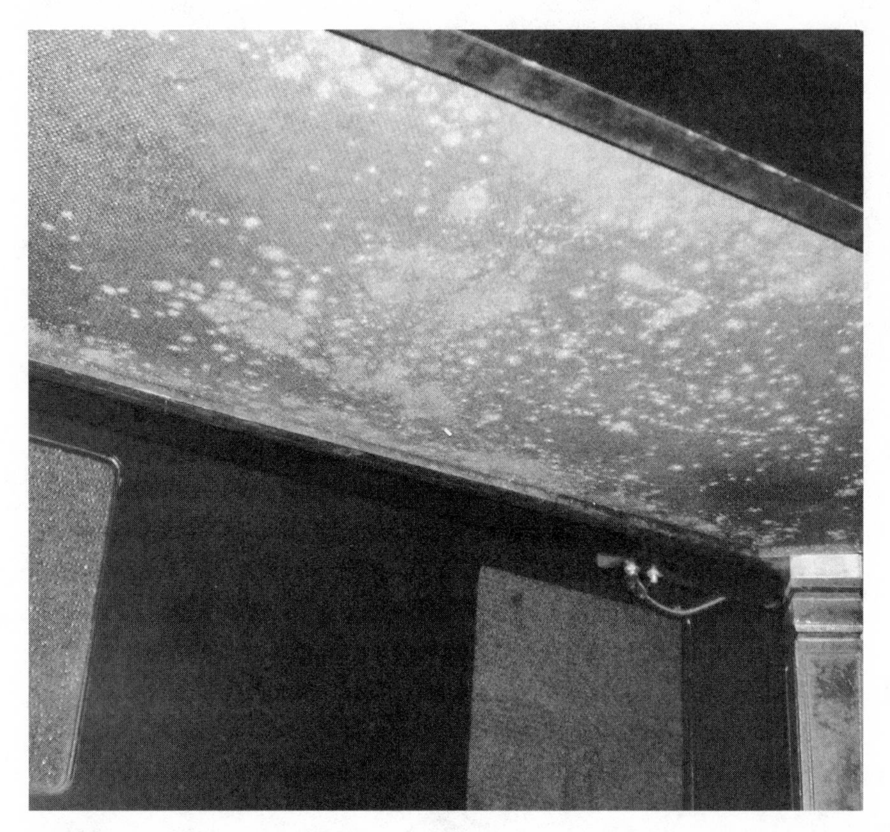

FIGURE 11.2. A moldy oldie. Mildew grew on the underside of this used piano bench while it was stored in a damp basement. The mildew was readily visible, if anyone had thought to look. The bench was then sold to a pianist, who experienced symptoms whenever he sat on the bench to play his piano. *May Indoor Air Investigations LLC*

One unlikely place where students and staff can have significant exposures to pesticides is in botanical collections, where specimens have been treated with chlorinated phenols, paradichlorobenzene, or napthalene.

OLD AND MOLDY

Antiques, secondhand furniture, and used books may have spent decades in damp basements or garages before being offered for sale. It is common to find the unfinished bottoms and backs of exquisitely finished pieces of furniture colonized by *Penicillium* or *Aspergillus* mold. Before a piece of furniture is taken into the shop and displayed for sale (or purchased), all surfaces, finished as well as unfinished, should be checked for discoloration that might signal mold growth.

Antique and secondhand rugs can also be full of mold growth as well as dog and cat dander.

PET STORES

Pet stores, obviously, can contain a variety of bioaerosols: feather fragments; dander from cats, dogs, and birds; algae and bacteria from fish tanks; insect and mite allergens from rodent cages; and even spores from mold subsisting on fish food and animal feed. Adequate filtration (at a minimum, MERV 6 to 8 in the mechanical system, with frequent filter changes, and perhaps even supplementary HEPA-filtered room air purifiers) will reduce the amount of particulate allergens. Unfortunately, most pet stores have to be kept warm, and ventilation is often restricted in an effort to reduce heating costs. Ventilation costs money, but improved air quality is worth the expense.

SOME PRACTICAL STEPS

- Whenever chemicals with potentially toxic fumes are handled, employees should wear the required personal protection, such as a rated mask or a charcoal respirator.
- Chemicals, including solvents and pesticides, should always be handled with the utmost care. Manufacturers' warnings and material safety data sheets (MSDS) should be accessible (and be read). Every business that handles potentially toxic chemicals, and this can include even simple cleaning compounds, should consider procedures to put in place in the event of a spill.
- If you work in a restaurant kitchen that has a rancid odor, investigate the grease trap. It may need to be cleaned out.
- Restaurants with powerful exhausts and nearby combustion equipment should be equipped with carbon monoxide detectors. If exhaust fans depressurize a building, makeup air may be needed.
- Clothes dryers should always be vented to the exterior.
- If you use a laundromat and are sensitive to laundry chemicals, including fragrances, consider drying your clothing at home rather

than using the commercial dryers, which may contain residual chemicals from fabric softener sheets.

- Spills of powdered detergents in laundromats or supermarkets should be thoroughly cleaned (minimizing aerosols), and residual dust levels should be kept at a minimum.
- Sensitized individuals should air out clothing that has been dry-cleaned before hanging it in a closet.
- If furniture has mold growth on unfinished surfaces, the surfaces can be wiped with rubbing alcohol—outdoors, and by someone wearing gloves and respiratory protection. Then, when dry, these unfinished surfaces can be sealed with either clear shellac or varnish to contain any residual irritating dust, and the furniture should be aired out before being brought back indoors. Furniture with mildew growth on a finished wood surface can be taken outside and wiped with a barely damp cloth and then polished. Don't apply anything to the surface that could damage the finish. If the furniture is valuable, check with an antiques professional before doing anything to it.
- If feasible, antique rugs should be cleaned professionally before being used or sold.
- A moldy rug that is being removed for cleaning or disposal must be handled with great care, to prevent the dispersal of potentially allergenic particles. Sensitized individuals should either leave the space or wear respiratory protection (at least a NIOSH N95 mask) while the rug is being moved, and surfaces should be HEPA-vacuumed after the rug is gone. Moldy wall-to-wall carpets should be removed by professionals, under containment conditions (see chapter 14).
- If washing or dry cleaning might damage an antique Oriental rug, compressed air can be blasted through the rug to blow out the dust. This should be done outdoors—and carefully, to avoid damaging the rug. Keep in mind, though, that this cannot remove all the allergens.
- People with mold sensitivities should avoid touching or disturbing books or other objects that smell musty or have visible mildew.
- Anyone handling moldy materials should wear respiratory protection.

CHAPTER

12

Before Nine and After Five

Recreation and Travel

Before we go to work in the morning, after we return from work in the evening, and on weekends, we relax in our homes or exercise at a local health club. On the way to and from work or school, we commute in cars, buses, or trains. When we go on trips for business or pleasure, we travel in airplanes and stay in hotels and motels. Any one of these spaces may be the source of indoor air quality problems, whether we are on land, at sea, or in the air.

LARGE RESIDENTIAL COMPLEXES

In my book *My House Is Killing Me!* I discuss indoor air quality problems in single-family homes and other small residential buildings.[1] It is worth mentioning here, however, that in *large* residential buildings, problems can flow down with water (leaks spreading because of gravity) and up with air (air flowing because of the stack effect; see chapter 4). Leaks that develop in units next to or above your unit can stain your walls or ceilings and cause mold growth in wall or ceiling cavities. Cooking odors, mold spores, cigarette smoke, and even pet dander can also travel from one apartment to another and from one floor to another. (Many nonsmokers call me because they hate the smell of cigarette or cigar smoke infiltrating their apartment from elsewhere in their building.) You may think that your apartment or dorm room is private, but as far as moving air and water are concerned, your domicile is just a brief delay in the fluid flow.

It is very difficult to prevent irritants, allergens, and contaminants from traveling on airflows, though changes in air pressure relationships may help. In the summer you can put a fan in one of your windows to increase the air pressure in your apartment. This isn't really feasible in an air-conditioned building, but you might talk to an HVAC technician familiar with the system to see if adjustments can be made to the AC or heat pump to increase the pressure in your apartment relative to the pressure in the common hallway. In the winter there isn't much to be done short of moving out, although an air-to-air heat exchanger, adjusted to supply more air than is being removed, may help.

The Greasy Noon

One woman who owned a unit in a deluxe condominium complex was annoyed every day around noon by the odor of fried onions that filled her apartment. Her neighbor routinely cooked onions for lunch. How did that odor find its way into the woman's apartment?

There were only two units per floor in each of the building towers, and each tower was served by its own elevator. At the woman's floor, air flowed out of the common hallway and into the elevator shaft through gaps between the elevator door and the door frame. The air pressure in the hallway was thus lower than the air pressure in the two condominium units, so air flowed out of each unit into the hallway through gaps around each unit's door. The neighbor's kitchen didn't have an adequate exhaust system, and soon after he started cooking onions, the odor would billow out from the gaps between his door and the door frame, fill the common hallway, and enter the elevator shaft with airflows.

The woman's heating system was located in a mechanical closet in her unit, adjacent to the elevator shaft. The system had no ducted return, and the partition wall between the elevator shaft and the mechanical closet had a gap at the top. This meant that some of the return air for the woman's heat pump came from the elevator shaft. At noon that air was saturated with the smell of fried onions. Additional return air came from a ceiling plenum that may not have been completely separated from the neighbor's ceiling plenum, offering another avenue for the distribution of the smell. The smell of onions coming from her supply register was so strong that it was as if she had been cooking them in her own apartment. It wasn't pleasant to use the elevator around that time of day, either.

To eliminate the problem, the elevator and unit doors had to be gasketed.

The mechanical closet had to have an airtight ceiling to isolate it from the plenum, and a separate return open only to the woman's unit had to be installed. Finally, the wall between her mechanical closet and the elevator shaft had to be sealed, and the neighbor's kitchen exhaust had to be improved.

Piping Air

The space around plumbing pipes, called the *plumbing chase*, can allow air from a below-grade space to travel through the chase to the uppermost levels of the building. Combustion gases from car exhausts can rise up from underground garages through plumbing chases (as well as through elevator shafts) into habitable spaces above.

In older buildings the floors may not extend across the bottom of a chase at each level, so there may be substantial spaces for airflows around the pipes. In most newer buildings the concrete floor extends into the pipe chase, and the pipes pass through holes in the concrete. Still, these holes are larger in diameter than the pipes themselves, and air can thus flow through the gaps between the pipes and the concrete. These spaces can be sealed by filling them with injectable expanding foam.

Technically, in wood-frame buildings there is supposed to be a material called *firestopping* around the pipes to minimize airflow and slow the speed of fire through the chase. When firestopping is missing or has been removed to facilitate pipe access and repair, a pipe chase acts like a chimney. The walls can be opened up, and noncombustible materials can be installed at the floor or ceiling of every level of the building, to minimize airflows and also to save energy, for warmed air often flows up through the chase into the attic and then exfiltrates.

A Ring Explains Rain

I was asked to investigate a serious leak in a college dormitory that was staining the walls in two rooms and flooding a library located in the basement. Valuable books were water-damaged and turning moldy. The building manager met me in his office and led me first to the large, well-lit reading room. I could hear water dripping as we approached the rear right corner of the below-grade space, and I could see that all the bookshelves were draped with sheets of wet plastic. The carpet had been removed, and water was running down the walls and puddling on the floor. We then went upstairs to the two dorm rooms: one on the first floor used as a bedroom for guests and one above it on the second floor, occupied by two students. Both rooms had private bathrooms with extensive water staining on the bathroom ceilings and walls. What perplexed the manager most was that these stains seemed to dry up during school vacations.

The manager's supervisor in the university's facilities division wanted to fix the problem as quickly as possible. About the same time that I arrived, a plumber showed up to give an estimate for opening up two walls in one of the bathrooms to replace the pipes that he suspected were leaking. The manager, however, wanted to have a clearer picture of the source of the leakage before taking expensive corrective action that might not be effective.

I asked the manager to let me into the dorm room on the third floor, which had a bathroom above the other two bathrooms below. The occupant was a visiting professor from England, and he was away for the day. There was no staining on the walls, floor, or ceiling of that bathroom. Given the pattern of the stains in the bathrooms below, I suspected that the source of the leaks lay in this room.

Using a borescope I was able to look into the bathroom walls through some small access holes. I failed to observe any pipes with stains that might indicate leakage. While I was trying to figure out how to get a look at the pipes in the wall cavity behind the ceramic tiles above the tub without making holes in the tiles and plaster, something peculiar caught my eye: a ring that went neatly around the entire inside circumference of the tub except at the very back curve. The ring was about 3 inches above the tub overflow.

Soap combines with minerals in the water to produce an insoluble waxy film called *soap scum* that adheres to the walls of a tub. Every time you take a bath, more soap is deposited on the tub walls. If you lean back against the back of the tub, however, you minimize heavy soap-scum deposits where your skin touches the tub wall. I surmised from the pattern of the soap scum that the visiting professor took long deep baths and rested against the back of the tub, perhaps to read a book while he soaked. Unfortunately, most bathtubs aren't designed to be filled above the overflow, and the rubber gasket between the metal escutcheon plate and the actual overflow pipe is often not watertight.

When the water level rises high enough in a tub, water starts to pour into the overflow. To keep the water level as high as the soap ring suggested, the man would have had to have as much water running into the tub as was flowing out the overflow pipe, resulting in a constant stream of water out the overflow. The gasket was leaky, so water was flowing onto the concealed floor under the bathtub, spreading to the ceilings and walls below, and flowing down the pipe chase, ultimately raining onto the books in the basement reading room.

To test my theory, I filled the tub to the level of the overflow and plunged a large plastic waste paper basket into the tub bottom-end first, to simulate what happened when a body slipped into the water. The water level rose to nearly the level of the soap scum and immediately started to pour out the overflow. At my request the building manager was standing in the bathroom below, and within moments he shouted that water was trickling down the walls of the second-floor bathroom, precisely where the stains were located. Together we went to the first-floor bathroom; soon water was trickling down there as well.

The solution to this problem? Fix the gasket in the overflow of the third-floor tub, and ask the visiting professor to use a shower for washing and an easy chair for reading.

INDOOR EXERCISE

Until the Industrial Revolution, most people in this country lived on family farms and toiled in barns and fields. Even in the early years of the Industrial Revolution, before automation and mass production, people were still active at work, operating machines. Today our economy is primarily service oriented, and too many of us lead sedentary lives, spending our days staring at computer monitors. Carpal tunnel syndrome has replaced the aching back. According to the 1999–2000 National Health and Nutrition Examination Survey, "an estimated 64 percent of U.S. adults are either overweight or obese."[2] Our forefathers got plenty of exercise from their work, but today most of us get our exercise by working out. And guess where that happens? Mostly indoors, in buildings where we jog on machines, lift weights, and swim in pools, inhaling more and more indoor contaminants as our respiration rates increase.

Your Local Unhealth Club

Health clubs are often carpeted, and many are located below grade. Unless below-grade spaces used for this purpose are kept consistently warm in winter and dehumidified in summer, problems with microbial growth are likely to result. Exterior maintenance is also important. An exercise club that I occasionally frequent (but less frequently lately!) is a one-story building with many roof leaks. When the rainwater misses a bucket, it soaks into the carpet, leading to microbial growth in the carpet dust.

Many hotels have exercise spaces located adjacent to indoor pools. Pool water must be filtered and treated with bactericides and algaecides, because by their very nature (warm and wet) pool areas are subject to bacterial and algal growth. In addition, people shed bacteria and yeast from their bodies into the water. The disinfectant most commonly used is sodium hypochlorite, a version of chlorine bleach. Bleach releases chlorine gas (Cl_2), irritating to those who are sensitized. (Chlorine gas, toxic and denser than air, was first used as a poison gas by Germany during World War I. The gas sank into the trenches where soldiers crouched.) It is also essential to control the acidity, called the pH, of pool water, because pH affects the amount of chlorine gas present. The higher the acidity (or the lower the pH), the greater the release of chlorine gas from the breakdown of sodium hypochlorite.

Studies have shown that not only the chemicals that are added to pool water but also the chemicals that are in the air above the pool surface can have an adverse health impact on swimmers, lifeguards, personal trainers who work in exercise rooms near pools, and anyone else who spends extended time in or around indoor pools. Pool water is a soup containing human effluent (including urine, protein from skin, and amino acids from sweat) that combines with chlorine from the sodium hypochlorite to produce chloramine (NCl_3), a toxic, carcinogenic compound also formed when bleach and ammonia are mixed.

In one study chloramine levels in air above indoor swimming pools were found to be as high as 0.57 milligram per cubic meter.[3] (This concentration is equivalent to 0.11 part per million, slightly above the exposure level of 0.1 ppm that is sometimes recommended.)[4] Three people who had worked around indoor swimming pools for years developed asthma. Their symptoms improved when they were away on holiday; when they returned to work, so did their wheezing and coughing. When exposed experimentally to chloramine at a concentration slightly less than what was found in the indoor air, these workers experienced asthma symptoms, proving that their illness was occupational.

Since people who work in indoor pool facilities may develop occupational asthma, the water must be monitored for disinfectant levels, and these areas must be ventilated to control the concentration of chlorine and chloramine. (The European Union recommends an exchange rate of about 5 air changes per hour [ACH], though at one pool studied 1.5 ACH was adequate.)[5]

Indoor pools can cause other building and indoor air quality problems. In a YMCA building in Boston, chlorine from the pool accelerated the rusting of the steel reinforcement bars in the concrete roof and led to the collapse of the building's roof structure. I investigated one indoor pool located in a space that was pressurized with respect to the exterior and adjacent rooms, which forced warm moist air from the pool room up into the attic space above, where the moisture condensed on the cold sheathing and rotted the wood. (Pool enclosures should be kept at a slightly negative air pressure, to prevent the flow of moist air into wall cavities or adjacent rooms.)

The dew point of air in swimming pool enclosures can range from 60 to 70°F, and moisture can condense on cold surfaces, leading to concealed mold growth on walls. To minimize the likelihood of condensation, perimeter walls should be kept about 5°F above the dew point.[6] Some pools have roll-out vinyl covers which are constantly exposed to moist conditions and which therefore suffer considerable mold growth as well as infestations of mold-eating mites. Pool areas with microbial growth often have a characteristic sour or musty odor, which may be masked by the chlorine.

Hot tubs and whirlpools in spas can be hot spots for microbial growth (including colonization on the covers, whether made of vinyl or wood), in par-

Studies have found that many competitive swimmers (in one report, as many as 60 percent) experience respiratory symptoms when exposed to chlorine or chlorine-containing compounds such as chloramine.[1] Since a number of swimmers report that they have fewer symptoms, if any, in outdoor pools, it makes sense for those who are sensitized to the chemicals found in the water in indoor pools and the air above the water's surface to do most of their swimming outdoors.[2]

1. J. Potts, "Factors Associated with Respiratory Problems in Swimmers," *Sports Medicine* 21, no. 4 (1996): 256–61.

2. L. Fjellbirkeland et al., "Swimming-Induced Asthma," *Tidsskrift for den Norske Laegeforening* 115 (30 June 1995): 2051–53.

Legionella pneumophila, unknown prior to the Philadelphia Legionnaires' Convention in 1976, is now known to be common in the environment. It can be found in plumbing systems, outdoor waterfalls, and spas. In 1997 an outbreak of Legionnaires' disease occurred in Christiansburg, Virginia, at a display of a hot tub in a home improvement store. The CDC determined that twenty-two people were infected, two of whom died. Many of the victims said they had stood near the tub for more than thirty minutes. *L. pneumophila* was growing in the water filter in the hot tub, and customers inhaled the bacteria in droplets aerosolized from the frothing water.[1]

1. Reuters, "CDC to Issue Hot Tub Guidelines," *Boston Globe,* 31 January 1997.

ticular the bacterial species *Legionella pneumophila,* which causes Legionnaires' disease (see chapter 1). In 1994 fifty cases of Legionnaires' disease were traced to the sand filter in a Bermuda cruise ship's whirlpool spa.[7] In 2003 another cruise ship reported three cases of Legionnaires' disease, including one fatality, caused by exposure to *Legionella* bacteria in the potable water system.[8]

Jinxed Rinks

In an enclosed ice-skating arena, the air over the ice is stratified, with cooler, denser air settling near the ice and warmer, less dense air "floating" above. (In winter, a heating system may warm the air for the audience, but the air near the ice is cold.) If the exhaust from an ice-grooming machine is discharged near the ice surface, combustion products, including nitrogen dioxide (NO_2) and carbon monoxide (CO), are cooled and become denser, potentially forming an invisible cloud of polluted air that hangs over the ice and surrounds the skaters.

There have been quite a few reports of hockey players, figure skaters, and even spectators being sickened by combustion products from ice-resurfacing machines. In March 1996 an arena in Seattle had to be evacuated after the CO level, measured by fire department personnel called to the scene, was found to be 354 ppm—more than ten times the suggested permissible limit. Sixty-seven people suffering from nausea and dizziness were taken to hospital emergency rooms and later released.[9]

The exhaust pipes of most ice-grooming machines are raised so that the combustion products mix with and are diluted by the warmer air farther above the ice. In addition, sophisticated catalytic converter systems for the exhaust

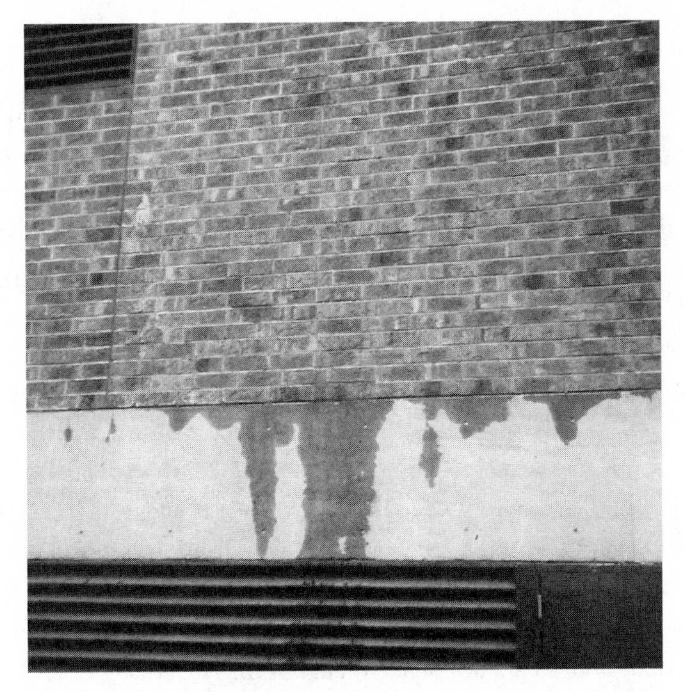

FIGURE 12.1. Excess moisture at a pool. This is the outside of a building on a cold, dry winter day. The building housed a large indoor pool. The air pressure inside the building was greater than the air pressure outside, so warm, moist air was moving from the pool area into the wall cavity behind the brick. Water condensed on the back of the brick, dripped down the wall, and exited at the crack between the concrete and the brick. Stains of efflorescence are visible on the concrete. *May Indoor Air Investigations LLC*

of ice-resurfacing machines are available. In one ice-skating arena, such a system, along with additional combustion controls, reduced the level of carbon monoxide in the air by 57 percent and the level of nitrogen dioxide in the air by 87 percent.[10] And in some states, arena owners are required to monitor the air quality inside these structures by testing regularly for CO and NO_2.

GETTING FROM HERE TO THERE

Unless you are on a bicycle or electrically powered bus or train, traveling between two points requires a fuel-powered vehicle of some kind and an engine to burn the fuel.

Fuels

Most of the fuels used in automobiles, buses, trains, and planes are liquids, such as gasoline and diesel, and consist of hydrocarbons, many of which are volatile organic compounds (see chapter 5). In automobiles, exposure to fuel VOCs can occur when hoses leak or when there is incomplete combustion because an engine needs tuning or repair. Automobile and truck exhaust contains carbon monoxide, nitric oxide, and incompletely burned fuel. Driving in slow-moving heavy traffic can increase exposures to unburned fuel components such as benzene, considered a carcinogen. (A 1997 study undertaken in Los Angeles found an outdoor level of benzene of 3 to 7 micrograms per cubic meter of air and a level in vehicles of 10 to 22 mcg/m^3 of air.)[11]

The chemical methyl-*tert*-butyl ether (MTBE) is added to gasoline as an antiknock compound. This chemical additive can account for as much as 15 percent of the gas you pump into your car. MTBE is being phased out of use, for several reasons. First there were mounting complaints among consumers that the odor of this chemical made them feel ill. Then traces of MTBE began to show up in drinking water, raising significant concerns about health risks.[12] When chemicals are found in drinking water, it is often difficult to pinpoint the source of the contamination, because there are so many possible sources. In this case, however, scientists knew that MTBE in the drinking water could only come from gasoline, because the chemical has no use other than as a fuel additive. Some other chemical must now be added to gasoline to provide the needed antiknock capacity. For the moment, ethyl alcohol appears to be the most promising and least toxic possibility. (Few people are likely to complain about ethyl alcohol residues in water, since this is the same alcohol found in vodka!)

Exhaust from diesel engines also contains soot (see chapter 7). Most school buses run on diesel fuel, so children and bus drivers can be exposed to fine particulate matter produced by combustion in diesel engines (including soot), particularly when several buses are idling in front of a school. A study undertaken in Connecticut showed that children riding in school buses were exposed to high levels of particulates, "as much as five to fifteen times higher than background levels of fine particulate matter." Another study, done by the Natural Resources Defense Council in 2001, "estimates that 23–46 children per million may develop cancer from the excess diesel exhaust on a 1–2 hours daily bus ride."[13]

A study undertaken in California has shown that the concentration of particulate matter is higher outside an automobile than inside.[14] Looking more closely at this relationship, though, reveals that automobile door and window seals are more efficient at preventing larger particles, rather than smaller particles, from entering the interior. Concentrations of smaller particles inside a car are closer to the concentrations of these particles outside (60 to 80 percent). And these smaller particles are more respirable. (The California study also found that vehicles in non-carpool lanes in which trucks were present had pollutant concentrations that were 30 to 60 percent higher than in vehicles in carpool lanes.) And gaseous pollutants consist of molecules that are far smaller than even the smallest particulates, so they enter the car with air infiltration; the concentrations of outside gaseous pollutants, therefore, are similar inside and outside a car.

We live in an automobile-dependent society, so it is difficult to avoid exposures to gasoline fumes and vehicle exhaust. We also depend on airplanes for longer-distance travel. Combustion gases and the fumes from jet fuel (or, in winter, the odor of glycol de-icing solutions) will sometimes enter the cabin when a plane is parked at or near the gate. The rooms in a hotel located at the airport may also smell of jet fuel if the wind is carrying these vapors toward the building.

Indoor Four-Door

A vehicle is usually on the move, but it is still an indoor environment that supplies conditioned (heated or cooled) air for its passengers. The air conveyance system in most cars contains two heat exchangers: one for heating and one for cooling. To supply heat, hot water from the engine block is circulated through the heating coil, and air is blown over the coil. To supply cooling, refrigerant is pumped from a compressor (which operates off the engine fan belt) to the evaporator coil, and the air blown over this coil is cooled. A single blower controls the airflow in either the heating or the cooling mode, and the two coils are next to each other, one downstream from the other.

The surface of the cooling coil in an automobile is no different from the surface of any other air-conditioning coil. Dust can accumulate on the coil when the blower is operating, and the dust can be moistened by water that has condensed when the air is cooled to its dew point, leading to microbial growth. Few pre-2000 vehicles have filters in the heating and cooling system, though after 2000, more and more manufacturers included options for these "cabin air filters." In my opinion, no heating or cooling system, wherever it is located, should ever be operated without efficient and readily accessible filtration (with a minimum MERV rating of 6; see chapter 7). Check to see if your vehicle is equipped with a cabin air filter, because this is an important item that may be omitted from the manufacturer's suggested maintenance schedule. The filter should be changed at least annually. Some of the filters are accessible from the passenger side of the interior, and others must be accessed from under the hood. If you have a hood-accessible filter, make sure that it does not get wet after driving in the rain, or it will get moldy.

As always, wherever there is biodegradable material such as cellulose or dust, microorganisms will proliferate if the conditions are suitable. Automobile carpeting may be dampened by wet shoes or by rainwater entering through some unintended opening in the car's body. The carpeting can then begin to stink as bacteria or fungi grow in the damp carpet dust. I purchased a 1993 Jeep Grand Cherokee that developed an odor reminiscent of an old wet sponge. The smell drove me crazy because I *knew* it was caused by microbial growth, but I couldn't find the source. The odor seemed strongest toward the back of the car. I removed the carpet and pad from the cargo area and found that the pad reeked. I threw both the carpet and pad away, and the smell went away, too.

I still couldn't figure out how water had gotten into the cargo area. Then one day, after a particularly heavy rainstorm, I found the answer. I opened the lift gate at the back, and a small puddle of water appeared on the floor near the lock latch. Apparently the license plate holder was loose, and there was a gap at the gasket that was supposed to be watertight. Water leaked in through the lift-gate door and drained out of the bottom through the latch mechanism and onto the latch plate. The water then flowed onto the cargo area floor. When the carpet and pad were still in place, the water seeped invisibly under the pad and soaked into the fibers. The repair was simple: eliminate the gap in the gasket by tightening the license plate holder. Yet this small leak had caused an air quality problem that nearly ruined my enjoyment of the new car.

Fortunately, most cars are subjected to temperatures hot or cold enough (depending on the climate) to minimize microbial growth. Nonetheless, any vehicle with carpeting that gets wet on a regular basis is a potential source of allergens and microbial volatile organic compounds (MVOCs).

Some vehicles, such as RVs (recreational vehicles), are like carpeted hotels on wheels, with beds, tables, chairs, kitchenette cabinets, and bathrooms. The widespread use of synthetic materials such as plastic in these vehicles creates the potential for all kinds of solvent off-gassing. In addition, these vehicles contain furniture fabricated with particle board, which off-gasses formaldehyde. Because RVs are relatively airtight, the concentrations of VOCs and formaldehyde can be irritating, particularly for people who are hypersensitive to such chemicals.

New-Vehicle Smells

Most people have pleasant associations with the characteristic odor of new car interiors, caused by off-gassing of solvents and other chemicals from vinyl plastics, adhesives, and sealants. Some people think that new-car smell and windshield fogging are both caused by plasticizers such as dioctyl phthalate off-gassing from vinyl. This isn't necessarily the case. The odor associated with new vinyl is caused primarily by the off-gassing of xylene and other solvents. If present in high enough concentrations, these vapors can even condense onto cooler surfaces, including the windshield. In an effort to prevent windshield fogging, car manufacturers generally try to keep concentrations of all of these chemicals low enough that condensation does not occur.

In a study undertaken in 1998 for Australia's Commonwealth Scientific and Industrial Research Organisation, researchers analyzed the volatile organic compounds in three new cars and found more than thirty chemicals, including vapors from residual solvents such as xylene, toluene, ethylbenzene, trimethylbenzene, and five-carbon to twelve-carbon hydrocarbons (C_5H_{12} to $C_{12}H_{26}$).[15] In one car the initial concentration of total volatile organic compounds (TVOCs) was 64 milligrams per cubic meter of air. These concentrations dropped significantly over time. After six months the levels were about 1.5 mg/m^3, and after two years the levels were about 0.4 mg/m^3. For comparison, the outdoor air next to the cars measured 0.1 mg/m^3. Still, owners of new cars should drive with windows open to flush these chemicals out.

At one time, TVOC concentrations in then-new buildings ranged from 20 to 40 milligrams per cubic meter, but as in new cars, these concentrations dropped over time.[1] Nonetheless, it is generally agreed that when TVOC concentrations are greater than 10 mg/m^3—whether in a building or in a car—people will suffer symptoms of sick-building syndrome, such as headaches, respiratory problems, mucous membrane irritation, and hoarseness. We may not think that we spend as much time in cars as in buildings, but for those of us who have a long commute to work or who drive for hours as part of our jobs, the car in a way *is* our office.

1. L. Ember, "Survey Finds High Indoor Levels of Volatile Organic Chemicals," *Chemical and Engineering News*, 5 December 1988.

New-car smell has been used as a marketing tool. One of the first artificial fragrances developed for cars was leather scent, a smell often associated with quality and wealth. Cars that no longer smell new can be treated with new-car-smell spray. The interior of an older car may also be wiped with cleaning compounds containing strong fragrances to give the car a "fresh" scent.

Some people aren't bothered by the chemicals in new and secondhand cars, but others have been forced to return a vehicle, at a significant financial loss, because they couldn't tolerate the off-gassing.

Respiration aboard Public Transportation

Soot and combustion products generated by traffic, as well as VOCs evaporating from fuels, may be present in the air in a bus or on a train. And a vehicle's heating or air-conditioning system may also be a source of bioaerosol. Exposure to these contaminants may be considerable for bus drivers and train conductors as well as for commuters. The best way to minimize transportation pollutants is to maintain the vehicle so that emissions of soot, unburned fuel, and other VOCs are as low as possible.

Air in the Air

One of the biggest improvements in air quality on airplanes has been the banning of smoking, at least on domestic flights in this country. That said, there have still been documented problems with air quality in airplanes, including the use of pesticides on flights to Australia and New Zealand as well as instances of vapors from hydraulic fluids and engine oils getting into a plane's ventilation system.[16] People who are highly allergic to mold, pets, or mites should be aware that there may be a fellow passenger sitting nearby or walking past whose clothing is peppered with allergens that are intermittently aerosolized. And there is always the concern that someone will catch a cold or the flu if a neighboring passenger sneezes and coughs.

Many people feel that they are more likely to become ill after flying in an airplane than after traveling by other means, and sometimes you will see people on airplanes wearing face masks, presumably to screen out microorganisms. Wearing a mask will also protect others from your germs if you travel with a cold; in Japan this is considered polite behavior. (A mask filters out particulates that may carry bacteria and viruses, but it also adds moisture to air you inhale. The relative humidity on airplanes can be as low as 5 to 15 percent, and breathing such dry air increases your likelihood of getting a cold.)[17]

A number of people recently became infected with SARS (Severe Acute Respiratory Syndrome, a lethal contagious disease) while traveling by air. Investigators found, however, that few cases could be directly attributed to transmission during air travel. According to Dr. David Heymann, chief of communicable diseases for the World Health Organization, "There were 35 flights on which SARS-infected people who were symptomatic with disease traveled. . . . We know, however, that on only four of those planes was there actually passage of the disease." Two of the individuals who became infected were flight attendants and fourteen were passengers seated within four seats of the SARS patient.[18]

An airplane is a sealed metal tube full of people. Years ago it was relatively cheap to heat fresh air that was pumped into the cabin, because fuel was less expensive. But today fuel is more costly, so about half the air in an airplane is recirculated, to save heating costs.[19] In 2000 some consultants recommended that the amount of fresh air supplied be halved from the 10 cubic feet per minute per person recommended by the Federal Aviation Administration to 5 cfm/person in order to save money. "But the notion that the industry would consider less fresh air," reported the *Wall Street Journal,* "has already created an uproar among flight attendants."[20] And, of course, reduced ventilation in any indoor environment means higher concentrations of carbon dioxide and any contaminants or infectious microbes that may be present. In 1994, however, *Consumer Reports* found that on 158 flights, only 1 out of 4 had a carbon dioxide concentration above 1,000 ppm (though the concentration may be higher if a plane is idling on the runway).[21]

DESTINATIONS

Hotels are cleaned more often than many other residential spaces; thus fragrances and irritating residues of cleaning compounds can be a problem for sensitized individuals. Hotel vacuum cleaners are rarely HEPA-filtered, so every time housekeeping vacuums the carpet, whatever is in the carpet can become suspended in the air. And most hotels and motels have ice machines and beverage vending machines on every floor or every other floor. These machines have compressors, coils, and fans that can become contaminated and circulate bioaerosol. In addition, condensation from cold surfaces in or on the machines can drip, supplying moisture for microbial growth in carpet or other dust.

In a newer hotel or motel, each room usually has its own fan coil or heat pump. In a large hotel there could be hundreds of such units, each of which should be kept clean, free of microbial growth, and adequately filtered (MERV 6 or 8; see chapter 7). It is hard, however, to keep so many units serviced properly, so they are often contaminated and thus produce the characteristic sweat-sock odor associated with microbial growth. In addition, many motels are of slab-on-grade construction. Often the rooms on the ground floor are characterized by a strong musty odor, commonly arising from mildew growth on dust in carpeting that is laid on concrete.

In warm and humid climates, when the air pressure is lower inside a motel room than outside the building, warm moist air infiltrates wall cavities, and water vapor migrates into interior drywall. When the walls are covered with vinyl wallpaper, the wallpaper creates a vapor barrier, and moisture trapped or condensing behind the wallpaper can lead to extensive fungal growth. MVOCs can diffuse through the wallpaper, and if the wallpaper seams become loose as a result of the fungal growth beneath, mold spores can enter the room on airflows.

Mold at the Hilton

One of the most dramatic examples of mold growth in a hotel or motel occurred at Hilton's Hawaiian Village in Honolulu.[22] The $100 million twenty-four-story Kalia Tower on Waikiki Beach opened in May 2001 with over four hundred guest rooms, and it closed a mere three months later after widespread fungal growth was found on walls and furniture. Numerous lawsuits ensued. One of the actions claimed that the bathroom exhaust removed more air than the ventilation system could supply. The building envelope wasn't airtight, so moist warm air infiltrated the wall cavities and leaked into the interior, creating conditions of high relative humidity indoors, conducive to mold growth. The repairs, initially estimated at $10 million, ended up costing $56 million and took approximately a year to complete. Carpeting, drapes, wallpaper, bedding, furniture, and even towels made the trip to the dumpster. Some of the hotel employees reported allergy problems, but apparently the exposures weren't long enough, either for employees or guests, for most of the people involved to develop chronic health problems.

Redecorating

The Kalia Tower was closed during the remediation and subsequent remodeling, but most hotels and motels cannot afford to shut down while undergoing cosmetic renovations. All too often, walls are painted and new carpeting installed in the absence of containment conditions and while the rest of the hotel is open for business. And after the work is completed, rooms are usually occupied before the carpeting and newly finished surfaces have off-gassed sufficiently.

In an ideal world, it would make sense for hotel management to attempt to isolate areas during remodeling and to flush out spaces after the work is done. But alas, financial considerations all too often outweigh indoor air quality concerns.

Sleep Tight, Don't Let the Bedbugs Bite

Bedbugs are making a comeback in the United States. The size of an apple seed, bedbugs hide during the day in small, dark, protected spaces, like cracks in floors and walls, behind baseboards, or in mattresses or box springs. A bedbug feeds on a sleeper's blood at night, sometimes consuming three times its weight in fluid in just ten minutes. Bedbugs do not spread diseases to human beings, but they do leave itchy marks, often on the arms. (Dust mites, which are microscopic and do not bite but can cause allergies, feed on shed skin flakes in mattresses, pillows, upholstered furniture, and carpets; see chapters 3 and 6.)

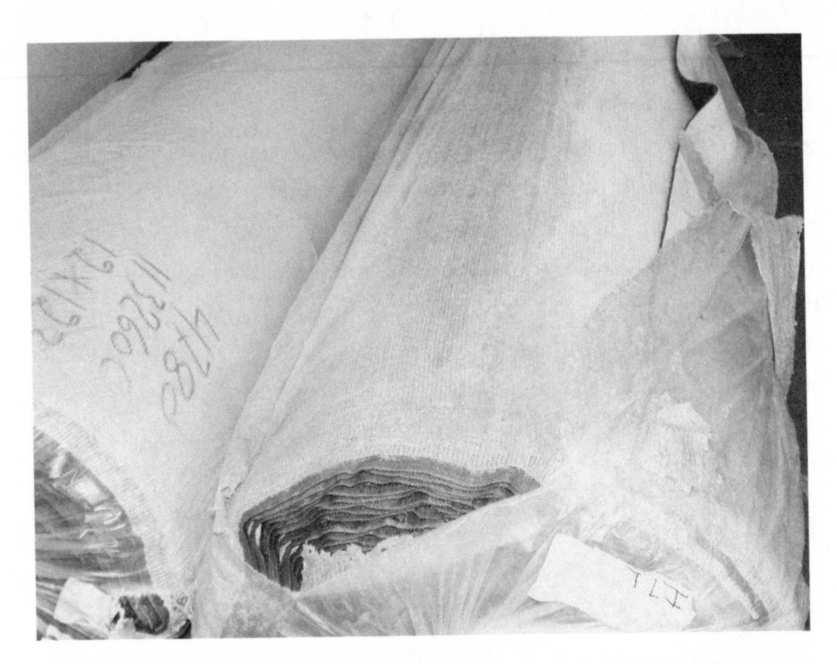

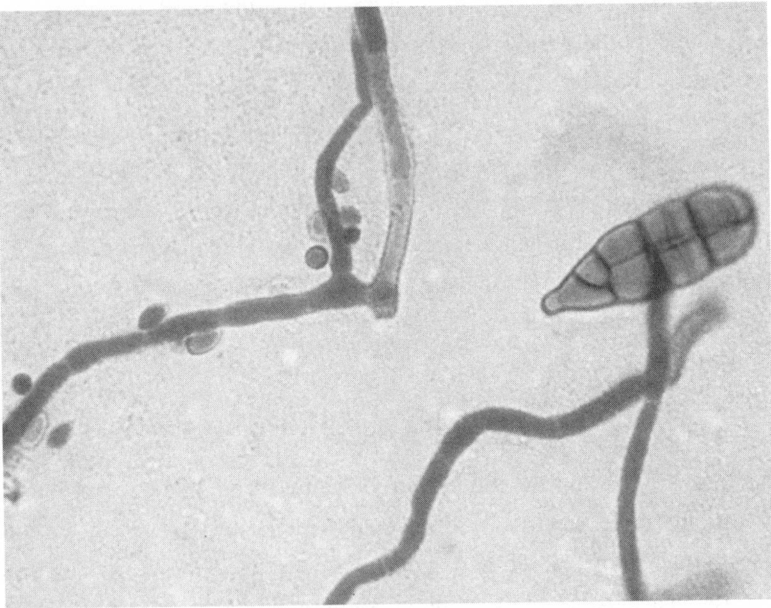

FIGURE 12.2. Doomed from the start. *Top panel:* Two rolls of new carpet, awaiting installation, sit on the floor in a hotel lobby. The plastic wrap on the roll at the right is torn, and there are water stains on the carpet backing, suggesting that the carpet had been sitting in a puddle of water. *Bottom panel:* This photomicrograph (a photograph taken through a microscope, in this case magnified about 500 times) depicts mold hyphae and two different types of mold spores that were found in the dust adhering to the carpet: a large *Alternaria* spore at the right, and several smaller oval and round *Cladosporium* spores at the left. This carpet was contaminated with mold before it was even installed. *Jeffrey C. May*

Bedbugs are carried in clothing, suitcases, and secondhand mattresses, bedding, and furniture. They can also live in birds' nests. In multilevel residential buildings, bedbugs can spread from one unit to another. To control these pests, their hiding places *(harborages)* must be found and treated by professionals. Mattresses can also be treated with steam vapor.

Hotels and motels seem particularly plagued by bedbugs. Even luxurious establishments can be stricken: Manhattan's Helmsley Park Lane Hotel was sued by a Mexican guest who claimed he was attacked by bedbugs while he was sleeping at the hotel![23]

SOME PRACTICAL STEPS

- For the sake of fire safety and indoor air quality, pipe openings in walls or floors that might be allowing infiltration of contaminants should be sealed.
- Never fill a bathtub above the bottom of the escutcheon plate.
- Avoid exercising in a musty-smelling health club, especially if the exercise space is below grade.
- If you have asthma and find that you wheeze when swimming in an indoor pool, swim outdoors whenever you can and talk to your doctor.
- Drivers, particularly of school buses, should minimize engine-idle time.
- If you notice a sweat-sock or musty odor emanating from an automobile's heating/cooling system, you can reduce your exposure to allergens by briefly running the blower on high with the windows open to air out the system. The system can also be removed and cleaned.
- Water-impervious mats that can be cleaned and replaced when worn should be placed over automobile carpeting that is likely to get wet.
- If the air on a bus seems stuffy, sit next to an operable window and open it for some fresh air.
- If you are a flight attendant, keep a log of any symptoms you experience that might be connected to the quality of the air within the

plane (pilots often get 100 percent fresh air, though outdoor pollutants can still enter the cockpit).

- If the smell of jet fuel bothers you, avoid staying in a hotel located near an airport.
- When booking a room in a hotel or motel, ask for one with operable windows.
- If you have mold sensitivities or allergies and your hotel room has a musty smell, ask to be moved to another room. If that's not possible, turn off the room's heating or air-conditioning system and lay sheets or towels down on the carpeting to serve as "runners"—pathways that you can walk on without excessively disturbing contaminated carpet dust.
- If you have mite, mold, or feather sensitivities, avoid feather pillows and quilts, even when traveling.
- If you are sensitive to paint solvents or dust, ask if renovation or remodeling work is going on in the hotel before you book a room there. You may want to consider staying elsewhere if such work is in progress.
- Regular vacuuming can aerosolize contaminants, so if you have dust or mold sensitivities, ask that housekeeping skip your hotel room while you are there. A room does not need to be vacuumed every day.
- If you are on a building's housekeeping staff and you have allergies or asthma, encourage the management to purchase HEPA-filtered vacuums, which can reduce aerosol problems.
- If you are affected by poor indoor air quality, carry a NIOSH N95 mask. If you are sensitive to hydrocarbons (see chapter 5), keep a charcoal vapor mask handy. And don't be embarrassed to use a mask when you need it.

PART

III

The Final Test

Grading the Air

If people who have always felt comfortable in their office space begin to experience headaches or other sick-building symptoms soon after the installation of new carpeting, one obvious possible source of the problem is chemical emissions from the carpet or the carpet adhesive. If musty or sour odors develop soon after a school building has experienced a flood, microbial growth has most likely occurred in carpeting or within wall cavities. A moldy ceiling tile, a patch of mold on a wall, or a soiled HVAC system (particularly one in which the lining material has been wet) are other obvious potential sources of allergenic bioaerosol. Any of these sources of contaminants could possibly be remediated before expensive air testing is undertaken.

If you are trying to unravel an indoor air quality puzzle, create a time line of events that occurred in the building before people began to experience symptoms, take a walk-through to look for obvious sources of trouble, and apply simple solutions to see if the IAQ complaints abate. If this approach doesn't solve the problem, then testing may be needed. Testing is most useful when there are no obvious sources or documented events that may have led to IAQ problems.

In chapter 13 I discuss some of the tests for gases and allergens that building occupants can perform themselves. In chapter 14 I discuss tests that are generally done only by IAQ professionals. IAQ professionals who collect samples of air and dust must have a basic understanding of building science, the workings of mechanical systems, and potential sources of allergens and irri-

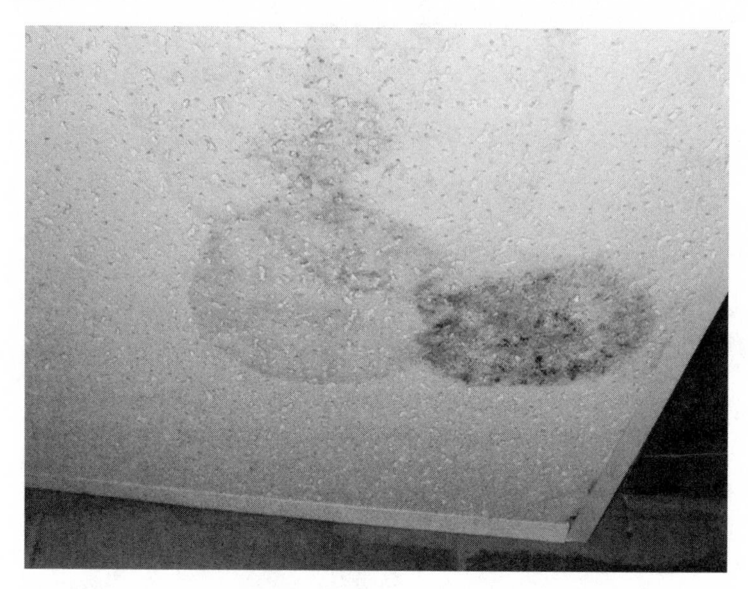

Stained and moldy ceiling tiles like these are often ignored, but they can be a source of allergens. *May Indoor Air Investigations LLC*

tants. For that matter, *anyone* who undertakes an air quality test, whether the person is an IAQ professional or a building occupant, must have a clear sense of where to begin, and why.

Chapter 15 contains further IAQ information that may be useful to technically minded readers.

CHAPTER

13

Do It Yourself

This chapter is titled "Do It Yourself," but not everyone has the confidence or knowledge to conduct air quality testing. Still, there are a number of simple testing devices that building occupants can use to find possible sources of air quality problems.

If you choose to use such a device, make sure you know what the conditions should be during the testing period and what a numerical result may mean. In addition, always read manufacturers' directions thoroughly before you begin, because while many test kits are safe, others contain dangerous chemicals and require that you break glass seals.

MEASURING GASES AND VAPORS

Most of the tests that building occupants can use to measure gases and vapors are *passive devices:* they do not have pumps to move the air. Such devices may consist simply of tubes or badges that react with or adsorb chemicals from the air. (The Resource Guide lists several companies that sell passive testing devices.) Some passive testing devices are *direct-read* (the results can be read directly from the device), while others must be returned to a lab for analysis.

Carbon Dioxide

Concentrations. Carbon dioxide is usually present in the outdoor air at about 360 parts per million (the concentration depends mostly on nearby combustion sources such as chimneys and vehicular traffic). General recom-

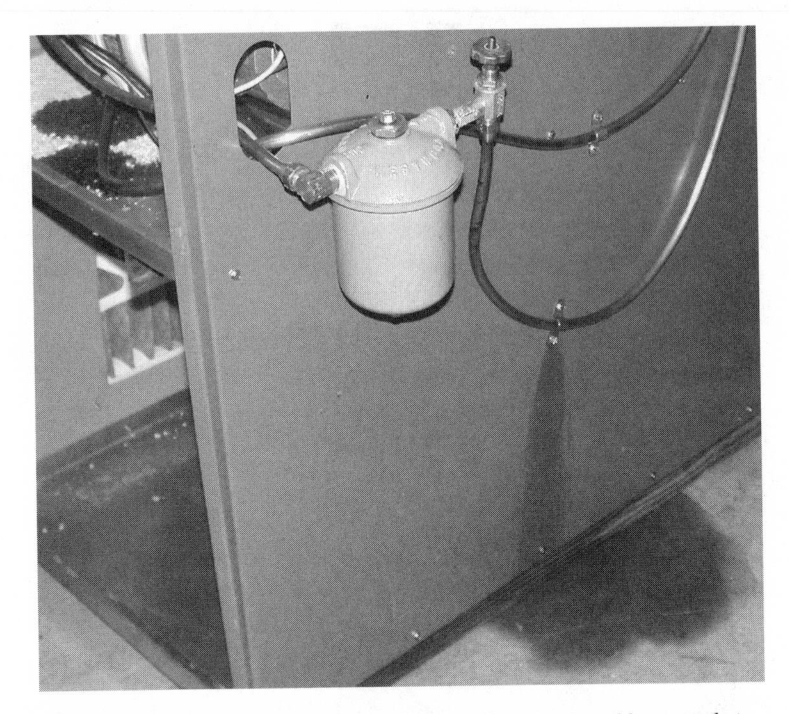

FIGURE 13.1. Oil leaks at a furnace. The origins of some IAQ problems are obvious. Here is a furnace with two visible oil leaks: the dark circular stains in the upper left and lower right corners of the photograph. The white object on the outside of the furnace is an oil filter with copper tubing entering and leaving. Oil is leaking from the safety valve at the right of the filter, then dripping down the oil line and the side of the furnace and pooling on the floor. The second leak (upper left corner) is from the oil burner (not visible in the photograph). Instead of repairing the leak, a heating technician placed an absorbent compound (the stained white granules) under the dripping line to soak up the oil. Leaks like these are easy to repair and if left unaddressed can lead to hydrocarbon vapors in the air (see chapters 5 and 14). *May Indoor Air Investigations LLC*

mendations for indoor concentrations range from 600 to 1,000 ppm (see chapter 5). In the EPA's BASE (Building Assessment, Survey, and Evaluation) Study, fifty-six randomly selected non-complaint (not "sick") office buildings were found to have indoor CO_2 concentrations in the range of 449 to 1,092 ppm, with a mean of 665 ppm.[1] In other studies, subjects in controlled environments were exposed to CO_2 in concentration ranges of 10,000 to 40,000 ppm (1 to 4 percent of air). Participants experienced fatigue during exercise as well as changes in blood chemistry, but no serious long-term health effects were noted.[2] The concentration of CO_2 that is considered by NIOSH to be "immediately dangerous to life or health" (IDLH) is 50,000 ppm, or 5 percent of the air. This concentration could never be reached in a nonindustrial environment, unless a tank of carbon dioxide ruptured.

What you can do. If your office seems stuffy and you are concerned about carbon dioxide levels, you can buy a device called a *direct-read diffusion tube* to measure the CO_2 concentration. This device is small and contains chemicals, including a dye that changes color when exposed to CO_2. The tube is designed to be hung in place for up to eight hours, and the CO_2 concentration can then be read from a scale on the glass surface of the tube. Keep in mind that these tubes are associated with a large margin of error—plus or minus 15 percent or more (up to 25 percent). In addition, they measure the *average* CO_2 concentration over the specific time period rather than the *maximum* CO_2 concentration that might be present over that time period. Still, a diffusion tube is one way for you to start addressing your IAQ concern. (Just be very careful to follow the directions when working with glass tubes.)

Carbon dioxide concentration is a measure of the ventilation provided for a space. If the CO_2 in your workspace is high (well over 1,000 ppm), find out how fresh air is being delivered and whether the ventilation can be increased. Though you cannot directly measure the volume or flow rate of fresh air yourself, ASHRAE recommends that ventilation systems be designed to provide 20 cubic feet of fresh air per minute per person for offices and 15 cfm/person for schools. Note that since the occupancy of any space varies, so do its ventilation requirements. It would be wasteful, for example, to ventilate an auditorium for its allowed number of occupants if no one is seated in the audience.

Carbon Monoxide

Concentrations. The ASHRAE recommendation for maximum indoor carbon monoxide concentrations in nonindustrial buildings is 9 parts per million, and the OSHA permissible exposure limit (PEL) for CO for the industrial workplace is 50 ppm (see chapter 5).

Some CO detectors sound an alarm whenever an elevated level of CO is present; other CO detectors sound an alarm and also have a light-emitting diode (LED) display that indicates the CO concentration, expressed numerically in parts per million. Keep in mind, though, that few if any CO alarms of less-than-professional quality will detect the gas at the ASHRAE limit of 9 ppm. In fact, one alarm commonly available at hardware stores only registers CO levels from 30 to 999 ppm. In other words, the purpose of most readily available CO detectors is to measure rapid increases in CO concentrations that might quickly lead to serious health symptoms, rather than long-term low concentrations that could still have health consequences as a result of chronic exposures. To measure lower CO concentrations (2 to 25 ppm), a short-term passive direct-read testing device can be used (*short-term* meaning that the device is left in place for several hours).

What you can do. Where carbon monoxide exposures are likely to occur, buying a CO detector is a sensible step. Most hardware stores sell plug-in CO detectors. Correct placement of the detector is important, so follow the manufacturer's directions carefully. In smaller buildings with a basement heating system, such as an oil- or gas-fired boiler, I suggest that one CO detector be installed close to the basement ceiling, because any CO present will be carried in the hot air that leaks out of the boiler and then rises. In any building, a CO detector should be installed close to the ceiling of any occupied space located near a boiler room or mechanical closet, whether in a basement or on any other level of the building. In areas of a building that are remote from combustion sources, it does not matter how high off the floor the detector is placed, because any CO present will be more evenly mixed in the air. Finally, any alarm-type CO detector should be placed within earshot.

Formaldehyde

Concentrations. As you remember from chapter 3, formaldehyde is an irritating, pungent, and carcinogenic gas.[3] The OSHA PEL for formaldehyde in industrial settings is 0.75 part per million.[4] The ASHRAE guideline for acceptable indoor levels of formaldehyde in nonindustrial buildings is less (0.1 ppm).

Formaldehyde is a possible product of incomplete combustion (see chapter 5). The most common indoor sources of formaldehyde, however, are pressed-wood products and furniture finishes that contain formaldehyde-based resins (see chapter 3). In older homes with solid-wood furniture, formaldehyde levels are below 0.1 ppm. In homes containing construction materials and many pieces of furniture made of pressed-wood products, the levels can be greater than 0.3 ppm.[5] Formaldehyde emissions from sources vary with temperature and relative humidity. The higher the RH and temperature, the stronger the emission rate.

What you can do. Passive test kits that measure formaldehyde concentrations usually cost under $100. One type of kit consists of a sealed glass vial containing an accurately weighed amount of a white powder (sodium bisulfite) that combines chemically with formaldehyde in the air. The vial is uncapped, left open for about five days, then sealed and mailed to a lab for analysis.

Nitrogen Dioxide

Concentrations. The indoor concentration of nitrogen dioxide in offices is generally close to the outdoor concentration, unless there are indoor combustion sources. In a German study of fourteen offices, the average concentration of NO_2 was 14.7 parts per billion.[6] The World Health Organization guideline for NO_2 in indoor ice arenas is 213 ppb. (In a study that measured concentrations of NO_2 at 332 ice arenas in nine countries, the mean concentration was found to be 228 ppb.)[7] Nitrogen dioxide concentrations above 300 ppb can make asthma symptoms worse (see chapter 5).

What you can do. Some passive monitors measure average nitrogen dioxide concentrations over several days, but measuring concentrations of NO_2

In 1996 the EPA calculated that the total formaldehyde emissions outdoors in Connecticut were just over 2,000 tons per year. Major sources included on-road heavy-duty diesel vehicles (180 tons/year); on-road light-duty gasoline trucks (293 tons/year); on-road light-duty gasoline vehicles (282 tons/year); off-highway diesel vehicles (807 tons/year); and off-highway gasoline four-stroke vehicles (121 tons/year). Two surprising sources were motorcycles (11 tons/year) and the open burning of forest fires and wildfires (185 tons/year). Softwood drying kilns won the contest, if one could call it that, with the lowest emission of formaldehyde (0.09 ton/year).[1]

1. EPA, "Air Toxics in New England: Formaldehyde Emissions Breakdown for Connecticut (1996)," www.epa.gov/region01/eco/airtox/ct_pollutants/form.html.

TABLE 13.1. Air quality index (AQI) for outdoor levels of ozone

Index value	Level of health concern
51–100*	Moderate
101–150	Unhealthy for sensitive groups
151–200	Unhealthy
201–300	Very unhealthy
301–500	Hazardous

Source: Adapted from EPA, "Air Quality Index: A Guide to Air Quality and Your Health," table on 5–6, www.epa.gov/airnow/aqibroch/aqi.html.

* An AQI of 100 for ozone generally corresponds to an ozone level of 0.08 part per million (averaged over eight hours).

for several shorter periods is a more accurate indicator of sporadic, potentially higher-level exposures. For short-term measurements, an active sampler is needed, which probably requires the hiring of an indoor air quality professional. NO_2 concentrations should be monitored periodically in buildings such as indoor skating rinks or offices attached to warehouses, where gas-powered (propane, natural gas) or gasoline-powered equipment or vehicles routinely operate indoors, particularly if combustion odors are noticeable.

Ozone

Concentrations. The National Ambient Air Quality Standard for ozone concentrations in the outdoor air is 0.08 part per million (averaged over eight hours). The FDA recommends that ozone-producing devices create a maximum ozone concentration indoors of no more than 0.05 ppm.

Unless there are indoor sources of ozone, the ozone concentration outdoors is greater than the concentration indoors, partly because ozone is constantly being generated by the action of sunlight on oxygen and other gases and vapors in the atmosphere, and partly because ozone is very reactive (it combines chemically with other substances): once ozone has infiltrated a building, it begins to combine with other VOCs present in the indoor air as well as with substances on or close to the surfaces of walls, floors, and ceilings. Thus the indoor ozone concentration falls below the outdoor concentration.

Some people think that low levels of ozone can purify the air. But ionizing purifiers do not eliminate formaldehyde or many of the VOCs that can be present indoors. In addition, ozone does not get rid of particulates (mold spores, pollen).[8] Ozone will eliminate some odors, but it can combine with other vapors to create irritants (see chapter 5). In fact, the use of ozone can create particulates through chemical reactions between ozone gas and VOCs.[9]

What you can do. I am not aware of any inexpensive ozone-testing instruments; however, a small and fairly inexpensive passive ozone indicator, called the *OzoneWatch,* is available (see the Resource Guide). This indicator can be placed in an environment for an hour to measure levels of ozone up to 140 ppb (or 0.14 ppm), with an error margin of plus or minus 15 percent. The OzoneWatch can be used to test ozone concentrations in ambient air outside and inside, as well as ozone concentrations in rooms where copiers and ionizing "air purifiers" are operated.

An elevated concentration of ozone can often be detected by those who are familiar with the odor of this gas. If you do not know what ozone smells like, sniff a piece of clothing that has been washed (with fragrance-free detergent, please!) and hung out in the sun to dry, or smell the air coming out of an ozone-generating purifier or an ionizing "air purifier," which generally emits ozone along with ions (charged molecules).

Radon

Concentrations. As you remember from chapter 5, a level of radon in air greater than 4 picocuries per liter (pCi/L) is considered to be above the EPA's action level, and further testing or remediation is needed.

What you can do. Radon test kits are available at most hardware and building-supply stores. All radon test kits must be sent to a lab for analysis. When you buy a radon test kit, you prepay for the analysis and report.

The placement of a radon test kit can affect the test results. A kit placed on a basement floor or at a foundation crack may give a much higher reading than a kit placed above the floor or several feet away from the crack, because air containing radon enters the building from the soil surrounding the foundation walls and floor. (See the Resource Guide for information regarding the EPA's recommendations for radon-testing protocol.)

Levels of radon in air can fluctuate from one day to the next, from 3 pCi/L to over 100 pCi/L, because the rate at which air containing radon enters a building depends on how much the air pressure in the soil exceeds the air pressure in the below-grade space (see chapter 5). If you get a high reading during one test, it is definitely worth repeating the test. Because the levels of radon in air can vary so dramatically, the results of an Alpha-Trak radon test kit (see the Resource Guide) that can be left in place for over a month are more meaningful than the results of a kit that stays in place for only forty-eight hours.

MEASURING RELATIVE HUMIDITY AND TEMPERATURE

Ranges. Relative humidity outdoors can range from 100 percent down to about 10 percent. The indoor range in a building with the windows open can be similar to the outdoor range, but in the BASE study of fifty-six buildings, indoor RH was found to be in the range of 9 to 55 percent, with a mean (average) of 33 percent.[10]

What you can do. If you feel that your workspace is too warm or too cool, or too humid or too dry, for comfort, you can buy a thermo-hygrometer, available in many hardware stores. A *hygrometer* measures RH, and a *thermo-hygrometer* measures temperature as well as RH. Older hygrometers have a dial face. The actual moisture sensor in many of the older dial instruments was a tautly stretched blond human hair (hair adsorbs and loses water vapor, depending on the RH). Newer thermo-hygrometers have a digital display. Thermo-hygrometers costing much less than $40 are too inaccurate to be useful. Even $40 instruments can provide readings that are above or below the actual RH by as much as 15 percent.

As you now know, elevated RH can be conducive to mold growth. Keep in mind that where there is mildew growth indoors, on a wall at a foundation or at the exterior perimeter of a building, more than likely the RH at the mildewed surface is higher than the RH at the center of the room. The RH should therefore be measured at both locations.

DETECTING MOLD

A settle-plate test kit, available at home- and building-supply stores, can be used to determine the presence of airborne mold spores. The kit consists of a sterile petri dish with nutrient agar (gelled water containing nutrients for mold); mold spores settle out of the air (hence the name of the test) and stick

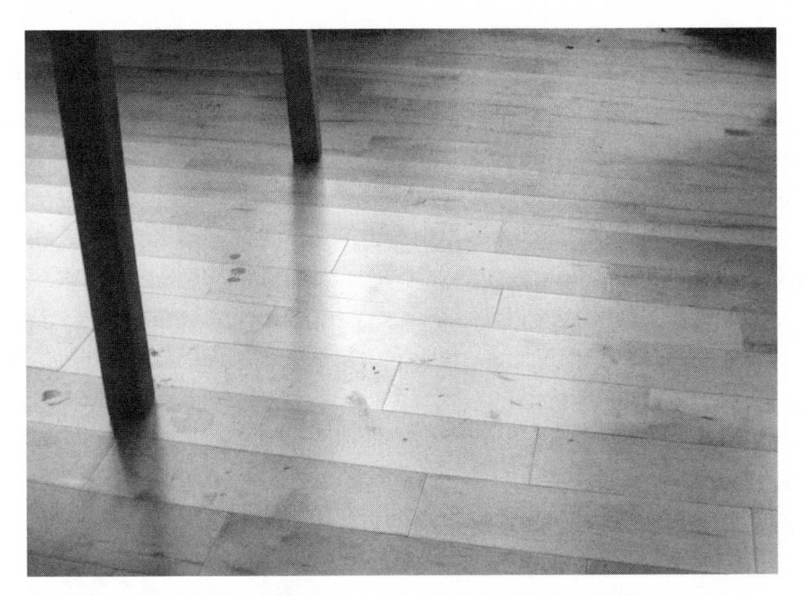

FIGURE 13.2. Warped floorboards. When wood flooring is installed, the moisture content of the wood must be in equilibrium (in balance) with the relative humidity in the room; otherwise the boards will either shrink (if the air is drier) or swell and expand (if the air is more humid). Moisture can also enter wood flooring from below. In this photograph, birch flooring was installed over concrete, and there is no vapor barrier between the concrete and the soil below. Moisture diffused from the soil through the concrete into the floorboards, which then swelled after installation and warped (cupped): each board is now higher at the edges than at the center. *May Indoor Air Investigations LLC*

to the agar. To conduct a settle-plate test, you place the sealed dish in the area you want to test, remove the cover, and leave the dish open for a set period of time (usually at least an hour). You then cover the dish and either allow it to incubate at room temperature or send it to a lab for incubation and analysis.

In my opinion, the results of settle-plate tests are not always a reliable measure of mold problems, for several reasons.

First, some people leave the dishes open for a few minutes, while other people leave them open for days. The longer a petri dish remains open, the more airborne spores the dish can collect. If you leave an open petri dish anywhere long enough, it will collect mold spores, since they are always present in air. One man proudly told me that he had left a petri dish open for seventy-two hours. It is no surprise that the dish became overgrown with mold colonies.

Second, larger spores settle out of air more quickly than smaller ones do, so a petri dish tends to collect the larger spores, particularly if open for less than an hour. Yet the smaller mold spores are more likely to cause health problems, because they remain airborne longer and are more respirable.

Third, the lab report on the mold growth that occurred in the petri dish may not be altogether helpful. Depending on the season and direction of airflows, many of the mold spores may have entered the building from the exterior, and thus the growth in the petri dish may not represent the potential for exposure to mold growing inside the building. Moreover, some molds grow more readily than others in petri dishes, so the absence of a colony in the dish does not mean that the mold spores are absent from the air. And finally, only culturable (living) mold spores germinate in the agar, whereas even dead spores can cause indoor air quality problems (see chapter 8).

Settle-plate testing is generally useful only if colonies of spores typical of damp building environments (such as *Penicillium* and *Aspergillus* species) are found indoors but not outdoors, and this means that the outdoor air must always be tested at the same time.

DETECTING DUST MITE, COCKROACH, AND PET ALLERGENS

Concentration ranges for dust mite, cockroach, and pet allergens are discussed in chapter 14. People frequently hire indoor air quality professionals to test for these allergens in office and commercial buildings, but you don't really need a professional. Inexpensive and easy-to-use test kits are readily available from laboratories (see the Resource Guide). Such kits consist of a filter bag that is attached to a vacuum cleaner to trap the dust. The bag is then returned to the lab for analysis.

SOME PRACTICAL STEPS

- Consider using some of the inexpensive measuring devices mentioned in this chapter.
- All buildings with combustion equipment or underground parking garages should have carbon monoxide detectors.

CHAPTER

14

Call in a Professional

Indoor air quality professionals (IAQPs) who sample dust and air generally use complicated and delicate measuring instruments, refer to puzzling regulatory limits, and write reports with incomprehensible lists of contaminant concentrations. It is my hope that this chapter and the chapter that follows will help guide you through this fog.

DUST OR AIR?

There is a longstanding controversy in the scientific community concerning how best to test for particulate matter. Some think that the only way to assess personal exposures to particulates is to identify and measure the concentrations of aerosol (airborne particulates, rather than gases and vapors) through *air sampling*. Others think that measuring the contaminants in settled dust *(dust sampling)* is a meaningful substitute for aerosol measurements, which are often difficult to make because of the relatively small amount of aerosol usually present.

Air sampling can be short-term (minutes) or long-term (hours to days). There is no question that long-term air monitoring for the identity and changing concentrations of aerosol gives the fullest information about what contaminants are present and how their concentrations change over time. Because the aerosol concentrations may be low, long sampling times with high-volume, noisy air samplers may be needed. For government-supported studies of outdoor air, this approach is suitable, but for commercial indoor investigations, the costs may be prohibitive. Since contaminants in dust are often the cause of indoor air quality problems, dust sampling for allergens or mold spores or short-term air sampling may be the least expensive and most rapid means to determine if there are reservoirs for aerosol present.

SAMPLING AIRBORNE AND SETTLED DUST FOR PARTICULATE MATTER

Particulate matter can be either *biogenic,* such as bioaerosol containing pollen, mold spores, and bacteria, or *nonbiogenic,* such as aerosol containing fiberglass or asbestos (see chapter 6). There are a number of ways in which IAQPs sample dust on surfaces as well as particulate matter in the air.

In *source sampling,* the suspected source of contamination is sampled. There are two common kinds of source sampling. In *bulk sampling,* a sample of the material that might be contaminated (such as drywall, paper, or wood) is removed carefully (to avoid spreading contaminants), packaged, and sent to a lab for analysis. In *surface sampling,* dust is removed from the surface of what may be a contamination source, using clear tape, sterile swabs, or wipes. Air and surfaces other than the contamination sources are also sampled, to gauge the spread of contaminants into the environment. Again, samples of surface dust can be collected on clear tape or with sterile swabs or wipes.

Aerosolized particulates can be captured with an active device that has a fan or vacuum pump to draw in air at a known rate (usually between 0.1 and 30 liters of air per minute) through some kind of filter or trap (a plastic or glass surface with a sticky coating). The sampling time is measured, and since the airflow rate is known, the total amount of air can be calculated (airflow rate × time) and a numerical value for the concentration be determined. Sampled dust may be weighed and analyzed either chemically or visually (by microscopy, to characterize the particles present), or both.

Sampling for Mold

As we have seen over and over again in this book, elevated indoor concentrations of mold spores in air can have a serious impact on the health of sensitized building occupants and may even lead to sensitization. Determining the presence of mold spores is thus an important component of any IAQ investigation. In chapter 8 we took a detailed look at the mold sampling reports from the McKinley school and at some of the pitfalls of mold testing. Here I look at some of the actual testing equipment that IAQPs use to test for mold as well as the aspects of mold testing and the results obtained that I believe are important.

The *Burkard Personal Air Sampler* and the *Allergenco MK-IV* are two of the many air-sampling instruments used to collect bioaerosol such as mold. The *Air-O-Cell® Cassette* is another commonly used device, but since it consists of a disposable plastic impactation trap (used to catch spores on a surface), it must be connected to a separate air pump. Whichever device is used, the particulates are examined by light microscopy for visual identification. In *total spore sampling,* hyphal fragments are also counted, and spores and hyphae are reported as counts or spores per cubic meter. Generally the spores are identified only by genus (plural *genera,* groupings in the system of biological classification) and not by species (there are usually many species within a genus), though in some cases the species can be determined. What cannot be determined visually through light microscopy is whether the spores are alive (culturable).

If impacted spores (spores that have been caught on a surface) are to be cultured (left over time to grow), they are usually trapped on a culture medium: an agar gel of water containing dissolved nutrients. This kind of sampling is called *culturable* or *viable,* and the most common device used by IAQPs for this purpose is the *Andersen Sampler,* which consists of a round metal holder just big enough to contain a petri dish. Above the dish is a metal plate with four hundred tiny, evenly spaced holes. A separate vacuum pump sucks air out of the base of the holder, under the petri dish. To equalize the air pressure, air rushes back into the holder through the sampler opening above the perforated plate and petri dish. As the air moves through the plate, it is divided up by the holes into four hundred fine airstreams that blow onto the surface of the petri dish, where airborne particulates impact and stick to the agar.

During sampling, the petri dish is exposed to an airflow of about 30 liters per minute, usually for about three to six minutes (though in a highly contaminated environment, sample times of less than a minute may be used). After exposure, the petri dish is covered, packaged up, and sent overnight to a lab, where it is placed in an incubating oven and left there for about a week. The mold colonies that grow are then counted and identified by species, if this

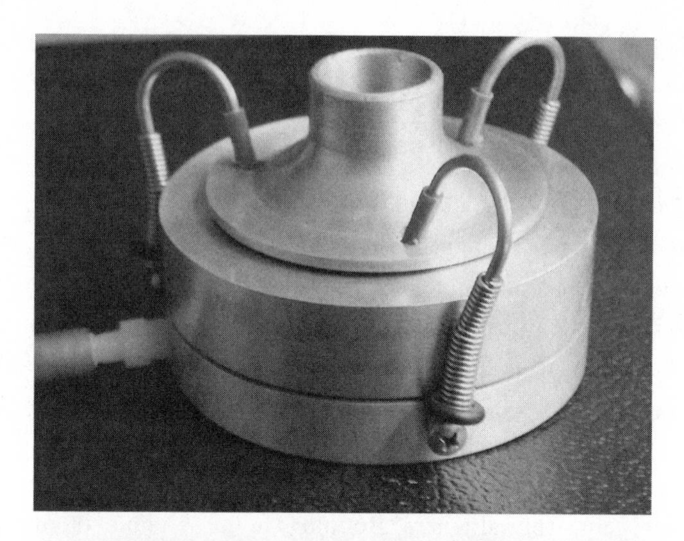

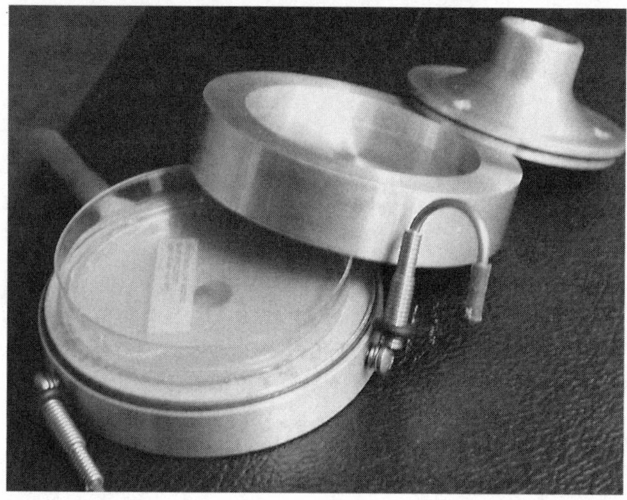

FIGURE 14.1. An Andersen N6 Sampler. The photograph at the top shows the Andersen N6 Sampler in operation. In the photograph below, the sampler is open and the petri dish is visible, sitting on the base. The perforated plate described in the text is resting at the edge of the petri dish. The vacuum pump is not present in either photograph.
May Indoor Air Investigations LLC

is part of the lab order. In my opinion, *whenever viable sampling is done, total spore sampling should also be done,* because as noted in chapter 8 the majority of spores found indoors are not viable (alive), yet they may still be allergenic or even toxic.

There are over seventy-five thousand known species of mold, but many fewer species, such as those of the genera *Aspergillus, Cladosporium, Penicillium, Alternaria, Fusarium,* and *Stachybotrys,* seem to be associated frequently with damp buildings and human health symptoms (see chapters 1 and 6).[1] If testing and speciation (the identification of species) confirm an outdoor absence but an indoor presence of the species *Stachybotrys chartarum, Aspergillus versicolor, A. flavus, A. fumigatus,* or *Fusarium moniliforme,* the American Industrial Hygiene Association recommends that "urgent risk management decisions" be made.[2] All of these mold species are toxigenic (capable of producing mycotoxins) and potentially allergenic. In addition, *Aspergillus* species can be pathogenic (causing disease), though infection is usually associated with people whose immune systems are compromised. In chapter 15 I describe some of the fungi commonly found in buildings.

Sampling for Bacteria

Most of the bacteria found in a typical indoor environment are shed with skin flakes from the skin and clothing of the occupants, though in some damp environments, bacterial growth can be elevated, and aerosolization of bacteria and bacterial toxins can be an exposure issue. As discussed in chapters 7 and 11, humidifiers, sprays, and indoor fountains are potential locations of bacterial growth.

Sampling for bacteria is often undertaken with the same device used to sample for mold: an Andersen Sampler. But the nutrients and chemicals in the petri dish are specifically chosen for their ability to suppress the growth of fungi and enhance the growth of bacteria. In the EPA's BASE Study, a study of IAQ in one hundred randomly chosen U.S. office buildings, total counts of bacteria in winter and summer averaged about 280 colony-forming units per cubic meter of air indoors and about 470 cfu/m^3 outdoors.[3]

Bacterial endotoxin. As noted in chapter 6, endotoxin is a toxin found in the bacterial cell walls of Gram-negative bacteria. Such bacteria are not found in significant concentrations in typical indoor environments unless there are contaminated reservoirs such as humidifiers, chronically damp carpeting, or surfaces water-damaged from flooding.

Both air and dust can be sampled for endotoxin. In both cases, samples are trapped by impaction (collision) on an endotoxin-free filter and sent to a laboratory for analysis. The concentration of endotoxin is measured in endotoxin units (EU), whereby 1 EU is the equivalent of 1 nanogram (a billionth of a gram) of a reference standard solution (a solution that contains a known concentration of endotoxin to which unknown endotoxin concentrations of other solutions can be compared). Outdoor concentrations of endotoxin are typically under 3 EU per cubic meter of air, and in buildings without IAQ problems, indoor levels are close to outdoor levels.

Exposure to elevated levels of endotoxin can cause fatigue, a feeling of tightness in the chest, airway obstruction, and coughing, among other symptoms. (Exposures in manufacturing and farming to concentrations above 50 EU/m^3 of air can cause acute health effects.) The American Conference of Governmental Industrial Hygienists has established what it calls a *relative limit value* (recommended limit) for endotoxin concentrations in indoor environments. In buildings where occupants experience symptoms that may be associated with endotoxins, the relative limit value is ten times the outdoor concentration; in buildings where no symptoms are experienced, it is thirty times the outdoor concentration.[4] Unfortunately, because of the nature of the sample analysis procedures, measurements of endotoxin levels, particularly if low, are imprecise.

Sampling for Other Bioaerosol

In addition to mold and bacterial allergens, bioaerosol can also include mite, cat and dog, and cockroach allergens.

Mite allergens. Air sampling for dust mite allergens is not particularly useful, because the fecal pellets, which contain most of the allergens, are fairly large (10 to 25 microns in diameter) and settle out of air within minutes. Still, the concentrations of HDM (house dust mite) allergens in dust can easily be determined and are important to measure, because if the dust is disturbed and aerosolized, even for a short period of time, HDM allergens can be inhaled by those who are sensitized. As mentioned in chapter 13, dust from a cushion or carpet can be vacuumed into a special filter supplied by a lab and then returned for a calculation of concentrations, measured in micrograms (millionths of a gram) per gram of dust (mcg/g).

Most physicians accept the following guidelines for concentrations of allergens from the dust mite species *Dermatophagoides pteronyssinus* and *D. farinae:*

—Less than 2 mcg/g of dust = low
—2 to 10 mcg/g of dust = moderate
—More than 10 mcg/g of dust = high[5]

Moderate levels are likely to cause allergy symptoms in those already sensitized and may even lead to sensitization. High concentrations create increased risk of acute asthma attacks.[6] In the EPA BASE Study mentioned earlier, researchers tested carpet and floor dust from ninety-three buildings for HDM allergens and detected the allergens in about half the buildings.[7] Approximately half the dust samples contained allergens in the low range, and less than 1 percent of the samples contained allergens in the high range.

Unfortunately, even if dust in a building is tested for HDM allergens and the concentrations are found to be low, there may still be high concentrations of allergens from other types of mites. There are about ten species of mites common in damp buildings to which occupants could be sensitized. Most of these mites eat mold, so they produce fecal pellets containing both mite and mold allergens. But few physicians or labs have the ability to test for these allergens.

Cat and dog allergens. As you remember from chapter 3, people can transport cat and dog dander into a building on their clothing, so dander and cat and dog allergens can be present even if the pets are not. Pet allergens can be measured in air, because the dander is smaller than dust mite fecal pellets and thus remains airborne longer. Nonetheless, the simplest way to measure the presence of cat and dog allergens is through dust sampling.

Cat and dog allergens are measured in micrograms per gram of dust. Guidelines for cat allergens are listed below (there are as yet no exposure guidelines for dog allergens):

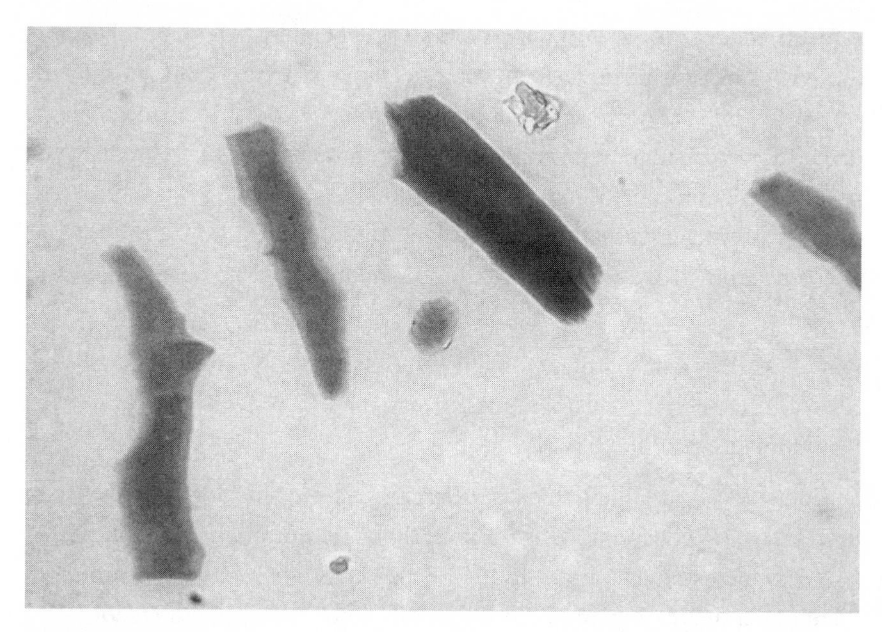

FIGURE 14.2. Dog dander (light microscopy 500×). The four long dark shapes are poodle dander particles, collected from the air by a Burkard personal sampler. The particles originate from the skin and hair of the animal and are coated with dog allergen. The dark spherical object at the center of the photograph is either a *Penicillium* or *Aspergillus* mold spore. *May Indoor Air Investigations LLC*

—Less than 1 mcg/g of dust = low
—1 to 8 mcg/g of dust = moderate
—More than 8 mcg/g of dust = high

Exposure to a high concentration of cat allergen is considered a risk for sensitization.

Let's look at some measurements of dog and cat allergens:

—In the EPA BASE Study, testing of carpeted floor dust from ninety-three office buildings detected cat allergens in over 90 percent of the buildings. About 75 percent of the buildings in the study had low levels of cat allergens, and less than 1 percent had high levels.[8]
—In a Swedish study of twenty-two day care centers, cat and dog allergens were detected in all the centers. The median concentration of cat allergen was 1.6 mcg/g (a moderate level), and the maximum con-

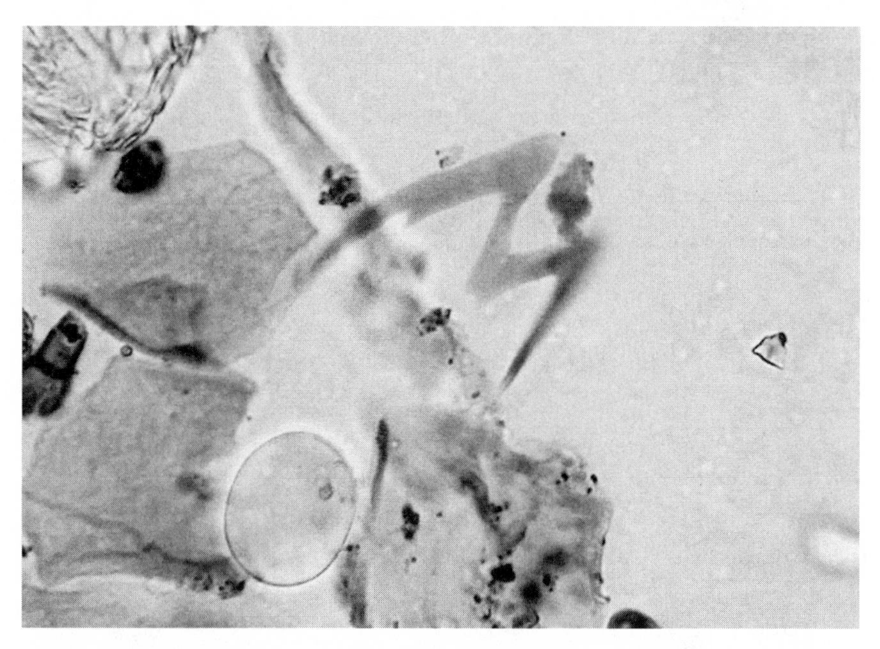

FIGURE 14.3. Rabbit dander (light microscopy 600×). The M-shaped particle in the middle of the photograph is rabbit dander. Immediately to the left are two human skin scales, one above the other. The large oval particle just to the right of the lower skin scale is probably a starch granule. To the left of and between the two skin scales, at the edge of the photograph, is a fragment of a mold spore. I collected this dust sample from a couch in a finished basement. The family didn't own a rabbit, but three years earlier guests and their pet rabbit had stayed in the basement. The animal was long gone, but the dander with its allergens remained. *May Indoor Air Investigations LLC*

centration was about 23 mcg/g (a high level). Median concentration of dog allergen was 4.3 mcg/g, and the maximum concentration was 21 mcg/g.[9]

—In another Swedish study, researchers found dog and cat allergens in all fifty-seven samples taken from classrooms and children's clothing, but dog owners had more dog allergens in their clothing than cat owners had cat allergens.[10]

—Concentrations of dog allergens greater than 10 mcg/g were found in 40 percent of upholstered seats sampled in public places.[11] The study concluded that upholstered seats in public buildings, as well as on public transportation vehicles such as buses and trains, represent potential reservoirs of dog allergens.

—In facilities used for dog shows, dog allergens were measured at 2,100 mcg/g of dust.[12]

—The following concentrations (mean and range) of dog, cat, dust mite, and cockroach allergens were found in samples taken from twelve public elementary schools in Baltimore:[13]

Allergen	Mean	Range
Dog	1.44 mcg/g	(0.1 to 9.6 mcg/g)
Cat	1.66 mcg/g	(0.2 to 12 mcg/g)
Dust mite	0.38 mcg/g	(0 to 11.9 mcg/g)
Cockroach	1.49 units/gram	(0 to 8 units/gram)

Cockroach allergens. Concentrations of cockroach allergens, found in cockroach excretions and body parts, are usually measured in units of allergens per gram of dust (U/g), though they may also be expressed in micrograms per gram of dust. Exposure to cockroach allergens between 2 and 8 U/g can create an increased risk of developing sensitization or experiencing asthma symptoms.

Cockroach allergens are present in homes as well as in other buildings where food is served (see chapters 8 and 11), including schools. In a study conducted in Tampa, Florida, researchers found cockroach allergens in fifteen day care centers, in concentrations similar to those found in Tampa-area homes.[14] In Brazil, cockroach allergen levels were higher in elementary school classrooms than in day care centers and preschools.[15] Several high school classrooms in New York City contained cockroach allergens above the threshold level, 2 U/g.[16] In chapter 8 I mentioned that in a study of schools in Baltimore, 69 percent of the buildings contained measurable levels of roach allergens in dust.[17] In that study, the allergen levels were higher in food-related areas (median, 5.8 U/g; maximum, 591 U/g) than in classrooms. And in England, 65 percent of the classrooms sampled contained cockroach allergens in concentrations greater than 2 U/g.[18] In British hospitals, on the other hand, cockroach allergens were below the detection limit in the dust samples taken.[19]

Proteases

Scientists are working on developing methods to measure the concentrations of *proteases* in air. (Many of the most potent allergens from insects are proteases.) Proteases are enzymes that facilitate the creation (synthesis) and digestion (breakdown) of proteins—the metabolic process that is the hallmark of life. Even enzymes themselves are proteins, as are the muscles and all the organs of the body. It should be no surprise, then, that the immune system is primed to detect foreign enzymes and alert the body to the presence of a potentially hostile invader. In fact, upon contact with its host or nutrient niche, any propagule (something that propagates or grows, like a mold spore, bacterium, or yeast cell) secretes enzymes to facilitate its own survival.

Scientists have discovered protease detectors on the exterior membranes of cells in blood vessels, connective tissue, skin, and the lung. These detectors alert the cells to the presence of the foreign enzymes. When stimulated, these detector molecules, called *protease-activated receptors (PARs),* are responsible for a host of cellular and ultimately physiological reactions associated with the inflammation caused by many familiar allergic respiratory diseases.

Proteases, like all enzymes, are essential components of the bacteria and spores that we inhale indoors. In a recent paper Charles E. Reed, M.D., and Hirohito Kita, M.D., reviewed much of the research and current thinking on PARs. They concluded that "proteases from mites and fungi growing in damp water-damaged buildings may be the basis for the increased prevalence in these buildings of rhinitis, asthma and other respiratory diseases."[20]

What Is It?

When I look with a light microscope at a sample of dust from a building or at the particulates that I collect from an indoor air sample, I am always amazed at the variety of sizes and shapes of the particles and awed by the challenge of identifying them, understanding what might be on their surfaces, and locating the sources of all of these potential contaminants. Fortunately, some of the biogenic particles, such as pollen and mold spores, are fairly easy to distinguish. On the other hand, some nonbiogenic particles are difficult, even impossible, to identify with a simple light microscope, because they can originate from an almost infinite number of interior and exterior sources (though more sophisticated optical, chemical, and X-ray techniques can be used, if necessary, to identify specially prepared samples). In addition, because they are often random fragments, they can be of any size and shape. Fortunately, most of these particles are benign.

Rust is one nonbiogenic particle that is usually easy to identify, because the particles are either yellow or orange, and they have a characteristic shape or pattern, though they are often produced in a variety of sizes, from less than 0.5 micron to 3 or 4 microns. Rust can come from any number of outdoor and indoor sources, but one indoor source that would concern me would be a rusty reservoir in a mechanical system that contains microbial growth—or any reservoir in a mechanical system, for that matter, contaminated with microbial growth (see chapter 7).

I investigated one building in which the air was extraordinarily free of particulates because of efficient media filtration, but I as well as others nevertheless found the air allergenic. The only particles I found in my sampling were respirable rust crystals that originated from a humidifier contaminated with bacteria. Inhaled, small particles can be irritating in and of themselves, but the concentration of these rust particles was so low that it is highly unlikely that they alone could have been a problem. It is more likely that allergens from the biological "brew" in the humidifier were adhering to the rust crystals, and that the rust was acting as a *surrogate* (substitute) allergen (like the starch granules contaminated with latex allergens from rubber gloves mentioned in chapter 10).

In another office, workers were complaining that they found black dust on their desks every morning when they came to work. Some of the workers also said they were suffering allergy and asthma symptoms. The black dust consisted of mold growth laced with fiberglass fibers. The fibers were coming from the surface of the deteriorating fiberglass insulation that lined the interior of the ducts, and mold was growing in the settled dust in the insulation.

In chapter 6 it was useful to define particulates as either biogenic or nonbiogenic, but definitions can be tricky things. On the one hand, we need words to define objects and ideas. On the other hand, as soon as we label something with a word, we have identified what it is and, equally important, what it is not. This can be limiting. The categories *biogenic* and *nonbiogenic* are not as separate as the definitions suggest.

Rust particles, fiberglass fibers, and drywall dust can be coated with fungal enzymes and mycotoxins as well as with bacterial endotoxin. If moldy drywall is disturbed, contaminated paper and gypsum fragments can become aerosolized and be inhaled (see chapters 3 and 6). Soot particles arising from combustion in cooking equipment, heating systems, jar candles, and car and truck engines operating in underground garages can acquire allergens if the particles come into contact with mold or bacteria growing inside a mechanical system.[21] Studies have shown that soot particles carry cat allergens in homes where there are cats. Pollen allergens have also been found on soot particles.[22] And soot is respirable (see chapter 6), so the particles can penetrate deep into the lung, carrying allergens with them.

An IAQ investigator finding rust, soot, plaster dust aerosol, or fiberglass fibers within what are considered typical indoor concentrations might overlook the fact that these particulates could be acting as allergen surrogates, for which there are few available tests. That is why I maintain that quantitative findings are not the sole measure of indoor air quality; one must also take into account the health complaints of those who may have been exposed.

What Approach to Take?

A traditional scientific approach to testing for particulates entails gathering numerous air and dust samples in many areas of one or more buildings, comparing these samples with samples taken outdoors or from areas that have not been a source of complaints, and, in the case of mold spore testing, performing statistical analyses on comparisons of the concentrations. While such studies provide invaluable knowledge about building conditions that increases everyone's understanding of IAQ problems, such comprehensive testing, like long-term continuous air sample monitoring, is usually too costly for the typical IAQ investigation. In addition, this approach often does not point to specific causes of airborne contamination and thus does not necessarily help define effective remediation strategies.

And such studies can even be misleading. For example, many IAQ investigators, physicians, and scientists believe that as long as the indoor level of any particular species of mold is less than the outdoor level, there is no problem. Clearly, a very elevated indoor level of a microbe, one typically associated with damp buildings, as compared with the outdoor level of this microbe is an indication of a contamination problem. But if the indoor level is below the outdoor level, sensitized individuals who spend extended time in the building can still suffer from consistent exposures to the bioaerosol and experience symptoms. And even if indoor sources of particulate contaminants are not disturbed, indoor levels of bioaerosol may still be lower than outdoor levels one day yet higher the next, depending on differences in conditions in the interior and at the exterior of the building (such as pressure differentials and airflows). Concentrations of allergens outdoors, and thus indoors, can also fluctuate with season and weather.

As we saw in chapters 2 and 7, allergens such as pollen and mold spores can be carried indoors in air flowing through open windows or infiltrating through construction openings and gaps. In a small building with operable windows, spores and pollen are carried into the building on air moving through the windows, and the ratio may be near 1 to 1 (the level of allergens indoors may be nearly the same as the levels of allergens outdoors). The ratio of particulates indoors to particulates outdoors also depends on the size of the particulates. In a relatively tight office building with efficient filtration in the HVAC system, indoor concentrations of large aerosolized particles may be much lower than outdoor concentrations. But smaller particles (ultrafines; see chapter 6), such as soot and the particles in smoke and haze, will find their way indoors and be circulated through the building on airflows, and the indoor concentrations of these smaller particles may be close to the outdoor concentrations. It is nonetheless important to take air samples outdoors as well as indoors when measuring the concentrations of bioaerosols (and possibly even VOCs, if there are exterior sources), to gain a clearer understanding of the potential sources of contaminants found within the building envelope.

I wish that more IAQPs would analyze and identify the samples of particulate matter that they take, rather than just send them out to a laboratory for this purpose. An IAQP can look at the entire area (100 percent) of the sample he or she gathered, looking for any particles that could be causing allergic symptoms—mold spores, pet dander, clumps of bacteria, insect droppings, and so on. When a sample is sent to a laboratory, however, the technician may scan only a certain number of representative portions of a slide (15 percent of the area is not uncommon) and look only for what the client asked the lab to look for (usually mold spores). For spores occurring in clumps, very large errors can be associated with counting methods that analyze only 15 percent of the total area of a sample. If a clump is in the uncounted area (85 percent of the sample), the concentration can be grossly underestimated.

For the technician to search for a number of potential allergens, additional samples may be required. This process can increase the cost of the testing to the point where choices must be made about what categories of allergens to look for, thus narrowing the focus of the investigation.

Measuring Total Particulate Aerosol

There are two ways in which IAQPs commonly measure total particulate aerosol by direct reading (as opposed to laboratory analysis). One method, described in chapter 6, uses laser light to count the number of particulates in different size ranges in air that is drawn by a pump into a *particle counter.* Another instrument, called an *aerosol mass monitor,* continuously collects particles on an oscillating (vibrating) quartz crystal, to determine the mass of aerosol. (The frequency of the quartz crystal's oscillation, which can be measured, depends on the mass of the particles that collect on the crystal.)

A third way of measuring particulates requires laboratory analysis. Particles are separated into size ranges and collected onto filters. In the EPA BASE study of one hundred U.S. office buildings, PM_{10} (see chapter 6) ranged from 3.0 to 35.4 micrograms per cubic meter (with a mean of 11.4 mcg/m^3), and $PM_{2.5}$ ranged from 1.3 to 24.8 mcg/m^3 (with a mean of 7.2 mcg/m^3).[23] Outdoor concentrations of PM_{10} ranged from 5.8 to 102.9 mcg/m^3 (with a mean of 23.1 mcg/m^3), and outdoor concentrations of $PM_{2.5}$ ranged from 4.5 to 47.4 mcg/m^3 (with a mean of 14.7 mcg/m^3). For comparison, the American Conference of Governmental Industrial Hygienists limit for "nuisance dust" (nonhazardous dust) in industrial environments varies from about 3 milligrams per cubic meter to 15 mg/m^3—hundreds of times greater than the typical dust particle concentrations noted in the EPA study (1 milligram is equal to 1,000 micrograms).

The numbers of total particulates indoors and outdoors vary greatly and depend on many factors, including the extent of any activity that may be going on as well as air movements. If IAQ testing has been done in the building in which you work and measurements were taken of total particulate aerosol (either counts or mass), look at the report to see if measurements were taken both indoors and outdoors, as well as under differing conditions, so as to recognize varying levels of activity.

From the measurements I have taken, indoor counts of particulates greater than 0.3 micron in size varied from about 100,000 to over 1,000,000 per cubic foot of air and depended largely on the outdoor concentrations of particles in that size range. When I adjusted my particle counter to measure only particles greater than 3 microns in size, the numbers counted were far smaller, ranging from about 1,000 to 6,000 per cubic foot of air. (These particles consisted mostly of skin scales shed by people indoors.) In other words, as smaller and smaller particles are included in the instrument's measurements, the number of particles detected increases. These observations lead to at least two conclusions: first, that smaller particles are suspended in air for much longer periods of time than larger particles are; and second, that smaller particles tend to originate from outdoors because they move with airflows into a building (though in one smoking room with a strong cigarette odor but no visible smoke, I measured over 10,000,000 particles greater than 0.3 micron in size per cubic foot of air!).

SAMPLING THE AIR FOR GASES AND VAPORS

To measure concentrations of volatile organic compounds in offices using passive devices, long sampling times (days) may be needed. The results can be misleading, however, because they do not necessarily acknowledge that VOC concentrations may be high only intermittently; in addition, highly volatile chemicals might be adsorbed and then reevaporate from the sampling device. An IAQP therefore usually uses an active sampling device to trap the contaminants. The setup can consist of one or more sample tubes, filled with an adsorbant such as Tenex® or charcoal, and attached by tubing to a vacuum pump that pulls air at a known flow rate through the tubes. The contaminants adhere to the adsorbant. After a fixed period of time the tubes are removed, sealed, and sent to a lab, where they are analyzed by gas chromatograph/mass spectrometer (GC/MS, discussed in the following section).

Another device used for VOC sampling consists of a stainless steel container (available in different sizes) with a valve, called a SUMMA® can. The lab that supplies the SUMMA® can cleans the interior surface, evacuates all the air, and closes the valve. The can is transported to the site and placed in the testing location. The valve is then partially opened, and because there is a vacuum in the can, room air flows into the container. When the air pressure in the can and room are about equal, the valve is closed and the container is sent back to the lab, where the air itself is directly analyzed, again by GC/MS.

The lab may report the concentration of individual VOCs or the concentration of the sum of all the VOCs present—the TVOC concentration.

The TVOC concentration can also be measured by a hand-held device called a *photoionization detector,* though this instrument, which uses an air pump and has a digital readout, is more appropriate for industrial environments, where the TVOC concentration is usually higher than it is in offices.

Not Always Exact Science

Identifying gases and vapors in a laboratory is a scientific endeavor, but it is not always "exact science," regardless of how sophisticated or costly the instruments used.

The *mass spectrometer (mass spec* or *MS)* separates molecules by mass and identifies them by breaking them up into pieces and then looking at the pattern of the pieces. If you think of a molecule as a sentence containing words, each made up of ordered letters, then the mass spec is a device that breaks up the sentence and its words into syllables and then identifies each syllable.

To extend this metaphor, a pure substance consists of only one sentence pattern. In the early days of mass spectroscopy, chemists knew the syllables of any pure-substance sentence and could recognize the sentence pattern (the substance) from a collection of the syllables present. The modern mass spectrometers in use today have a computerized library containing the fragmentation patterns of hundreds of molecules. For identification purposes, the MS computer program can compare the fragmentation patterns of an unidentified molecule (the unknown) with the known patterns in the library.

Unfortunately, air containing a mixture of vapors and gases is not a pure substance, so analyzing contaminated air is like having many different sentence patterns on the page. Breaking these sentences down into syllables and rearranging them back into sentences is a bit of a guessing game. Thus, if a mixture of substances is analyzed, a modern mass spectrometer may give *probable* identifications, rather than exact identifications, of the contaminants that may be present.

One way to improve the results is to separate the gaseous mixture before analyzing it in a modern mass spectrometer, so usually a sample (either air from a SUMMA® can or vapor from a Tenex® or heated charcoal adsorbant) is first injected into a gas chromatograph, to separate the components in a mixture. A *gas chromatograph (GC)* consists of a long, thin coiled tube, usually filled with a porous substrate, installed within a heated oven. A carrier gas flows continuously through the tube, and a sample from the mixture is injected into the stream of gas. Much as runners in a marathon begin the race in a clump and then separate as they move, the molecules of the mixture begin to separate as they flow along through the tube with the carrier gas. The rate at which the molecules move through the chromatograph depends on many variables, including the flow rate of the carrier gas, the temperature of the oven, and the properties of the molecules and how strongly they adsorb to the substrate filling the column.

Ideally the molecules will divide up into groups of like molecules, but in reality the molecules do not always separate completely in this way, and thus the smaller groupings may still be mixtures of different kinds of molecules. Nonetheless, these groupings (some of which may be pure) contain fewer kinds of molecules than the original mixture did, and so the molecules are easier to identify.

When the gas chromatograph and mass spectrometer are used in tandem, the analysis is called a *gas chromatograph/mass spectrometer (GC/MS) analysis.*

Combustible Gas Detectors

If ignited when mixed in the right proportions, combustible gases, which include the fuels methane and propane as well as vapors from flammable solvents such as alcohol and acetone, can burn in air. These gases add to the total volatile organic compounds that people are exposed to indoors. A *combustible gas detector* is used by IAQPs (and sometimes by building occupants) to try to locate a source of leaking combustible gas or of strong odors such as sewer gas.

This instrument makes a ticking sound and has a sensor at its tip that responds to a variety of gases and vapors. If the concentration of one of these gases or vapors increases as the sensor is moved from one location to another, the ticking rate increases. When the detector is very close to the source of the emission, the ticking becomes a siren screech. The lowest concentrations detected by one manufacturer's combustible gas detector are about 500 parts per million for hydrocarbon gases, 50 ppm for acetone and methanol, 5 ppm for hydrogen sulfide, and 1 ppm for gasoline. Unfortunately, most combustible gas detectors are very insensitive to carbon monoxide, even at a concentration of 100 ppm. Some detectors are also sensitive to water vapor, so the instrument's ticking may lead the investigator to a pot of water boiling on a stove!

A friend who provided my company with Internet services once complained to me that she was having debilitating headaches at work. She was convinced these were symptoms of sick-building syndrome (see chapter 1), because the pain went away on weekends. I offered to check out her workspace, which consisted of several rooms on the second floor of a typical two-story business block, with retail shops on the first floor and a variety of offices upstairs.

I did not detect any particular odor in her office; nonetheless, I began to check around the space with my combustible gas detector for sources of odors and combustible gases. I removed a drop ceiling tile. The instrument's ticking rate seemed to increase in the ceiling plenum and got faster still the closer I moved to the outside building wall. At the outer wall, I could actually smell some odors from the retail space below where fragrances were used, suggesting that airflows were moving from one level to the next inside wall cavities.

The boiler for the building was located in a locked basement room beneath the fragranced retail space, so I asked someone from maintenance to accompany me to the boiler room. I will never forget the sight that greeted us when we unlocked the door and peered into the dark cavern. I turned on my flashlight and began to descend the stairs to what I thought was the boiler-room floor, when I realized that the "floor" was actually the surface of a room-sized murky pond. The partially submerged boiler stood like a rusty steel heap in the center. The only way I could have gotten to the boiler was with a canoe.

The odor of sewer gas was so overwhelming that the two of us turned around, shut the door, and relocked it. Somehow, water from the sewer system had backed up into the boiler room and never drained out. In addition, water from a boiler leak had probably been adding to the pond. Gases and vapors were floating from this little horror into the wall cavities and infiltrating the upstairs office. As soon as the boiler room was cleaned out and the leaks repaired, my friend's headaches went away.

Tracking Airflows

Using smoke to determine how air moves from one space to another can be useful in tracking down the sources of odors, which are, after all, gases or vapors. Smoke from a cigarette cannot serve this purpose, however, because the smoke is warm and rises, and this movement disturbs or reroutes the airflow you are trying to track. There are a variety of smoke pencils available that produce *neutral density smoke,* smoke that is not warm and that neither rises nor sinks. Some smoke pencils contain strong chemicals and must be used with caution. I generally recommend that only IAQPs use smoke pencils.

Some precautions: The stream of particulates from a smoke pencil can set off a smoke detector. In addition, smoke testing should *never* be done before any kind of aerosol testing (testing for airborne particulates), because the smoke particulates can affect the results.

WHAT ABOUT STANDARDS?

Standards and guidelines may delineate the difference between "safe" and "dangerous" levels of contaminants. Standards can be enforced by law, whereas guidelines are only recommendations, usually determined by consensus among relevant stakeholders. The whole process of defining standards and setting guidelines can be fraught with opposing political and economic interests.

Limits for Gases and Vapors

Nonprofit organizations such as the Association of Industrial Hygienists of America (AIHA) and the American Conference of Governmental Industrial Hygienists (ACGIH), along with federal agencies such as the Occupational Safety and Health Administration (OSHA), have been setting guidelines and standards for manufacturing, industrial, and mining environments for decades.

To promote public health, regulatory bodies want lower concentrations for acceptable limits of gases and vapors. To keep the costs of controlling pollution down, industries want higher concentrations for acceptable limits, and sometimes companies sue regulatory authorities to have standards lowered. In addition, in many cases other stakeholders (unions, insurance companies) also participate in creating guidelines and standards. Regulatory standards and guidelines for acceptable limits of gas and vapor concentrations are thus usually compromises between the effects these contaminants can have on people's health and the costs associated with reducing the likelihood of emissions into the air.

The guidelines and standards set by the various organizations for concentrations of certain gases and vapors sometimes differ so much that it can be difficult to make sense of the numbers. For example, the ASHRAE guideline for carbon dioxide concentrations for office workers is about 800 ppm, while the OSHA PEL for industrial workers is 5,000 ppm—more than six times greater. Why are high CO_2 levels safer for industrial workers than for office workers? Are industrial workers less susceptible to experiencing fatigue in their work environments? Do the differing standards and guidelines suggest that elevated levels of gases and vapors are expected to be present in certain manufacturing environments, while similar levels of these chemicals are not expected to be present in office spaces?

"Limits" for Bioaerosol

There are no standards or even guidelines for determining "safe" and "dangerous" indoor concentrations of microbes such as mold, yeast, and bacteria, because these organisms exist naturally in the outdoor environment and so may also exist in buildings. In addition, people's sensitivities to cellular components in microbial growth can differ by factors of over a thousand, unlike people's reactions to carbon monoxide, which are more consistent; and CO levels are more predictable and thus easier to measure. (As noted in chapter 11, the only bioaerosol for which there is an exposure guideline is the bacterial enzyme called *subtilisin,* exposure to which has caused allergic sensitization and occupational asthma.)

Creating standards and guidelines also depends on measurement, which is a difficult task with bioaerosol. Microbes are living organisms, and each living cell may contain toxins as well as dozens of potentially allergenic components. The concentrations of all the individual components cannot easily be measured. In addition, in any given environment in which fungal or bacterial growth is present, the concentrations of airborne allergens and contaminants from these organisms can vary drastically, depending on whether (and when) the sources of the growth are disturbed. And particulate bioaerosol can settle out of the air but be reaerosolized if disturbed.

IN THE END, WHY TEST?

If a number of people are suffering from sick-building syndrome or building-related illnesses and commonsense steps have not helped, then air and dust sampling should be undertaken to find the sources of the bioaerosol, vapors, or gases that may be contributing to poor IAQ. The results of such testing can dictate appropriate remediation efforts as well as help us become aware of the relationships between what we do inside a building and IAQ problems.

TVOC concentrations in the range of 1 to 10 mg/m^3 can lead to sick-building symptoms among building occupants (see chapter 5). What does this mean, really, in terms of the choices we make? Imagine allowing a single drop of solvent (about 40 mg) to evaporate into the air of a small office that is 3 meters by 2 meters by 2.5 meters in size, or 15 cubic meters (about 555 cubic feet). Assuming an even mixing of the solvent vapor and air as well as very little air exchange (ventilation), the concentration of VOC in the air will be 40 mg divided by 15 m^3, or 2.6 mg/m^3—within the range of concentrations that might cause sick-building symptoms. So if someone applies nail polish, sprays fragrance into the air, or uses a cleaning agent containing solvent in a small, poorly ventilated room, VOC concentrations can quickly reach the point where people may experience sick-building symptoms (and chemically sensitized individuals may feel ill). And VOC concentrations can also rise in adjacent spaces as the vapors are carried along with airflows. Someone down the hall may not smell the nail polish, fragrance, or cleaning agent but may still experience the physiological effects caused by the VOCs.

In other words, it doesn't take much liquid solvent evaporating into a space to create what some would perceive as an IAQ problem. (Recall the events at the University of Massachusetts Boston described in chapter 1.) And unfortunately, in most circumstances where solvents are used, the equivalent of hundreds of drops may evaporate. So in the end, whether or not IAQ testing has been conducted, building occupants must take care not to introduce contaminants within the building envelope.

REMEDIATION

To help building occupants better understand testing processes and testing reports, I have focused in this chapter on professional IAQ testing. But remediation—the removal of known biogenic and nonbiogenic contaminants such as mold, lead paint, and asbestos (see chapter 6)—often follows testing. Significant remediation should be undertaken *only* by trained individuals, usually professionals, using containment that complies with applicable local, state, or federal regulations in order to protect workers and building occupants. (See the Resource Guide for information on remediation.)

One of the most important steps to take when hiring a professional remediator is to research, thoroughly and in advance, the company's credentials, because not everyone doing this kind of work has the training and expertise required. Several schools in Connecticut and Virginia hired a "professional" to remediate mold problems. The man used a process he called the Microb Phase Treatment. The "remediator" supposedly claimed that he could apply his product to combat mold growth without interrupting the school day: classrooms could be reoccupied two hours after he had cleaned.[24]

The EPA brought charges of fraud against the man because of his dealings with several schools in Connecticut, though the warrant for his arrest noted that he had been providing mold remediation services for approximately ten years to schools, hotels, and other facilities, not only in Connecticut but also in New York, New Jersey, South Carolina, and Virginia. The warrant summarized some of the details of the man's schemes: he generated testing reports, but testing equipment was not found in his place of business or storage facility; he allegedly generated false laboratory reports, including reports that confirmed he had successfully remediated IAQ problems; his diploma for a Master's of Engineering degree and his certification as an environmental inspector seemed to have been fabricated; his claim that he held a Ph.D. was unsubstantiated; and according to the warrant, he asserted falsely that he had received EPA research grants, as well as EPA approval for his product. The warrant states that the man admitted that his mold-combating product was a mixture of isopropyl alcohol and some soap solution that he prepared in his garage.[25]

In major remediation projects, remediators use air scrubbers (portable, high-flow commercial HEPA-filtered air cleaners) and negative air machines (HEPA-filtered blowers) to remove particulates from the air. In addition, negative air machines exhaust the air to the exterior, thus depressurizing the space.

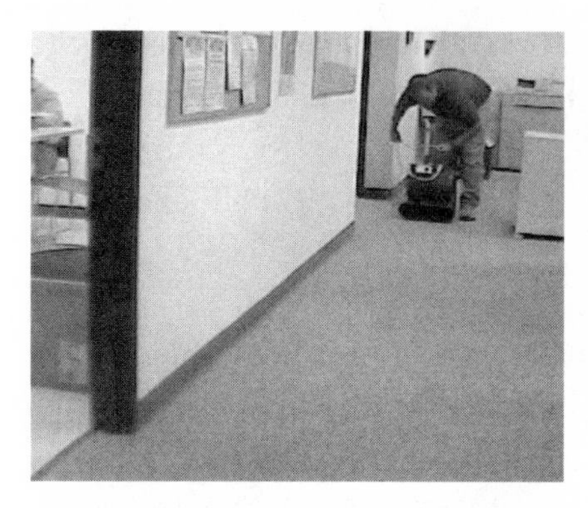

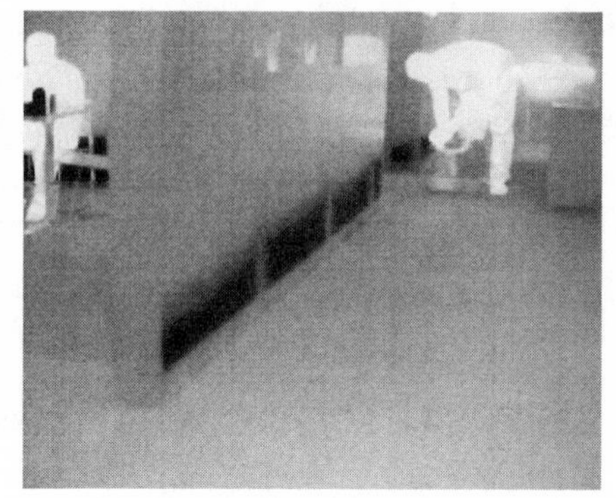

FIGURE 14.4. Concealed dampness. Water flooded this floor, and a remediation company was hired to dry out the space. The photograph on the left was taken in visible light and shows someone sitting at a desk (extreme left) as well as a remediator (upper right corner). The remediator is leaning over an air mover (blower), used to dry the floor and wall. The photograph on the right was taken with an infrared camera, which is sensitive to heat radiation rather than visible light. Water from the floor had soaked up into the drywall. The color is darker at the bottom of the wall, where moisture was evaporating (evaporation lowers the temperature of surfaces). The people appear white, because they are "hot" compared with the wall. An infrared camera is a valuable tool for remediators, because it can show surface temperature patterns, many of which are caused by excess moisture. To confirm that the pattern is moisture based, the remediator takes moisture-meter readings. *Lew Harriman, moistureDM.com*

TRUST YOURSELF

One of the ironies of indoor air quality investigations is that professionals who are sampling the dust and air are often unaffected by indoor pollutants. In addition, most testing is initially undertaken by the "defendant" (property management, school superintendent, or hospital administration) rather than the "plaintiff" (a building occupant suffering from poor IAQ). The conditions surrounding the testing and the methodology used therefore deserve scrutiny.

Do not let testing results that declare that the air is "safe" undermine your trust in yourself. Your body is your best IAQ instrument. If you as well as some of your co-workers experience symptoms when inside the building and feel better when away from the building, there is most likely an IAQ problem. Somehow, someone should be hired who can find a solution.

SOME PRACTICAL STEPS

- To determine if there is a cockroach infestation in your building, set out sticky traps near water and food sources.
- Be careful not to introduce VOCs into your interior environment.
- If IAQ testing has been conducted in your building and the test results have been made public, explore in greater detail the nature of the tests undertaken and the equipment used to test the air and dust. Confer with an IAQP or an industrial hygienist, as well as an appropriately trained or experienced environmental physician, on the meaning and implications of the IAQ testing report.
- If remediation is to be done in your building, be sure the remediators are trained, that they set up containment, and that they follow applicable state and federal laws.

CHAPTER

15

More Data for Techies

Readers who like "the numbers" can review the testing results connected to the McKinley school (see chapter 8). In this chapter I provide additional samples of data from indoor air quality studies. These figures may be similar to what you will read in air quality testing reports.

VOLATILE ORGANIC COMPOUNDS

The most common volatile organic compounds found in the EPA's BASE study of fifty-six non-complaint buildings are listed in table 15.1. These VOCs were always found in higher concentrations indoors than outdoors, sometimes by a factor of as much as ten. Still, each concentration is below a level that would be considered responsible for sick-building symptoms (see chapter 1). Even the TVOC concentration of all the volatile organic compounds listed in the table is less than 0.1 mg/m^3. This figure probably explains why these were "non-complaint" buildings.

CIGARETTE SMOKE

As noted in chapter 5, where smoking is permitted, cigarettes are responsible for many of the chemicals in indoor air. Table 15.2 lists some of the hundreds of vapors and gases present in cigarette smoke.

TABLE 15.1. Concentrations and sources of some common volatile organic compounds found in fifty-six "non-complaint" buildings

Compound	Median concentration (mg/m3)	Potential sources
Acetone	0.029	Nail polish remover, printers, photocopiers, solvents, cleaning fluids
Toluene	0.009	Synthetic carpet, wood floor finishes, cigarette smoke, printers, photocopiers
Limonene	0.0071	Citrus fruits, "lemon-scented" cleaning compounds
Xylenes	0.0052	Gasoline, marker pens, photocopiers, printers
2-butoxyethanol	0.0045	Water-based paints, cleaning compounds
N-undecane	0.0037	Solvent-based paints, photocopiers, carpet (polypropylene fibers)
Benzene	0.0037	Cigarette smoke, wood floor finishes
1,1,1-trichloroethane	0.0036	Typewriter correction fluid, cleaning solvents, shoe polish, spot remover
N-dodecane	0.0035	Solvent-based paints, photocopiers, wax on wood flooring
Hexanal	0.0032	Kitchen cabinets, particle board, solvent-based paints, photocopiers
Nonanal	0.0031	Particle board
N-hexane	0.0029	Flooring

Source: Adapted from J. Spengler et al., eds., *Indoor Air Quality Handbook* (New York: McGraw-Hill, 2001), tables 31.4, 31.7–10; J. Girman et al., "Individual Volatile Organic Compound Prevalence and Concentrations in 56 Buildings of the Building Assessment, Survey, and Evaluation (BASE) Study," in *Proceedings of Indoor Air 1999, the 8th International Conference on Indoor Air Quality and Climate,* Edinburgh, Scotland, 8–13 August 1999.

TABLE 15.2. A few of the vapors and gases in cigarette smoke

Compound	Emission (mg/cigarette)
Acetaldehyde	4–5
Acrolein	1.25 (sidestream)*
Benzaldehyde	0.08
Benzene	0.3–0.5 (sidestream)
Formaldehyde	0.7 (sidestream)
Toluene	1

Source: Adapted from Spengler et al., eds., *Indoor Air Quality Handbook,* table 31.4, p. 31.7, and table 32.5, p. 32.7.

* A sidestream is the smoke that comes off the burning tip of the cigarette rather than the smoke that is inhaled.

BIOAEROSOL

Tables 15.3 and 15.4 are based on data from over eleven hundred bioaerosol samples collected from eighteen states over a nine-month period and then sent to a laboratory for analysis. Over nine hundred of the samples were taken from commercial and residential buildings; the rest were taken from outdoors. Table 15.5 lists mold genera found in seventy-two samples of contaminated building materials.

TABLE 15.3. Frequency of occurrence and average cfu/m^3 of indoor bioaerosols

Observed	Frequency	Average cfu/m^3
Total	100	157
Cladosporium	77	92
Yeast	56	52
Sterile hyphae	56	29
Bacteria	52	28
Penicillium	50	48
Aspergillus	33	20
Alternaria	17	30
Curvularia	7	20
Acremonium	30	8
Epicoccum	3	8
Geotrichum	3	18
Phoma	2	7
Fusarium	2	16
Paecilomyces	2	9
Dendryphiella	2	5
Drechslera	2	13
Absidia	2	1
Chaetomium	2	6
Nigrospora	2	10
Actinomycetes	1	3
Monocillium	1	17
Cunninghamella	1	11
Monilia	1	5
Rhizopus	1	5
Trichoderma	1	10
Gilmaniella	1	3
Hansfordia	1	3
Hyalodendron	1	3
Mucor	1	8
Stemphylium	1	5
Botrytis	1	2
Pleospora	1	4
Humicola	1	23
Pithomyces	1	10
Unidentified	1	6
Stachybotrys	1	3
Ulocladium	1	4
Basipetospora	<1	2
Gliocladium	<1	5
Oidiodendron	<1	2
Aureobasidium	<1	8

Source: L. Robertson, "Monitoring Viable Fungal and Bacterial Bioaerosol Concentrations to Identify Acceptable Levels for Common Indoor Environments," *Indoor and Built Environment* 6 (1997): 295–300.

TABLE 15.4. Frequency of occurrence and average cfu/m³ of outdoor bioaerosols

Observed	Frequency	Average cfu/m^3
Total	100	860
Cladosporium	85	570
Sterile hyphae	76	87
Yeast	58	126
Penicillium	52	120
Bacteria	46	58
Alternaria	38	58
Aspergillus	27	277
Geotrichum	20	91
Curvularia	12	71
Fusarium	12	74
Epicoccum	8	17
Drechslera	6	62
Acremonium	6	43
Phoma	5	31
Trichoderma	2	35
Cunninghamella	2	21
Paecilomyces	2	22
Pleospora	2	35
Basipetospora	2	15
Nigrospora	2	22
Monilia	1	89
Monocillium	1	56
Ulocladium	1	10
Botrytis	1	22
Phomopsis	1	24
Pithomyces	1	3
Rhizomucor	1	9
Rhizopus	1	7
Mucor	1	14
Humicola	1	14
Stachybotrys	1	7
Actinomycetes	1	106
Absidia	1	36
Aureobasidium	1	12
Chrysosporium	1	36
Gonatobotrys	1	24
Gliocladium	1	35

Source: Robertson, "Monitoring Viable Fungal and Bacterial Bioaerosol Concentrations."

DESCRIPTIONS OF SOME FUNGI FOUND INDOORS AND OUTDOORS

The fungi listed below may be included in an IAQ report.[1] Note, however, that fungal spores found in indoor air may come from an outdoor source. Similarly, testing may not detect spores from a mold growing inside the wall cavity of a building. In other words, air testing results can be very useful, but they are not necessarily definitive.

TABLE 15.5. Principal mold genera isolated from seventy-two samples of mold-affected building materials

Genus	Samples (%)*
Penicillium	68
Aspergillus	56
Chaetomium	22
Ulocladium	21
Stachybotrys	19
Cladosporium	15
Acremonium	14
Mucor	14
Paecilomyces	10
Alternaria	8
Verticillium	8
Trichoderma	7

Source: S. Gravesen et al., *Microfungi in Water Damaged Buildings* (Horsholm: Danish Building Research Institute, 1997).

*Percentage of samples in which genus is found.

The descriptions I am providing are minimal; you may wish to obtain further information about particular molds, including their potential effects on health.

—*Acremonium* species require wet growing conditions and are found on damp or wet walls or wallpaper, as well as in humidifier water.

—*Alternaria* species cause leaf-spot diseases on living plants, in the process producing copious spore masses. The spores are thus more numerous in outdoor air than in indoor air, though spores can be found indoors in settled dust. These fungi are sometimes found on damp building materials. Once I discovered paper colonized with *Alternaria* mold; the paper had been placed on recently washed, still damp carpeting, and then covered with cardboard boxes. Allergy to *Alternaria* species is common; some species are toxigenic (can produce mycotoxins; see chapter 1). The colonies can range from dark olive green to gray and black in color.

—Ascospores and basidiospores are types of spores, rather than genera of fungi, but many total-spore-count reports include counts for these groups. Ascospores are produced by cup fungi (which look like shallow cups) and sponge mushrooms (which have a sponge-like appearance). Basidiospores are produced by crop rusts, grain smuts (fungi that attack crops), mushrooms, and bracket fungi (which decay wood and look like shelves growing out of trees or logs). Spores reported as ascospores or basidiospores are typically from the outdoor air. When they are found indoors, it is usually because they are abundant outdoors (although basidiospores of the dry-rot mushroom *Serpula lacrymans* may be associated with the growth of this fungus on structural wood indoors).

—*Aspergillus* species (there are more than 150 known) are common worldwide. Some species grow in house dust under relatively dry conditions (as low as 75 percent relative humidity; see chapter 4); other species grow on damp walls and building materials that have become wet. Some species do not require visible dampness in order to grow and produce spores. I have often found *Aspergillus* mold growing on the unfinished wood surfaces (bottoms and backs) of antiques that had been stored in damp spaces. Many species of *Aspergillus* are toxigenic. A few are even known to cause infections of the airways, lungs, ears, and nails (e.g., *A. fumigatus*). The presence of *Aspergillus* species in health facilities is therefore of great concern. *Aspergillus* spores are small enough (between 2 and 10 microns) to remain airborne over long periods of time and to be respirable (see chapter 6). Colonies may be blue, green, white, or black in color, and they are powdery, so spores are readily aerosolized.

—*Aureobasidium* species require wet conditions for growth and are therefore found on wet wood and window frames as well as on bathroom walls and ceilings, shower curtains, and tile grout. *Aureobasidium* can grow as both a mold and a yeast (the yeast form is favored under very high moisture conditions). When the mold grows on wood, it can penetrate the paint and cause dark spots. The colonies can be cream to pink in color and darken to brown as they age.

—*Chaetomium* species thrive in wet conditions and are common in building materials (drywall, wood) and cardboard as well as mattresses and upholstered goods that have been wet for a period of time. *Chaetomium* species are among the most aggressive agents of deterioration of cellulose (paper, cotton, and canvas). These fungi were known to decimate military supplies such as tents and rucksacks during World War I and World War II, and thus preventing their growth was the object of concerted study by military scientists. Colonies growing on paper may be gray-brown or black in color, sometimes appearing as very tiny raised dots.

—*Cladosporium* species (there are over five hundred known) are common worldwide, so spores are present in the outdoor air, particularly during the warmer summer months, when the mold is growing on plants and leaves. Spores may enter indoor air via infiltration (see chapter 4) or come from indoor sources. These fungi grow on organic materials (wood, textiles, dust) in water-damaged buildings and on surfaces next to windows dampened by condensation (especially the species *C. sphaerospermum*). I often find *Cladosporium* mold growing in damp fiberglass lining material inside air-conditioning fan coils. Colonies are usually dark green or black in color. *Cladosporium* "mildew" (mold), common on foundation walls, is often mistaken for *Stachybotrys* mold (see below), which requires wetter conditions for growth.

—*Epicoccum* species degrade dead plants and are thus more commonly found outdoors than indoors, except in the fall, when spores can infiltrate buildings and be found in dust. *Epicoccum* mold has been found indoors, however, growing on damp paper. Colonies tend to be bright orange or reddish, becoming covered with a granular mass of dark brown spots.

—*Fusarium* species require wet growing conditions and attack cereal seeds such as barley and corn. They can also be found on damp building materials as well as in humidifier water. Some species produce mycotoxins—a real concern in animal feed, because the consumption of infected corn can affect animals' reproductive organs. In the indoor environment, *Fusarium* mold can be found in persistently wet boot mats as well as drain traps. Colonies are fast-growing, ranging in color from white to pink to lavender.

—*Paecilomyces* species require wet conditions and are found growing in humidifier water and on damp floors and walls. The mold has caused diseases in dogs, cattle, and other animals. Colonies of the most common species, *P. varioti*, are golden brown in color. Other less common species may have red, white, or violet colonies.

—*Penicillium* species (there are over 250 known) grow on damp building materials (wallpaper, wallpaper glue, and drywall) and moist dust. (*Penicillium* spores indoors can also originate from citrus fruit covered with blue-green colonies of *P. digitatum* or *P. italicum*.) Many species produce mycotoxins or musty odors (microbial volatile organic compounds, or MVOCs; see chapter 3). The antibiotic penicillin is derived from the most common species, *P. chrysogenum*. Some white cheeses, like Brie and Camembert, are made with *P. camemberti*, whereas blue-veined cheeses are made with *P. roqueforti*. The spores of *Penicillium* species are mostly between 2 and 10 microns in size, allowing them to penetrate deep into the lung if inhaled. Colonies of *Penicillium* are typically bluish green and powdery, so they are readily aerosolized.

—*Pithomyces* spores are not common indoors except in the fall (suggesting an outdoor source), although this mold can grow on paper or ceiling tiles. Settled spores can also be found in carpet dust, particularly if carpets are not vacuumed frequently in the fall. Some *Pithomyces* species produce mycotoxins. *P. chartarum* produces the mycotoxin sporidesmin, which causes facial eczema in sheep and cattle. If foraging animals consume enough sporidesmin, they become jaundiced; some even die from liver damage. In New Zealand, major outbreaks have been noted in sheep and in cattle.[2] Colonies of *Pithomyces* are white and cottony, soon becoming peppered with black spores.

—*Stachybotrys* species require wet growing conditions and will flourish on paper and paper products, including drywall and cardboard, that have remained damp for days to weeks. Commonly referred to as toxic black mold, the species *S. chartarum* and *S. chlorohalonata* are capable of producing mycotoxins such as tricothecenes and roridan. These species can grow on wet hay. Animals that eat hay contaminated with these mycotoxins can sicken and die. *Stachybotrys* spores are usually 8 to 12 microns in size and tend to settle out of the air more quickly than *Aspergillus* and *Penicillium* spores do. In addition, the spores are formed in sticky clumps; therefore, individual *Stachybotrys* spores are not readily aerosolized.

— *Trichoderma* species grow on potted-plant soil, on water-saturated wood and wooden furniture, and sometimes in the dust in soaked fiberglass insulation and on wet air-conditioning filters. Some species can produce mycotoxins as well as MVOCs. To create the faded appearance of "stonewashed" jeans, the pants are placed in a vat containing an enzyme of *Trichoderma* mold. The enzyme degrades the cellulose surface of the cotton fabric (cellulose is a structural component of plants and is found in cotton and paper). Enzymes from *Trichoderma* species are also used in the production of beer and wine. Spores of *Trichoderma* are mostly 2 to 12 microns in size; however, they are sticky and tend not to become airborne as easily as the spores of *Aspergillus* and *Penicillium*. Colonies of *Trichoderma* are fast-growing and cottony, becoming punctuated with grass-green tufts where the spores are produced.

— *Ulocladium* species grow on drywall or wallpaper that has been saturated by flooding. Sometimes mistaken for *Stachybotrys* mold, *Ulocladium* colonies can be dark brown to black in color.

To understand IAQ testing reports, it is useful to have some numbers and descriptions to serve as a basis of comparison. I hope this chapter has provided you with some of the information you need. As always, if you have questions or concerns, it's a good idea to consider arranging for a personal consultation with an indoor air quality professional.

CONCLUSION

This conclusion is hard for me to write, because I'm not ready to end the book. I have covered a lot of ground (and air), and yet I feel that I have only begun to discuss the story of poor indoor air quality—all the science involved and the full impact on human health. But as I sit at my desk, fretting about how to conclude, my gaze falls upon the stack of telephone directories sitting on a shelf across the room. I suddenly realize that if I were to say all that I want to say, this book would be thicker than that pile of directories. And even then the book would not be complete, because the field of IAQ is a contentious and unsettled frontier, in which research is ongoing, new theories are being proposed, and scientists from academia and from industry do not agree. Unfortunately, people who are suffering from IAQ problems can't afford to hold their breath while these conflicts are resolved.

Ever since the energy crisis of the 1970s, we have been constructing buildings that are ever more airtight and well insulated, in order to reduce fuel consumption. We have come to accept that the inside of a building is necessarily isolated from the outside environment. Windows are now thought to be a breach in the building envelope. The authors of the NIOSH Health Hazard Evaluation of Brigham and Women's Hospital (see chapter 10) stated that windows that open can "have a significant negative impact on the indoor environment."[1] This opinion, though justifiable in its context, underscores the importance of mechanical ventilation systems. But all too often, unfortunately, building ventilation is inadequate, whether owing to poor design or maintenance of the system or to a deliberate reduction in the fresh air supply.

According to the indoor building comfort guideline defined by ASHRAE, as long as 80 percent of the people in a building are satisfied and only 20 percent dissatisfied, acceptable conditions for thermal comfort have been met. We assume and accept, then, that even in the best case, 20 percent of a building's occupants will typically be uncomfortable when it comes to temperature. But we should not accept such a guideline when it comes to indoor air quality. Even if only 5 percent of a building's occupants are experiencing symptoms that may be caused by poor IAQ, we should be concerned.

About 7 percent of the U.S. population have asthma, over 10 percent may have chemical sensitivities, and 25 percent have allergies. Yet there are no guidelines or standards for acceptable indoor levels of microorganisms (mold, yeast, bacteria, and actinomycetes) and their numerous by-products (see chapter 14). In addition, in most sick buildings the concentration of any given volatile organic compound is below OSHA's permissible exposure limit (PEL).

A PEL is derived by toxicologists through experiments using laboratory animals such as rodents. We may not think that we conduct tests using human subjects, yet in a way our everyday "trials" with poor IAQ are comparable to just such exposure experiments. We seal the windows of buildings and then fill the air inside with solvents, pesticides, and other chemicals. We set up humid microenvironments inside that are conducive to microbial growth. Then we move children and adults in and watch what happens. The results are becoming predictable but are all too often ignored. In laboratory experiments we believe what the rodents "tell" us. Why don't we believe these human subjects who tell us they are suffering?

People who have a history of allergies or asthma or heightened sensitivities to indoor contaminants may suffer symptoms before the rest of us do, but eventually more and more of us may begin to suffer from environmentally induced illnesses. Joellen Lawson of the McKinley school (see chapter 8) called her watchdog organization the Canary Committee—an apt name because Joellen and others like her are the canaries in the coal mine: harbingers for the rest of us. We have two choices. We can either blame, isolate, or medicate those who are suffering, or we can study the causes and sources of IAQ problems and clean up our indoor environments.

Joellen Lawson said that "many of the health and career decisions I made in 1998 would have been dramatically different had I comprehended the connection between my illness and work environment."[2] I believe that, in the end, education, understanding, and compassion are vital in illuminating the road from suffering to health.

RESOURCE GUIDE

This list of resources is intended to help readers gather information and make up their own minds as to which organizations, products, publications, and services may help them deal with indoor air quality questions and concerns. Inclusion in this list does not constitute an endorsement by the author or the publisher.

Organizations

- American Academy of Allergy, Asthma, and Immunology (AAAAI) (Milwaukee, Wisc.; 414-272-6071; www.aaaai.org). Provides information on allergies, as well as on pollen and mold spore levels, supplied by seventy-five counting stations in the United States and two in Canada. The website has a geographical list of allergists.
- American Association of Heating, Refrigerating, and Air-Conditioning Engineers (ASHRAE) (Atlanta, Ga.; 800-527-4723; www.ashrae.org). Provides educational opportunities, publications, and consensus guidelines and "ASHRAE standards."
- American Conference of Governmental Industrial Hygienists (ACGIH) (Cincinnati, Ohio; 513-742-2020; www.acgih.org). Offers educational opportunities and over four hundred publications, publishes its own journal, and trains mold consultants and remediators through its Learning Center.
- American Indoor Air Quality Council (AIAQC) (Glendale, Ariz.; 800-

942-0832; www.indoor-air-quality.org). Promotes IAQ awareness and education and offers a number of professional certifications.

- American Industrial Hygiene Association (AIHA) (New York; 703-849-8888; www.aiha.org). Offers publications, educational opportunities, and accreditation for laboratories via its Environmental Microbiology Proficiency Analytical Testing (EMPAT) program. Represents the industrial hygiene profession in public policy.
- American Lung Association (800-586-4872; 212-315-8700; www.lungusa.org). Fights lung diseases and promotes tobacco control. Check the website for local chapters.
- American Public Health Association (APHA) (Washington, D.C.; 202-777-APHA; www.apha.org). Promotes public health and equity in health status.
- Association of Energy Engineers (AEE) (Atlanta, Ga.; 770-447-5083; www.aeecenter.org). Offers publications and provides information on energy efficiency, facility management, plant engineering, and environmental compliance. Certifies IAQ professionals, among others.
- Association of Specialists in Cleaning and Restoration (ASCR) (Millersville, Md.; 800-272-7012; www.ascr.org). Represents more than twenty thousand cleaning and restoration professionals. Maintains a technical library and offers educational opportunities and professional training as well as various products.
- Asthma and Allergy Foundation of America (AAFA) (Washington, D.C.; 202-466-7642; www.aafa.org). Has chapters in a number of states and offers lectures and educational programs for people who have allergies or asthma.
- Carpet and Rug Institute (CRI) (Dalton, Ga.; 800-882-8846). Carpet manufacturers' organization that disseminates information on carpets.
- Centers for Disease Control and Prevention (CDC) (Atlanta, Ga.: 404-639-3534, 800-311-3435; www.cdc.gov). Lead federal agency for protecting human health and safety. Investigates and monitors health problems, conducts research, works for sound public health policies, and provides training and leadership in the health field.
- Center for Health, Environment, and Justice (CHEJ) (Falls Church, Va.;

703-237-2249; www.chej.org). Organizes people to work for a healthy, sustainable future.

- Children's Environmental Health Network (CEHN) (Washington, D.C., and Berkeley, Calif.; 202-543-4033 and 510-526-0081; www.cehn.org). Works to protect children and fetuses from environmental health hazards.
- Connecticut Foundation for Environmentally Safe Schools (information@pollutionfreeschools.org; www.pollutionfreeschools.org). Provides information and connection to a nationwide network of IAQ organizations committed to pollution-free school buildings.
- Environmental Protection Agency (EPA) (Washington, D.C.; 202-272-0167; www.epa.gov). Works to protect human health and the environment. Supports research and provides education and publications (refer to the publications list below as well as to the EPA publication website, www.epa.gov/iaq/pubs/). Map of regional offices available on the EPA website.
- Healthy Kids (Newton, Mass.; 617-965-9637; www.healthy-kids.info/aboutus.lasso). Dedicated to a better understanding of the needs of students with asthma and other chronic conditions, and to the improvement of health policies and practices in schools.
- Healthy Schools Network, Inc. (Albany, N.Y.; 518-462-0632, 212-482-0204; www.healthyschools.org). Promotes the development of policies, regulations, and funding for healthy school facilities.
- Indoor Air Quality Association (IAQA) (Rockville, Md.; 301-231-8388; www.iaqa.org). Offers courses for remediators and investigators and lists Internet resources on its website.
- Indoor Air Quality Information Clearing House (800-438-4318). The EPA's indoor air quality information hotline.
- Institute of Inspection, Cleaning, and Restoration Certification (IICRC) (Vancouver, Wash.; 360-693-5675; www.iicrc.org). Certifies carpet cleaners and publishes "industry standards" for the profession (refer to the publications list below).
- National Air Duct Cleaners Association (NADCA) (Washington, D.C.; 202-737-2926; www.nadca.com). Disseminates information, sets "industry standards," and encourages ethical practices in the duct-cleaning industry.

- National Institute of Occupational Safety and Health (NIOSH) (Atlanta, Ga.; 404-639-3534, 800-311-3435; www.cdc.gov/niosh/homepage.html). Provides leadership in preventing work-related illnesses and injuries; offers educational and training programs and publications; and funds research. Under its Health Hazard Evaluation (HHE) program (www.cdc.gov/niosh/hhe/), NIOSH offers workplace studies that determine whether hazardous materials or harmful conditions are present. HHE studies are conducted at no cost to the complainant. Many HHE reports are available on the website.
- Occupational Safety and Health Administration (OSHA), U.S. Department of Labor (Washington, D.C.; 800-321-6742; www.osha.gov). Aims to ensure the safety and health of every worker in the United States by setting and enforcing standards; providing training, outreach, and education; establishing partnerships; and encouraging continual improvement in workplace safety and health.
- Restoration Consultants (Sacramento, Calif.; 916-736-1100; www.restcon.com). Trains mold consultants and remediators.

Products

- *Air purifier with gooseneck:* IQAir (877-715-4247; www.iqair.us).
- *Allergy products* (including steam vapor machines, HEPA vacuums, and air purification systems): Home Environmental (781-862-2873; www.homeenv.com).
- *Carpet covering* (self-adhering clear plastic): Pro-Tect Associates, Inc. (800-545-0826; www.pro-tect.com).
- *Cockroach allergen test kit:* DACI Laboratory, Johns Hopkins University Asthma and Allergy Center (Baltimore, Md.; 800-344-3224; www.hopkinsmedicine.org); and P&K Microbiology Services, Inc. (Cherry Hill, N.J.; 866-871-1984; www.stl-inc.com/labs/P&K/P&K_index.htm).
- *Combustible gas detectors:* Professional Equipment (800-334-9291; www.professionalequipment.com).
- *Dehumidifiers:* Therma-Stor Products (800-533-7533; www.thermastor.com).
- *DennyFoil* (a paper–aluminum foil laminate that can be used to temporarily cover surfaces): Denny Wholesale (561-750-3705; www.dennywholesale.com).

- *Dust mite allergen test kit:* DACI Laboratory, Johns Hopkins University Asthma and Allergy Center (Baltimore, Md.; 800-344-3224; www.hopkinsmedicine.org); and P&K Microbiology Services, Inc. (Cherry Hill, N.J.; 866-871-1984; www.stl-inc.com/labs/P&K/P&K_index.htm).
- *Carbon dioxide direct-read diffusion tube:* BGI Inc. (Waltham, Mass.; 781-891-9380; www.bgiusa.com); and SKC Inc. (Eighty Four, Pa.; 800-752-8472; www.skcinc.com).
- *Filters (heating and air conditioning):* Research Products Corporation (608-257-8801; www.Aprilaire.com).
- *Formaldehyde test kit:* SKC Inc. (Eighty Four, Pa.; 800-752-8472; www.skcinc.com).
- *Moisture meter* (Tramex): Professional Equipment (800-334-9291; www.professionalequipment.com).
- *Nitrogen dioxide test kit:* SKC Inc. (Eighty Four, Pa.; 800-752-8472; www.skcinc.com).
- *Ozone gas passive indicator* (OzoneWatch): *IQ*Air (877-715-4247; www.iqair.us).
- *Pet allergen test kit:* DACI Laboratory, Johns Hopkins University Asthma and Allergy Center (Baltimore, Md.; 800-344-3224; www.hopkinsmedicine.org); and P&K Microbiology Services, Inc. (Cherry Hill, N.J.; 866-871-1984; www.stl-inc.com/labs/P&K/P&K_index.htm).
- *Radon test* (Alpha-Trak): National Safety Products, Inc. (877-412-3600; http://testproducts.com).
- *Vents (ridge and soffit):* Headrick Building Products, Inc. (678-513-7242; www.headrick.net).

Publications

- *Basic Information about Indoor Air Quality,* Environmental Protection Agency (www.epa.gov/iaq/ia-intro.html).
- *Building Air Quality: A Guide for Building Owners and Facility Managers,* Environmental Protection Agency and National Institute for Occupational Safety and Health, 1991.
- *Casualties of Progress: Personal Histories from the Chemically Sensitive,* edited by A. Johnson (Brunswick, Maine: MCS Information Exchange, 2000).
- *Causes of Indoor Air Quality Problems in Schools,* by C. Bayer, S. Crow, and

J. Fischer, Energy Division, Oak Ridge National Laboratory, for the U.S. Department of Energy, January 1999.

- *A Citizen's Guide to Radon,* EPA publication available through the Indoor Air Quality Information Clearing House (800-438-4318; www.epa.gov/iaq).
- *Damp Indoor Spaces and Health* (Washington, D.C.: Institute of Medicine of the National Academies, 2004).
- "Fungal Contamination as a Major Contributor of Sick Building Syndrome," by D. Li and C. Yang, *Sick Building Syndrome* (San Diego, Calif.: Academic Press, 2004).
- *Green Guide for Health Care,* convened by the Center for Maximum Potential Building Systems, sponsored by Hospitals for a Healthy Environment and the New York State Energy Research and Development Authority (www.gghc.org).
- *Guidance for Clinicians on the Recognition and Management of Health Effects Related to Mold Exposure and Moisture Indoors,* by E. Storey et al., University of Connecticut Health Center, Division of Occupational and Environmental Medicine, 2004 (http://oehc.uchc.edu/clinser/MOLD%20GUIDE.pdf).
- *Guidelines and Recommendations for Ventilation, Construction, and Renovation of Hospitals,* Environmental Protection Agency (www.cdc.gov/ncidod/hip/Guide/construct.htm).
- *Guidelines for Environmental Infection Control in Health-Care Facilities,* by L. Sehulster and R. Chinn, Centers for Disease Control and Prevention (www.cdc.gov/mmwr/preview/mmwrhtml/rr5210a1.htm).
- *Guidelines on Assessment and Remediation of Fungi in Indoor Environments,* New York City Department of Health and Mental Hygiene, Bureau of Environmental and Occupational Disease Epidemiology, 2000 (www.ci.nyc.ny.us/html/doh/html/epi/moldrpt1.html).
- *Gulf War Syndrome,* by A. Johnson (Brunswick, Maine: MCS Information Exchange, 2001).
- *Handbook of Pediatric Environmental Health,* American Academy of Pediatrics, 1999 (www.aap.org).
- *The Healthy House,* by J. Bower (Bloomington, Ind.: Healthy House Institute, 2001).

- *Humidity Control Design Guide,* by L. Harriman et al., American Society of Heating, Refrigerating, and Air-Conditioning Engineers, Inc., 2001.
- *IAQ Guidelines for Occupied Buildings under Construction,* Sheet Metal and Air Conditioning Contractors' National Association, Inc., 1995.
- *IICRC S001 Carpet Cleaning Standard,* Institute of Inspection, Cleaning, and Restoration Certification, 1997.
- *IICRC S520 Standard and Reference Guide for Professional Mold Remediation,* Institute of Inspection, Cleaning, and Restoration Certification, 2003.
- *Indoor Air Quality and HVAC Systems,* by D. Bearg (New York: Lewis Publishers, 1993).
- "Indoor Air Quality: Tools for Schools," EPA action kit offering parents and educators a practical plan for solving IAQ problems in school buildings, available through the Indoor Air Quality Clearing House (800-438-4318; www.epa.gov/iaq).
- *Integrated Pest Management (IPM) in Schools,* Environmental Protection Agency (www.epa.gov/pesticides/jpm/).
- *Mold Remediation in Schools and Commercial Buildings,* Environmental Protection Agency (www.epa/mold/mold_remediation.html).
- *The Mold Survival Guide: For Your Home and for Your Health,* by J. May and C. May (Baltimore, Md.: Johns Hopkins University Press, 2004).
- "Molds, Toxic Molds, and Indoor Air Quality," by P. Davis, *CRB Note* 8 (March 2001) (www.library.ca.gov/crb/01/notes/v8n1.pdf).
- *Mould Guidelines for the Canadian Construction Industry,* Canadian Construction Association, 2004 (www.cca-acc.com/documents/electronic/cca82/cca82.pdf).
- *My House is Killing Me! The Home Guide for Families with Allergies and Asthma,* by J. May (Baltimore, Md.: Johns Hopkins University Press, 2001).
- *Radon-Specific Publications and Resources,* Environmental Protection Agency (www.epa.gov/radon/pubs).
- *Your Car Can Be Hazardous to Your Health: The Book Automakers and Politicians Prefer You Not Read,* by B. Rudusky (AuthorHouse, 2002).

Services

Laboratories that will analyze dust samples from carpets and other surfaces:

- Aerotech Laboratory, Inc. (Phoenix, AZ; 800-651-4802; www.aerotech labs.com). Also sells testing supplies.
- American Industrial Hygiene Association (www.aiha.org). Offers a list of labs accredited by its EMPAT (Environmental Microbiology Proficiency Analytical Testing) program.
- DACI Laboratory, Johns Hopkins University Asthma and Allergy Center (Baltimore, Md.; 800-344-3224; www.hopkinsmedicine.org).
- Northeast Laboratory (Winslow, Maine; 800-244-8378; www.NeLab Services.com).

ABBREVIATIONS

AAFA	Asthma and Allergy Foundation of America
AC	air conditioning
ACGIH	American Conference of Governmental Industrial Hygienists
ACM	asbestos-containing material
ACT	asbestos composite tile
AHERA	Asbestos Hazard Emergency Response Act
AIHA	American Industrial Hygiene Association
ASHI	American Society of Home Inspectors
ASHRAE	American Society of Heating, Refrigerating, and Air-Conditioning Engineers
BASE	Building Assessment, Survey, and Evaluation
BRI	building-related illness
CDC	Centers for Disease Control and Prevention
cfu	colony-forming unit(s)
CRI	Carpet and Rug Institute
CS	chemical sensitivity
EIFS	exterior insulation and finish system
EPA	U.S. Environmental Protection Agency
EPDM	ethylene-propylene-diene monomer
ETS	environmental tobacco smoke
EU	endotoxin unit
FDA	U.S. Food and Drug Administration

g	gram
GC	gas chromatograph
GC/MS	gas chromatograph/mass spectrometer
GRAS	generally regarded as safe
HDM	house dust mite
HEPA	high-efficiency particulate arrestance
HUD	U.S. Department of Housing and Urban Development
HVAC	heating, ventilation, and air conditioning
IAQ	indoor air quality
IAQP	indoor air quality professional
IDLH	immediately dangerous to life and health
IICRC	Institute of Inspection, Cleaning, and Restoration Certification
IPM	integrated pest management
m^3	cubic meter
mcg	microgram
MCS	multiple chemical sensitivity
MERV	minimum efficiency reporting value
mg	milligram
MNA	Massachusetts Nurses Association
MS	mass spectrometer
MVOC	microbial volatile organic compound
NAAQS	National Ambient Air Quality Standards
NIOSH	National Institute for Occupational Safety and Health
ODTS	organic dust toxic syndrome
OSB	oriented strand board
OSHA	U.S. Occupational Safety and Health Administration
PAR	protease-activated receptor
pCi/L	picocurie(s) per liter
4-PC	4-phenylcyclohexene
PEL	permissible exposure limit
PM	particulate matter
ppb	parts per billion
ppm	parts per million
RH	relative humidity

RMV	Registry of Motor Vehicles
RTU	rooftop unit
RV	recreational vehicle
SARS	Severe Acute Respiratory Syndrome
SBS	sick-building syndrome
SEM	scanning electron micrograph
TCE	trichloroethylene
TVOC	total volatile organic compounds
U	units(s)
VCT	vinyl composite tile
VOC	volatile organic compound

NOTES

1 • POOR INDOOR AIR QUALITY

1. T. Palmer Jr., "Trouble in the Air Confounding U Mass, No Classes, Few Clues, and Unrest," *Boston Globe,* 1 February 1994.

2. T. Coakley, "U Mass Boosts Ventilation Level in Its Buildings," *Boston Globe,* 5 February 1994.

3. D. Edmondson et al., "Allergy and 'Toxic Mold Syndrome,'" *Annals of Allergy, Asthma, and Immunology* 94 (February 2005): 234–39.

4. K. Binkley, "Multiple Chemical Sensitivity? An Approach to Patients," *Allergy and Asthma Magazine,* spring 2004.

5. N. Ashford and C. Miller, *Chemical Exposures: Low Levels and High Stakes* (New York: John Wiley and Sons, 1998).

6. D. Bearg, *Indoor Air Quality and HVAC Systems* (New York: Lewis Publishers, 1993), 11.

7. J. Spengler et al., eds., *Indoor Air Quality Handbook* (New York: McGraw-Hill, 2001), 4.1.

2 • SHELTER IN THE STORM

1. J. Antó et al., "Long Term Outcome of Soybean Epidemic Asthma after an Allergen Reduction Intervention," *Thorax* 54 (August 1999): 670–74.

2. A. Sapkota et al., "Impact of the 2002 Canadian Forest Fires on Particulate Matter Air Quality in Baltimore City," *Environmental Science and Technology* 39, no. 1 (2005): 24–32.

3 • DISEASED DECOR

1. C. Hogue, "Regulators at Scene of Attacks," *Chemical and Engineering News,* 24 September 2001.

2. A. Ferro et al., "Source Strengths for Indoor Human Activities That Resuspend Particulate Matter," *Environmental Science and Technology* 38, no. 6 (2004): 1759–64.

3. S. Krimsky, *Hormonal Chaos: The Scientific and Social Origins of the Environmental Endocrine Hypothesis* (Baltimore: Johns Hopkins University Press, 2002).

4. I. Yu et al., "Evidence of Airborne Transmission of the Severe Acute Respiratory Syndrome Virus," *New England Journal of Medicine* 350 (22 April 2004): 1731–39.

5. F. LaMarte et al., "Acute Systemic Reactions to Carbonless Copy Paper Associated with Histamine Release," *Journal of the American Medical Association* 260 (8 July 1988): 242.

6. B. Wolverton et al., "Foliage Plants for Removing Indoor Air Pollutants from Energy Efficient Homes," *Economic Botany* 38 (1983): 224–28.

7. T. Godish, "Botanical Air Purification Studies under Dynamic Chamber Conditions," in *Proceedings of the 81st Annual Meeting of the Air Pollution Control Association,* Dallas, Tex., 1988.

8. D. Karimian-Teherani et al., "Allergy to *Ficus benjamina,*" *Bulletin de la Société des Sciences Médicales du Grand-Duché de Luxembourg,* no. 2 (2002): 107–13.

9. E. Erwin et al., "Animal Danders," *Immunology and Allergy Clinics of North America* 23 (August 2003): 469–81.

10. C. Saltoun et al., "Hypersensitivity Pneumonitis Resulting from Community Exposure to Canada Goose Droppings: When an External Environmental Antigen Becomes an Indoor Environmental Antigen," *Annals of Allergy, Asthma, and Immunology* 84 (January 2000): 84–86.

11. K. Rosenman et al., "Cleaning Products and Work-Related Asthma," *Journal of Occupational and Environmental Medicine* 45 (2003): 556–63.

5 • GASES IN THE SEA OF AIR

1. J. Last et al., "Ozone, NO, and NO_2: Oxidant Air Pollutants and More," *Environmental Health Perspectives* 102, suppl. no. 10 (December 1994): 179–84.

2. R. McConnell et al., "Asthma in Exercising Children Exposed to Ozone: A Cohort Study," *Lancet* 359 (2 February 2002): 386–91.

3. *Odor Thresholds for Chemicals with Established Occupational Health Standards* (Akron, Ohio: AIHA, 1989), 26.

4. J. Mah, *Non-Fire Carbon Monoxide Deaths Associated with the Use of Consumer Products, 1998 Annual Estimates* (Bethesda, Md.: U.S. Consumer Product Safety Commission), 1.

5. "National Ambient Air Quality Standards," *Code of Federal Regulations*, Title 40, Part 50.

6. J. Spengler et al., eds., *Indoor Air Quality Handbook* (New York: McGraw-Hill, 2001), 29.4, 29.13–16.

7. H. Koren, "Environmental Health Issues," *Environmental Health Perspectives* 103, suppl. 6, (1995): 235–42.

8. M. Matura et al., "Oxidized Citrus Oil (R-Limonene): A Frequent Skin Sensitizer in Europe," *Journal of the American Academy of Dermatology* 47 (November 2002): 709–14.

9. Z. Fan et al., "Ozone-Initiated Reactions with Mixtures of Volatile Organic Compounds under Simulated Indoor Conditions," *Environmental Science and Technology* 37 (1 May 2003): 1811–21.

10. J. Kleno and P. Wolkoff, "Changes in Eye Blink Frequency as a Measure of Trigeminal Stimulation by Exposure to Limonene Oxidation Products, Isoprene Oxidation Products, and Nitrate Radicals," *International Archives of Occupational and Environmental Health* 77 (May 2004): 235–43.

11. L. Mølhave et al., "Subjective Reactions to Volatile Organic Compounds as Air Pollutants," *Atmospheric Environment* 25a, no. 7 (1991): 1283–93.

12. Spengler et al., eds., *Indoor Air Quality Handbook*, 25.1–14.

13. D. Cortes et al., "Role of Dust Analysis in Complaint Resolution of Indoor Air Quality," in *Proceedings of Indoor Air 2002, the 9th International Conference on Indoor Air Quality and Climate*, Monterey, Calif., 30 June–5 July 2002.

14. Adapted from R. Hetes et al., "Office Equipment: Design, Indoor Air Emissions, and Pollution Prevention Opportunities" (Washington, D.C.: U.S. EPA, June 1995), table 1, p. 3 (assuming twenty sheets printed per minute).

15. Ibid.

6 • PARTICLES IN THE SEA OF AIR

1. G. Dolphin, "Minyak the Orangutan," *Indoor Environment Connections* 5 (June 2004).

2. *Damp Indoor Spaces and Health* (Washington, D.C.: Institute of Medicine of the National Academies, 2004).

3. J. Cox-Ganser et al., "Respiratory Morbidity in Office Workers in a Water-Damaged Building," *Environmental Health Perspectives* 113 (April 2005): 485–90.

4. L. Arlian et al., "Allergenic Characterization of *Tyrophagus putrescentiae* Using Sera from Occupationally Exposed Farmers," *Annals of Allergy, Asthma, and Immunology* 79 (December 1997): 525–29.

5. L. Arlian et al., "Serum Immunoglobulin E against Storage Mite Allergens in Dogs with Atopic Dermatitis," *American Journal of Veterinary Research* 64 (January 2003): 32–36.

6. T. Brasel et al., "Detection of Airborne *Stachybotrys chartarum* Macrocyclic Trichothecene Mycotoxins on Particulates Smaller Than Conidia," *Applied and Environmental Microbiology* 71 (January 2005): 114–22.

7. L. Dalton, "Chemical Analysis of a Disaster," *Chemical and Engineering News* 81 (20 October 2003): 26–30.

8. C. Hogue, "Regulators at Scene of Attacks," *Chemical and Engineering News*, 24 September 2001.

9. Dalton, "Chemical Analysis of a Disaster."

10. National Institute of Environmental Health Sciences, National Institutes of Health, "New Research Outlines Public Health Consequences of World Trade Center Disaster," NIEHS press release no. 04-10, 3 May 2004, www.niehs.nih.gov/oc/news/wtcnews.htm.

11. Dalton, "Chemical Analysis of a Disaster."

12. Associated Press, "EPA Hit with Ground Zero Lawsuit," 11 March 2004, www.cbsnews.com/stories/2004/03/11/health/printable605224.shtml.

7 • MENACE IN THE MECHANICALS

1. H. Eichel, "Mold in Mansion Tied to Renovation," *Charlotte Observer,* 12 July 2004.

2. Ibid.

3. Y. Zhu et al., "Concentration and Size Distribution of Ultrafine Particles Near a Major Highway," *Journal of the Air and Waste Management Association* 52 (September 2002): 1032–42.

4. A. Weber and K. Martinez, *HHE Report No. HETA-93-1110-2575, Martin County Courthouse and Constitutional Office Building, Stuart, Florida* (Washington, D.C.: NIOSH, May 1996).

5. S. Schooley, "Mold: A Living Construction Defect," HarrisMartin Publishing Perspectives, www.harrismartin.com/tour/pdfs/perspectives.pdf.

6. R. Bailey, "Martin County Courthouse—The Untold Story," *INvironment®* 3 (May 1997).

7. D. Menzies et al., "Effect of Ultraviolet Germicidal Lights Installed in Office Ventilation Systems on Workers' Health and Well-Being: Double-Blind Multiple Crossover Trial," *Lancet* 362 (29 November 2003): 1785–91.

8 • SCHOOLS

1. L. Cuddy, "Schools—The Perils of Permanent Marking Pens," *Green Teacher* (Toronto), December 1993/January 1994.

2. P. Eggleston and L. Arruda, "Ecology and Elimination of Cockroaches and Allergens in the Home," *Journal of Allergy and Clinical Immunology* 107, suppl. no. 3 (March 2001): S422–29.

3. S. Sarpong et al., "Cockroach Allergen (Bla g 1) in School Dust," *Journal of Allergy and Clinical Immunology* 99 (April 1997): 486–92.

4. W. Alarcon et al., "Acute Illnesses Associated with Pesticide Exposure at Schools," *Journal of the American Medical Association* 294, no. 4 (27 July 2005): 455–65.

5. EPA Region 6, South Central, "In the News—Children's Health: Update on Asthma Symptoms," 2002, www.epa.gov/region6/6xa/child_health_summit.htm.

6. "Statement of Joellen Lawson, Fairfield, CT," Senate Green School Hearing, 1 October 2002, http://epw.senate.gov/107th/Lawson_100102.htm.

7. Personal conversation with Joellen Lawson, December 2003.

8. J. Santilli, "Health Effects of Mold Exposure in Public Schools," *Current Allergy and Asthma Reports,* no. 2 (2002): 460–67.

9. C. Leslie, "Local PTA President Tells What She Learned from a School Crisis," *National Healthy Schools Training Manual* (Albany, N.Y.: Healthy Schools Network, 2002), 2.

10. J. Santilli and W. Rockwell, "Fungal Contamination of Elementary Schools: A New Environmental Hazard," *Annals of Allergy, Asthma, and Immunology* 90 (February 2003): 203–8.

11. Santilli, "Health Effects of Mold Exposure in Public Schools," 463.

12. M. Major, *Consultation Report for Town of Fairfield, Board of Education* (Connecticut Department of Labor, Division of Occupational Safety and Health, October 2000), appendix E, 6.

13. A. Verhoeff and H. Burge, "Health Risk Assessment of Fungi in Home Environments," *Annals of Allergy, Asthma, and Immunology* 78, no. 6 (June 1997): 544–56.

14. Associated Press, "School Officials Ponder Options to Deal with School Fungus," 18 October 2000.

15. Santilli, "Health Effects of Mold Exposure in Public Schools," 463.

16. *Initial HVAC & IAQ Evaluation, The McKinley School, Fairfield, Connecticut* (Turner Building Science, January 2001), 13.

17. J. Axelrod, "Kids Getting Sick from School," 5 June 2002. CBSNEWS.com.

18. Associated Press, "School Officials Ponder Options to Deal with School Fungus."

19. Leslie, "Local PTA President Tells What She Learned," 3.

20. Axelrod, "Kids Getting Sick from School."

21. Santilli and Rockwell, "Fungal Contamination of Elementary Schools."

22. Santilli, "Health Effects of Mold Exposure in Public Schools."

23. Personal conversation with Charlotte Leslie.

24. *Initial HVAC & IAQ Evaluation, The McKinley School,* appendix E.

25. T. Sakamoto et al., "Allergenic and Antigenic Activities of the Osmophilic Fungus *Wallemia sebi* [in] Asthmatic Patients," *Arerugi: Japanese Journal of Allergology* 38 (April 1989): 352–59; G. Reboux et al., "Role of Molds in Farmer's Lung Disease in

Eastern France," *American Journal of Respiratory and Critical Care Medicine* 163 (June 2001): 1534–39.

26. S. Gravesen et al., *Microfungi* (Viborg, Denmark: Special-Trykkeriet Viborg a/s, 1994), 154.

27. *Initial HVAC & IAQ Evaluation, The McKinley School,* 9.

28. Ibid., 26.

29. Major, *Consultation Report for Town of Fairfield, Board of Education,* appendix E, 11–12.

30. *Initial HVAC & IAQ Evaluation, The McKinley School,* 18.

31. A. Brophy, "$2.5 M Sought to Fix School in Fairfield," *Connecticut Post,* 12 April 2001.

32. M. Van Der Pol, "McKinley Work OK'd. Request for $2.5 Million Goes to RTM on Monday," *Fairfield Citizen News,* 4 May 2001.

33. A. Brophy, "School Solution May Be Too Late," *Connecticut Post,* 12 June 2001.

34. Canary Committee, "Mission Statement," www.canarycommittee.com.

35. C. Mong, "West Carrollton Not Alone in Air Issue," *Dayton Daily News,* 20 January 2002.

36. A. Dietz, "Public Poses Questions to Experts," *Cox News Service,* 31 January 2002.

37. S. Brennan, "Teacher: 'This Building Is Killing Me,'" *The News and Advance,* 9 May 2001.

38. C. Streuber, "Teacher Files Suit over Mold," *Beaufort Gazette,* 5 February 2003.

39. J. Moore, "Teachers: School Made Us Sick," *Carolina Morning News,* 7 February 2003.

40. Leslie, "Local PTA President Tells What She Learned," 3.

9 • NINE TO FIVE

1. J. Kral, "$170m Registry Move Gets Liftoff in Roxbury," *Boston Globe,* 22 May 1991.

2. T. Batten, "Union Official Urges Evacuation as 18 More at Registry Fall Ill," *Boston Globe,* 22 July 1994.

3. D. Armstrong and M. Vaillancourt, "Widespread Symptoms Hit Registry Workers," *Boston Globe,* 3 September 1995.

4. Ibid.

5. Ibid.

6. Private conversation with representative from the Ruggles building management company.

7. P. Howe and P. Langner, "Registry to Close Roxbury Offices, 'Sick Building' May Reopen in 6 Months," *Boston Globe,* 7 July 1995.

8. Private conversation with representative from the Ruggles building management company.

9. M. Grunwald, "Bank Ends Roxbury Project, Forecloses on Loan on Registry Buildings," *Boston Globe,* 9 October 1996.

10. H. Waldman, "Headaches, Coughing, and a Hard Fall," *Hartford Courant,* 1 September 2002.

11. H. Waldman, "Water Leaks and Lung Illness," *Hartford Courant,* 1 September 2002.

12. H. Waldman, "Moldy Building Becomes a Case Study," *Hartford Courant,* 1 September 2002.

13. "Additional Employee Adverse Health Effects Information," *Indoor Air Quality and Work Environment Study,* suppl. to vol. 1 (Washington, D.C.: U.S. EPA and NIOSH, November 1989), 29–35.

14. S. Lang, "Emissions from New Carpet Are Not a Health Problem, Cornell Study Finds," *Cornell University Science News,* March 1995.

15. Carpet and Rug Institute, "Carpet Industry Facts," www.carpet-rug.org.

16. K. Haneke, *4-Phenylcyclohexene, Review of Toxicological Literature* (Research Triangle Park, N.C.: Prepared by Integrated Laboratory Systems for the National Institute of Environmental Health Sciences, July 2002), i.

17. Carpet and Rug Institute, "Indoor Air Quality Testing Programs for New Carpet, Floor Covering Adhesives, and Carpet Cushion," www.carpet-rug.org.

10 • INFIRM INFIRMARIES AND COUGHING COURTHOUSES

1. *Some Industrial Chemicals,* IARC Monographs on the Evaluation of Carcinogenic Risk of Chemicals to Humans, no. 60 (Lyon, France: International Agency for Research on Cancer, 1994).

2. M. Kawamoto et al., *Health Hazard Evaluation Report HETA 96-0012-2652, Brigham and Women's Hospital, Boston, Massachusetts* (Washington, D.C.: NIOSH, September 1997).

3. R. Saltus, "Allergic Reactions Probed in Workers at Brigham & Women's," *Boston Globe,* 3 July 1993.

4. R. Saltus, "Five Brigham Operating Rooms Closed Due to Faulty Ventilation," *Boston Globe,* 29 July 1993.

5. R. Saltus, "Hospital Staffers Battle Mystery Malady, Airborne Irritants Are Targeted for Cleanup," *Boston Globe,* 21 November 1993.

6. Kawamoto et al., *Health Hazard Evaluation Report,* 20.

7. Ibid., 86.

8. J. Spengler et al., eds., *Indoor Air Quality Handbook* (New York: McGraw-Hill, 2001), 65.2, 65.5.

9. Saltus, "Hospital Staffers Battle Mystery Malady."

10. U. McFarling, "For Brigham Nurses, Health Woes Persist," *Boston Globe,* 23 July 1994.

11. D. Kong, "Lawsuit Is Filed over Air Quality, Brigham Hospital Contractors Named," *Boston Globe,* 24 February 1995.

12. A. Kramer, "Hospital to Undergo $8M Cleanup, Worker Ailments Spur Brigham," *Boston Globe,* 21 August 1995.

13. A. Johnson, ed., *Casualties of Progress: Personal Histories from the Chemically Sensitive* (Brunswick, Maine: MCS Information Exchange, 2000), 94.

14. D. Lewis, "Study Finds Workplace a Source of Ills for Women," *Boston Globe,* 18 November 1997.

15. A. Pham, "Former Quiet Caretaker Leads Union Charge," *Boston Globe,* 24 September 1996.

16. Ibid.

17. M. Shao, "Tab for Nurse Buyouts May Hit $5M at Brigham and Women's," *Boston Globe,* 25 September 1996.

18. Kramer, "Hospital to Undergo $8M Cleanup."

19. J. Ellement, "Courthouse Repairs Halted by Noxious Fumes, Fumes Sicken Employees, Halt Repairs at Suffolk Courthouse," *Boston Globe,* 30 June 1994; J. Ellement, "Ailing Courthouse to Be Aired Out," *Boston Globe,* 1 July 1994; J. Ellement, "Air Tests to Begin at Suffolk Court," *Boston Globe,* 23 August 1994; S. Murphy, "Suffolk Courthouse Workers Want Fresh Air and Answers," *Boston Globe,* 27 February 1995; J. Ellement, "Suffolk Court Workers File Lawsuit over Fumes," *Boston Globe,* 1 July 1995; J. Ellement, "5 Grand Jurors in Suffolk Courthouse Also Complain of Illness," *Boston Globe,* 3 November 1995; J. Ellement, "29 Courthouse Workers to Get $3M in Weatherproofing Case," *Boston Globe,* 13 January 1999.

20. OSHA, "Methylene Bisphenyl Isocyanate (MDI)," www.osha.gov/dts/sltc/methods/organic/org047/org047.html.

21. Pecora Corporation, "Duramen® 500," www.pecora.com (specification data sheet, no longer available on line).

22. Murphy, "Suffolk Courthouse Workers Want Fresh Air."

23. E-mail from Joan Parker, 6 January 2004.

24. J. Long, "Huntley Cops to Move out Because of Mold at Station," *Chicago Tribune,* 19 February 2002.

25. B. Schmitt, "70 Police Workers Ordered to Evacuate," *Free Press,* 4 April 2002.

26. T. Glanzer, "Mold Remains an Issue at Simsbury Town Hall," *Farmington Valley Post,* 20 February 2003.

27. K. Crummy, "Ailing Municipal Workers Call Hub City Hall a 'Sick Building,'" *Boston Herald,* 8 May 2001.

28. D. Hemmila, "Bad Chemistry: Nurses Sensitive to Respiratory Irritants Lead the Charge in Reducing Exposure to Chemical Hazards in the Workplace," *NurseWeek,* 11 April 2003, www.NurseWeek.com.

29. Associated Press, "Judge Orders Closing of 'Unsanitary' Jail," 7 July 2001.

30. M. Seuri et al., "An Outbreak of Respiratory Disease among Workers at a Water-Damaged Building—A Case Report," *Indoor Air* 10 (September 2000): 138–45.

11 • RETAIL SPACES

1. *Table B–1: Employees on Nonfarm Payrolls by Industry Sector and Selected Industry Detail* (Washington, D.C.: U.S. Department of Labor, modified 9 January 2004).

2. D. Slack, "Incoming Mayor Plans Shakeup in Somerville," *Boston Globe*, 3 January 2004.

3. B. Parker, "Thanks, Butt Goodbye," *Somerville Journal*, 21 January 2004.

4. B. Parker, "Smoking Ban Battle Still Smoldering in Somerville," *Somerville Journal*, 26 February 2004.

5. B. Hileman, "What's Hiding in Transgenic Foods?" *Chemical and Engineering News* 80 (7 January 2002): 20–23.

6. C. Lemière et al., "Isolated Late Asthmatic Reaction after Exposure to a High-Molecular-Weight Occupational Agent, Subtilisin," *Chest* 110 (1996): 823–24; A. Tripathi and L. Grammar, "Extrinsic Allergic Alveolitis from a Proteolytic Enzyme," *Annals of Allergy, Asthma, and Immunology* 86 (April 2001): 425–27.

7. J. Pepys, "Allergic Asthma to *Bacillus subtilis* Enzyme: A Model for the Effects of Inhalable Proteins," *American Journal of Industrial Medicine* 21 (1992): 587–93.

8. New York City Department of Health and Mental Hygiene, Bureau of Environmental Investigations, "Tetrachloroethylene (Perchloroethylene—'PERC') Fact Sheet," 2005, www.nyc.gov/html/doh/html/ei/eiperc.shtml.

9. E. Pellizzari et al., *Total Exposure Assessment Methodology (TEAM): Dry Cleaners Study* (Washington, D.C.: EPA, 1984).

10. H. Sosted et al., "55 Cases of Allergic Reactions to Hair Dye: A Descriptive, Consumer Complaint–Based Study," *Contact Dermatitis* 47 (November 2002): 299–303.

11. T. Leino et al., "Occupational Skin and Respiratory Diseases among Hairdressers," *Scandinavian Journal of Work, Environment, and Health* 24 (October 1998): 398–406.

12. C. Liden, "Occupational Dermatoses at a Film Laboratory," *Contact Dermatitis* 10 (February 1984): 77–87.

12 • BEFORE NINE AND AFTER FIVE

1. J. May, *My House Is Killing Me! The Home Guide for Families with Allergies and Asthma* (Baltimore: Johns Hopkins University Press, 2001).

2. *Prevalence of Overweight and Obesity among Adults: United States, 1999–2000* (Washington, D.C.: CDC, 2003).

3. K. Thickett et al., "Occupational Asthma Caused by Chloramines in Indoor Swimming-Pool Air," *European Respiratory Journal* 19 (May 2002): 827–32.

4. F. Gagnaire et al., "Comparison of the Sensory Irritation Response in Mice to

Chlorine and Nitrogen Trichloride," *Journal of Applied Toxicology* 14, no. 6 (1994): 405–9.

5. J. Spengler et al., eds., *Indoor Air Quality Handbook* (New York: McGraw-Hill, 2001), 67.4, 67.8.

6. L. Harriman III et al., *Humidity Control Design Guide for Commercial and Institutional Buildings* (Atlanta, Ga.: ASHRAE, 2001).

7. D. Jernigan et al., "Outbreak of Legionnaires' Disease among Cruise Ship Passengers Exposed to a Contaminated Whirlpool Spa," *Lancet* 347 (24 February 1996): 494–99.

8. C. Regan et al., "Outbreak of Legionnaires' Disease on a Cruise Ship: Lessons for International Surveillance and Control," *Communicable Disease and Public Health* 6 (June 2003): 152–56.

9. "Carbon Monoxide Poisoning at an Indoor Ice Arena and Bingo Hall—Seattle, 1996," *Morbidity and Mortality Weekly Report* 45 (5 April 1996).

10. Spengler et al., eds., *Indoor Air Quality Handbook*, figs. 67.1, 67.4.

11. C. Rodes et al., "Measuring Concentrations of Selected Air Pollutants inside California Vehicles" (Research Triangle Park, N.C.: Research Triangle Institute, December 1998), Executive Summary, Final Report.

12. "MTBE Odor Detects Gasoline Taint," *Chemical and Engineering News*, 9 December 1991, 21.

13. L. Hill, *Diesel Engines: Emissions and Human Exposure*, rev. ed. (Boston: Clean Air Task Force, 2005), 1, 2.

14. Rodes et al., "Measuring Concentrations of Selected Air Pollutants."

15. S. Brown and M. Cheng, "Volatile Organic Compounds (VOCs) in New Car Interiors" (Highett, Victoria, Australia: CSIRO Building, Construction, and Engineering, 2001), 2.

16. L. Bonvie and B. Bonvie, "Airline's Insecticide May Be Affecting More Than Bugs," *San Diego Union-Tribune*, 4 March 2001; D. Vergano, "Passengers Wait to Breathe Easy," *USA Today*, 29 September 2003.

17. E. Hunt and D. Space, "The Airplane Cabin Environment: Issues Pertaining to Flight Attendant Comfort," www.boeing.com/commercial/cabinair/ventilation.pdf.

18. Associated Press, "WHO: SARS Has Spread on Only Four Airline Flights," *Houston Chronicle*, 20 May 2003.

19. Hunt and Space, "Airplane Cabin Environment."

20. N. Keates, "How Safe Is Airplane Air?" *Wall Street Journal*, 9 June 2000.

21. "What's Happened to Airplane Air?" *Consumer Reports*, August 1994.

22. "Hilton Hawaiian Village," *Indoor Environment Connections*, June 2003.

23. G. Rising, "Bed Bugs," *Buffalo Sunday News*, 28 March 2004.

13 • DO IT YOURSELF

1. J. Spengler et al., eds., *Indoor Air Quality Handbook* (New York: McGraw-Hill, 2001), table 3.15, p. 3.24.

2. *Introduction to Indoor Air Quality: A Reference Manual* (Washington, D.C.: EPA, July 1991), 61.

3. National Cancer Institute, "Formaldehyde and Cancer: Questions and Answers," 30 July 2004, http://cis.nci.nih.gov/fact/3_8.htm.

4. *NIOSH Pocket Guide to Chemical Hazards* (Washington, D.C.: NIOSH, February 2004), www.cdc.gov/niosh/npg/npg.html.

5. EPA, "Sources of Indoor Air Pollution—Formaldehyde," www.epa.gov/iaq /formalde.html.

6. W. Bischof et al., "ProKlimA—History, Aim and Study Design," in *Proceedings of Indoor Air 1999, the 8th International Conference on Indoor Air Quality and Climate,* Edinburgh, Scotland, 8–13 August 1999, vol. 5.

7. Spengler et al., eds., *Indoor Air Quality Handbook,* 67.2, 67.2–3.

8. EPA, "Ozone Generators That Are Sold as Air Cleaners: An Assessment of Effectiveness and Health Consequences," www.epa.gov/iaq/pubs/ozonegen.html.

9. G. Sarwar et al., "Indoor Fine Particulates: The Role of Terpene Emissions from Consumer Products," *Journal of the Air and Waste Management Association* 54 (March 2004): 367–77.

10. Spengler et al., eds., *Indoor Air Quality Handbook,* table 3.15, p. 3.24.

14 • CALL IN A PROFESSIONAL

1. B. Flannigan et al., eds., *Microorganisms in Home and Indoor Work Environments: Diversity, Health Impacts, Investigation, and Control* (London: Taylor and Francis, 2001), 247.

2. H. Dillon et al., eds., *Field Guide for the Determination of Biological Contaminants in Environmental Samples* (Fairfax, Va.: AIHA, 1996), 58.

3. F. Tsai et al., "Concentrations of Airborne Bacteria in 100 U.S. Office Buildings," in *Proceedings of Indoor Air 2002, the 9th International Conference on Indoor Air Quality and Climate,* Monterey, Calif., 30 June–5 July 2002.

4. J. Macher, ed., *Bioaerosols: Assessment and Control* (Cincinnati: ACGIH, 1999).

5. J. Macher et al., "Concentrations of Cat and Dust Mite Allergens in 93 U.S. Office Buildings," in *Proceedings of Indoor Air 2002.*

6. Macher, ed., *Bioaerosols: Assessment and Control,* 22.5, 22.7.

7. Macher et al., "Concentrations of Cat and Dust Mite Allergens."

8. Ibid.

9. A. Munir et al., "Mite (Der p 1, Der f 1), Cat (Fel d 1), and Dog (Can f 1) Aller-

gens in Dust from Swedish Day-Care Centres," *Clinical and Experimental Allergy* 25 (February 1995): 119–26.

10. M. Berge et al., "Concentrations of Cat (Fel d 1), Dog (Can f 1), and Mite (Der f 1 and Der p 1) Allergens in the Clothing and School Environment of Swedish Schoolchildren with and without Pets at Home," *Pediatric Allergy and Immunology* 9 (February 1998): 25–30.

11. A. Custovic et al., "Domestic Allergens in Public Places II: Dog (Can f 1) and Cockroach (Bla g 2) Allergens in Dust and Mite, Cat, Dog, and Cockroach Allergens in the Air in Public Buildings," *Clinical and Experimental Allergy* 26 (November 1996): 1225–27.

12. H. Mussalo-Rauhamaa et al., "Dog Allergen in Indoor Air and Dust during Dog Shows," *Allergy* 56 (September 2001): 878–82.

13. S. Amr et al., "Environmental Allergens and Asthma in Urban Elementary Schools," *Annals of Allergy, Asthma, and Immunology* 90 (January 2003): 34–40.

14. E. Chu and A. Goldsobel, "House Dust Mite, Cat, and Cockroach Allergen Concentrations in Day Care Centers in Tampa, Florida," *Pediatrics* 110 (August 2002): 430–31.

15. V. Rullo et al., "Daycare Centers and Schools as Sources of Exposure to Mites, Cockroach, and Endotoxin in the City of Sao Paulo, Brazil," *Journal of Allergy and Clinical Immunology* 110 (October 2002): 582–88.

16. G. Chew, "New York City Public Schools: An Examination of Allergen Levels and an Assessment of the Prevalence and Severity of Asthma among Adolescents" (New York: Columbia University Mailman School of Public Health, 1999–2000), http://cpmcnet.columbia.edu/dept/niehs/pilot-projects/examination.html.

17. S. Sarpong et al., "Cockroach Allergen (Bla g 1) in School Dust," *Journal of Allergy and Clinical Immunology* 99 (April 1997): 486–92.

18. P. Eggleston and L. Arruda, "Ecology and Elimination of Cockroaches and Allergens in the Home."

19. A. Custovic et al., "Domestic Allergens in Public Places III: House Dust Mite, Cat, Dog, and Cockroach Allergens in British Hospitals," *Clinical and Experimental Allergy* 28 (1998): 53–59.

20. C. Reed and H. Kita, "The Role of Protease Activation of Inflammation in Allergic Respiratory Diseases," *Journal of Allergy and Clinical Immunology* 114 (5) (November 2004): 997–1008.

21. H. Ormstad et al., "Airborne House Dust Particles and Diesel Exhaust Particles as Allergen Carriers," *Clinical and Experimental Allergy* 28 (June 1998): 702–8.

22. Ibid.

23. L. Burton et al., "Airborne Particulate Matter within 100 Randomly Selected Office Buildings in the United States (BASE)," in *Proceedings of Healthy Buildings 2000*, Espoo, Finland, 6–10 August 2000, vol. 1, 157–62.

24. M. Powell, "Has Spring Sprung?" *Martinsville Bulletin,* 5 March 2004.

25. "Warrant for Arrest, Case Number 3:04.m229(56m), United States of America v. Ronald Schongar," United States District Court, New Haven, Conn., 12 July 2004.

15 • MORE DATA FOR TECHIES

1. Information for these descriptions came from six sources: B. Kendrick, *The Fifth Kingdom,* 3d ed. (Newburyport, Mass.: Focus Publishing, 2000); J. Webster, *Introduction to Fungi,* 2d ed.(Cambridge: Cambridge University Press, 1980); S. Gravesen et al., *Microfungi* (Copenhagen: Munksgaard, 1994); B. Flannigan et al., eds., *Microorganisms in Home and Indoor Work Environments* (London: Taylor and Francis, 2001); Environmental Microbiology Laboratory, "Fungi," www.emlab.com; and James Scott, assistant professor, Occupational and Environmental Health, Department of Public Health Sciences, Faculty of Medicine, University of Toronto.

2. R. Van der graaff, "Facial Eczema of Sheep and Cattle," *Agriculture Notes* (State of Victoria, Australia, Department of Primary Industries), May 1998.

CONCLUSION

1. M. Kawamoto et al., *Health Hazard Evaluation Report HETA 96-0012-2652, Brigham and Women's Hospital, Boston, Massachusetts* (Washington, D.C.: NIOSH, September 1997), 35.

2. "Statement of Joellen Lawson, Fairfield, CT," Senate Green School Hearing, 1 October 2002, http://epw.senate.gov/107th/Lawson_100102.htm.

INDEX

About the Author

Jeffrey C. May is principal scientist of May Indoor Air Investigations LLC, in Cambridge, Massachusetts, which specializes in identifying the causes of indoor air quality, mold, odor, and moisture problems in schools, offices, and residences. Over the past fifteen years May has investigated thousands of buildings and taken and analyzed over twenty thousand air and dust samples. He lectures nationally on indoor air quality and is the author of *My House is Killing Me! The Home Guide for Families with Allergies and Asthma* and the co-author of *The Mold Survival Guide: For Your Home and for Your Health,* both also available from Johns Hopkins University Press. May received his M.A. in organic chemistry from Harvard University.